Sports Medicine

Editors

VINCENT MORELLI
ANDREW J.M. GREGORY

PRIMARY CARE:
CLINICS IN OFFICE PRACTICE

www.primarycare.theclinics.com

Consulting Editor
JOEL J. HEIDELBAUGH

June 2013 • Volume 40 • Number 2

ELSEVIER

1600 John F. Kennedy Boulevard • Suite 1800 • Philadelphia, Pennsylvania, 19103-2899

http://www.theclinics.com

PRIMARY CARE: CLINICS IN OFFICE PRACTICE Volume 40, Number 2
June 2013 ISSN 0095-4543, ISBN-13: 978-1-4557-7145-5

Editor: Yonah Korngold
Developmental Editor: Donald Mumford

Primary Care: Clinics in Office Practice (ISSN: 0095–4543) is published quarterly by Elsevier Inc., 360 Park Avenue South, New York, NY 10010-1710. Months of issue are March, June, September, and December. Periodicals postage paid at New York, NY and additional mailing offices. Subscription prices are $216.00 per year (US individuals), $353.00 (US institutions), $108.00 (US students), $264.00 (Canadian individuals), $415.00 (Canadian institutions), $169.00 (Canadian students), $329.00 (international individuals), $415.00 (international institutions), and $169.00 (international students). Foreign air speed delivery is included in all *Clinics* subscription prices. All prices are subject to change without notice. POSTMASTER: Send address changes to *Primary Care: Clinics in Office Practice*, Elsevier Periodicals Customer Service, 11830 Westline Industrial Drive, St. Louis, MO 63146. Customer Service Health Sciences Division, Subscription Customer Service, 3251 Riverport Lane, Maryland Heights, MO 63043. **Customer Service: 1-800-654-2452 (U.S. and Canada); 314-447-8871 (outside U.S. and Canada). Fax: 314-447-8029. E-mail: journalscustomerservice-usa@elsevier.com (for print support); journalsonlinesupport-usa@elsevier.com (for online support).**

Reprints. For copies of 100 or more, of articles in this publication, please contact the Commercial Reprints Department, Elsevier Inc., 360 Park Avenue South, New York, NY 10010-1710. Tel. (212) 633-3812; Fax: (212) 482-1935; E-mail: reprints@elsevier.com.

Primary Care: Clinics in Office Practice is covered in *MEDLINE/PubMed (Index Medicus) and EMBASE/Excerpta Medica, Current Contents/Clinical Medicine, and ISI/BIOMED.*

Printed and bound by CPI Group (UK) Ltd, Croydon, CR0 4YY

Transferred to Digital Printing, 2013

Contributors

CONSULTING EDITOR

JOEL J. HEIDELBAUGH, MD, FAAFP, FACG
Clinical Associate Professor, Departments of Family Medicine and Urology, Clerkship Director, Department of Family Medicine, University of Michigan Medical School, Ann Arbor, Michigan; Ypsilanti Health Center, Ypsilanti, Michigan

EDITORS

VINCENT MORELLI, MD
Associate Professor, Department of Family and Community Medicine, School of Medicine, Sports Medicine Fellowship Director, Meharry Medical College, Nashville, Tennessee

ANDREW J.M. GREGORY, MD, FAAP, FACSM
Associate Professor, Departments of Pediatrics, Orthopedics and Rehabilitation, Vanderbilt University School of Medicine, Nashville, Tennessee

AUTHORS

JONATHAN A. BECKER, MD
Program Director, Primary Care Sports Medicine Fellowship, Jewish Hospital and University of Louisville; Associate Professor, Department of Family and Geriatric Medicine, University of Louisville, Louisville, Kentucky

ROBERT BRIAN BETTENCOURT, MD, CAQSM
Assistant Professor of Family Medicine and Sports Medicine, Team Physician, University of South Alabama, Department of Family Medicine, University of South Alabama College of Medicine, Mobile, Alabama

KENNETH M. BIELAK, MD, FACSM, FAAFP, MBA
Associate Professor, Associate Program Director, Primary Care Sports Medicine Fellowship, Department of Family Medicine, University of Tennessee Health Science Center, Graduate School of Medicine, University of Tennessee, Knoxville, Tennessee

BLAKE R. BOGGESS, DO
Assistant Professor, Department of Orthopedics, Duke University Medical Center, Morrisville, North Carolina

ERIC BOWMAN, DO
Sports Medicine Fellow, Division of Sports Medicine, Department of Pediatrics, Nationwide Children's Hospital, Dublin, Ohio

THOMAS MARK BRAXTON Jr, MD
Braxton Family and Sports Medicine, Jackson Purchase Medical Center, Mayfield, Kentucky

CRYSTAL BRIGHT, MD
Sports Fellow, Department of Family and Community Medicine, Meharry Medical College, Nashville, Tennessee

GABRIEL BROOKS, PT, DPT, MSPT, MTCH
Physical Medicine and Rehabilitation, Adolescent and Sport Medicine Clinic, Texas Children's Hospital, Houston, Texas

JEFFREY R. BYTOMSKI, DO, FAOASM
Associate Professor, Department of Community and Family Medicine, Duke University Medical Center, Morrisville, North Carolina

DOUGLAS J. CONNOR, MD
Clinical Instructor, Department of Orthopedics and Rehabilitation, Vanderbilt Sports Medicine, Vanderbilt University Medical Center, Nashville, Tennessee

AMY CORRIGAN, DO
Memorial Family Medicine Residency, South Bend, Indiana

CAROLYN DAVIS, PhD
Founder/Director of the Tennessee Institute for Performance and Sport Psychology, Core Faculty in the College of Social and Behavioral Sciences, Department of Counseling Psychology, Walden University, Minneapolis, Minnesota

ASHLEY FIELDS, MD, MPH
Department of Family and Community Medicine, Meharry Medical College, Nashville, Tennessee

BRIAN S. HARVEY, DO
Pediatric and Sports Medicine Physician, Salina Regional Health Center, Salina, Kansas

ALBERT HERGENROEDER, MD
Professor of Pediatrics, Chief, Adolescent Medicine and Sports Medicine Section, Baylor College of Medicine; Texas Children's Hospital, Houston, Texas

JULIE KAFKA, MD
Sports Medicine Fellow, Primary Care Sports Medicine Fellowship, Department of Family Medicine, University of Tennessee Health Science Center, Graduate School of Medicine, University of Tennessee, Knoxville, Tennessee

MEDHAT KALLINY, MD, PhD
Assistant Professor, Department of Family and Community Medicine, Meharry Medical College, Nashville, Tennessee

MARK E. LAVALLEE, MD, CSCS, FACSM
Co-Director, South Bend-Notre Dame Sports Medicine Fellowship Program, South Bend, Indiana; Chairman, USA Weightlifting, Sports Medicine Society, Colorado Springs, Colorado; Assistant Clinical Professor, Indiana University School of Medicine, Indianapolis, Indiana

DAVID G. LIDDLE, MD
Assistant Professor, Department of Orthopedics and Rehabilitation; Department of Internal Medicine, Vanderbilt Sports Medicine, Vanderbilt University Medical Center, Nashville, Tennessee

MICHAEL M. LINDER, MD
Director, Primary Care Sports Medicine Fellowship and Family Medicine Residency Program, Team Physician, University of South Alabama, Department of Family Medicine, University of South Alabama College of Medicine, Mobile, Alabama

VINCENT MORELLI, MD
Associate Professor, Department of Family and Community Medicine, School of Medicine, Sports Medicine Fellowship Director, Meharry Medical College, Nashville, Tennessee

JOHN MUNYAK, MD
Attending Physician, Sports Medicine, Department of Orthopaedic Surgery, Maimonides Medical Center; Team Physician, Brooklyn Nets Basketball, Brooklyn, New York

HEATHER O'HARA, MD, MPH
Assistant Professor, Department of Family and Community Medicine, Meharry Medical College, Nashville, Tennessee

MARI-ETTA E. PARRISH, RD, LDN, CSSD
Registered Dietitian, Baptist Sports Medicine, Sports Nutrition Liaison, Nashville, Tennessee

RENO RAVINDRAN, MD
Assistant Clinical Professor, Division of Sports Medicine, Department of Pediatrics and Family Medicine, Nationwide Children's Hospital, The Ohio State University College of Medicine, Dublin, Ohio

MIGUEL REYES Jr, MD
Musculoskeletal Radiologist, Department of Radiology, Medical Imaging of Dallas, Irving, Texas

RICHARD E. RODENBERG, MD
Program Director, NCH Sports Medicine Fellowship Program, Division of Sports Medicine, Assistant Clinical Professor, Department of Pediatrics, Nationwide Children's Hospital, The Ohio State University College of Medicine, Dublin, Ohio

RAMIN SADEGHPOUR, MD
Research Resident, Department of Orthopaedic Surgery, Maimonides Medical Center, Brooklyn, New York

AHMED SALEH, MD
PGY-3, Department of Orthopaedic Surgery, Maimonides Medical Center, Brooklyn, New York

KARI SEARS, MD
Memorial Family Medicine Residency, South Bend, Indiana

ALLEN K. SILLS, MD
Departments of Neurosurgery and Orthopedic Surgery, Vanderbilt University Medical Center, Franklin, Tennessee

JESSICA R. STUMBO, MD
Associate Program Director, Primary Care Sports Medicine Fellowship, Jewish Hospital and University of Louisville; Assistant Professor, Department of Family and Geriatric Medicine, University of Louisville; Centers for Primary Care, Louisville, Kentucky

KUMAR TAMMAREDDI, MD
Department of Sports Medicine, Meharry Medical College, Nashville, Tennessee

TOM TERRELL, MD, MPhil
Associate Professor, Assistant Director Sports Medicine Fellowship, Department of Family Medicine, University of Tennessee Health Science Center, Graduate School of Medicine, University of Tennessee, Knoxville, Tennessee

ROGER ZOOROB, MD, MPH, FAAFP
Frank S. Royal Sr. Professor and Chair, Department of Family and Community Medicine, Meharry Medical College, Nashville, Tennessee

Contents

Foreword: Common Injuries, Weekend Warriors, and Dedicated Athletes **xiii**

Joel J. Heidelbaugh

Preface **xv**

Vincent Morelli and Andrew J.M. Gregory

Treatment of Head Injuries **253**

Allen K. Sills

Sports-related brain injuries are increasing in incidence and may affect athletes from many different sports. Concussion is the most common form of sports-related head injury and is a form of mild traumatic brain injury. Evaluations of concussed athletes should include careful history, focused neurologic examination, balance testing, and cognitive testing. Postinjury management consists of avoiding aggravating factors until symptoms resolve. Return to play should not begin until all symptoms resolve, and then this should be done in a graduated fashion that avoids recreating symptoms. Research is ongoing concerning the maximum safe number of concussive injuries and any possible long-term sequelae.

Treatment of Neck Injuries **259**

Robert Brian Bettencourt and Michael M. Linder

Spinal cord injuries are uncommon in sports. Planning and practice for their occurrence, however, remains an essential component of Sideline Medical Team preparedness. Evaluation of cervical nerve injury, cervical cord injury, and cervical disc disease can be complex. Medical management, diagnostic imaging techniques and surgical recommendations in this setting continue to evolve. Most published guidance offers occasionally opposed expert opinion with sport participation after Cervical Cord Neuropraxia in the setting of Cervical Spinal Stenosis appearing particularly polarizing. Such conflicts can present challenges to clinicians in forming management and Return to Play decisions for the health of their athletes.

Back Pain in Adults **271**

Jonathan A. Becker and Jessica R. Stumbo

This article provides a summary of the many causes of back pain in adults. There is an overview of the history and physical examination with attention paid to red flags that alert the clinician to more worrisome causes of low back pain. An extensive differential diagnosis for back pain in adults is provided along with key historical and physical examination findings. The various therapeutic options are summarized with an emphasis on evidence-based findings. These reviewed treatments include medication, physical therapy, topical treatments, injections, and complementary and alternative medicine. The indications for surgery and specialty referral are also discussed.

PRIMARY CARE: CLINICS IN OFFICE PRACTICE

FORTHCOMING ISSUES

September 2013
Infectious Disease
Michael A. Malone, MD, *Editor*

December 2013
Orthopedics
George Pujalte, MD, *Editor*

RECENT ISSUES

March 2013
Cardiovascular Diseases
Robert D. Sheeler, MD, *Editor*

December 2012
Practice Management
Michelle Anne Bholat, MD, *Editor*

September 2012
Low Back Pain
Eron Manusov, MD, *Editor*

Foreword

Common Injuries, Weekend Warriors, and Dedicated Athletes

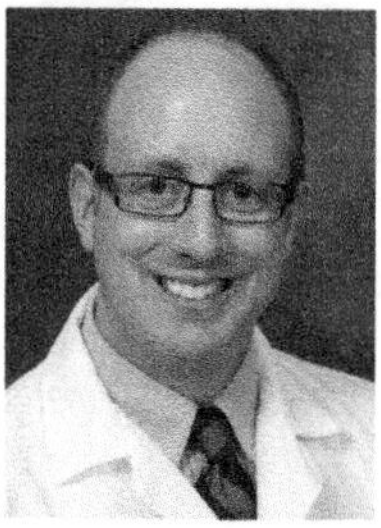

Joel J. Heidelbaugh, MD, FAAFP, FACG
Consulting Editor

Musculoskeletal injuries continue to rank as some of the most commonly encountered presenting complaints in primary care practices. Educational training in allopathic medical schools, nursing schools, and physician assistant programs often falls short of providing the necessary tools for appropriate cost-effective diagnosis and management of these conditions, while postgraduate residency training attempts to fill these gaps in knowledge. Moreover, we often provide ineffective counseling on prevention of injury and optimization of nutrition.

Osteopathic medicine, founded by Andrew Taylor Still in the nineteenth century as an alternative to standard medical practices, has at its core the concept of manipulation of bones and joints to treat a wide spectrum of diseases, not solely limited to orthopedic conditions. While students of osteopathic medicine are trained in osteopathic manipulative medicine, unfortunately most osteopathic physicians do not integrate this provision into daily practice. Sports medicine fellowships are popular and provide additional comprehensive training for clinicians who wish to dedicate a portion of their future practices to caring for athletes.

As decades pass, the field of "sports medicine" continues to evolve in both scope of training as well as across the backgrounds of the people who treat our patients and athletes. Most sports teams, ranging from those comprising young athletes to professional and Olympic level athletes, have multidisciplinary support systems comprising primary care clinicians, orthopedic surgeons, physical therapists, and sports psychologists, who provide expertise and guidance across a wide spectrum of care. It is highly important that primary care clinicians understand the roles that each specialist plays, so as to foster appropriate referrals within the health care system, as well as to provide the maximum standard of comprehensive primary care.

Prim Care Clin Office Pract 40 (2013) xiii–xiv
http://dx.doi.org/10.1016/j.pop.2013.04.001
primarycare.theclinics.com

This volume of *Primary Care: Clinics in Office Practice* provides outstanding evidence-based reviews on common injuries of the head, neck, spine, extremities, and major axial joints. The articles are written in a format that allows for facile integration of new knowledge into medical practice and teaching. Impressively, the articles also provide information on the prevention of common injuries as well as guides for timely rehabilitation. This volume provides an in-depth view into several topics that are rarely covered in the primary care literature. While few clinicians likely feel adept in providing education on standard nutrition for the athlete, or counseling relative to medicolegal or psychological aspects, the articles within this volume exceed the standard for common primary care knowledge.

Drs Morelli and Gregory, as well as the diverse cadre of authors who contributed to this volume, should be commended for developing a unique and comprehensive collection of articles of the highest standard that are easily translatable to daily practice. Whether it is the common injuries we encounter in our patients, ranging from those who are inactive to the proverbial "weekend warriors," or the dedicated athletes from school age to professional level, readers of this volume of *Primary Care: Clinics in Office Practice* can now better treat and counsel patients with musculoskeletal complaints in a multidisciplinary fashion.

Joel J. Heidelbaugh, MD, FAAFP, FACG
Departments of Family Medicine and Urology
Department of Family Medicine
University of Michigan Medical School
Ann Arbor, MI 48109, USA

Ypsilanti Health Center
200 Arnet Suite 200
Ypsilanti, MI 48198, USA

E-mail address:
jheidel@umich.edu

Preface

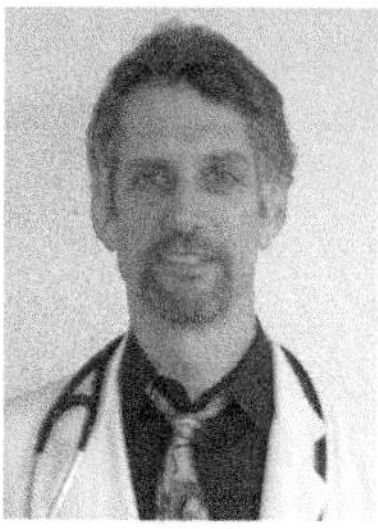 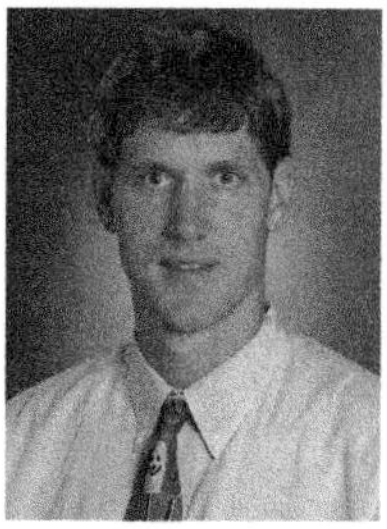

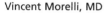

Vincent Morelli, MD Andrew J.M. Gregory, MD, FAAP, FACSM
Editors

As exercise has, over the last decades, become more and more a part of our daily lives, interest in wellness and sports medicine has experienced a concomitant dramatic rise. This heightened interest has spawned much new and often conflicting research, leaving in its wake an abundance of both valuable and misleading information. Our intent in this issue is to help the primary care sports medicine physician wade through this ever-rising sea of information in order to help them provide better care to patients and athletes at all levels of participation.

We highlight new and emerging trends in sports medicine, discuss controversial areas and therapies, and hopefully provide the primary care sports medicine physician with clinically relevant information. Although much scientific work has been done in these domains in recent years, more remains to be done. Our aim is to separate fact from fiction, to delineate the strengths, weaknesses, and limits of current medical literature, and to lay a clear path to direct future research. We hope that primary care sports physicians, primary care providers, residents, and medical students will find our work well written, well researched, and clinically relevant.

We are pleased and honored to serve as guest editors for this issue, and we feel privileged to have worked with such a distinguished group of collaborators. Many thanks to the contributing authors, who have worked painstakingly to make their articles both scholarly and relevant in the clinical setting. We also thank the Department of Family and Community Medicine at Meharry Medical College, the Family Medicine Department at Vanderbilt University, the Pediatrics Department at Vanderbilt University, and our publishers and editors at Elsevier for providing us with the support needed to complete this project.

Vincent Morelli, MD
Department of Family and Community Medicine
Meharry Medical College
1005 Dr D.B. Todd Boulevard
Nashville, TN 37208, USA

Prim Care Clin Office Pract 40 (2013) xv–xvi
http://dx.doi.org/10.1016/j.pop.2013.03.001
0095-4543/13/$ – see front matter

Andrew J.M. Gregory, MD, FAAP, FACSM
Department of Pediatrics
Orthopedics and Rehabilitation
Vanderbilt University School of Medicine
3200 MCE Medical Center East–South Tower
Nashville, TN 37232, USA

E-mail addresses:
morellivincent@yahoo.com (V. Morelli)
andrew.gregory@Vanderbilt.Edu (A.J.M. Gregory)

Treatment of Head Injuries

Allen K. Sills, MD[a,b,*]

KEYWORDS

- Concussion • Cognitive testing • Traumatic brain injury
- Chronic traumatic encephalopathy

KEY POINTS

- Concussion is a form of traumatic brain injury and appears to be increasing in incidence at all ages and levels of play.
- Concussion is no longer graded on a scale, but rather each event is assessed based on symptoms that are present at onset as well as on follow-up.
- It is helpful to have baseline evaluations of athletes prior to their participation so that future performance can be measured against this to ensure the brain has fully recovered after injury.
- Mainstays of postinjury management include avoidance of stimuli that aggravate symptoms. Return to activity cannot begin until all symptoms resolve. Once the athlete is asymptomatic, then a stepwise return to play can occur with progression based on continued lack of symptoms.
- Long-term effects of concussion remain to be better understood.

Neurologic injuries in athletes are increasing in incidence. These injuries are currently among the most common medical concerns in athletes, as they affect all ages and all levels of competition.[1] Concussions appear to be increasing in incidence across a wide variety of sports, with an estimated 1.6 to 3.8 million events per year in the United States alone. It is also estimated that up to 9% of high school athletes will suffer a concussion in any given year. This number does appear to be increasing, especially among high school athletes.[2,3] A recent annual survey suggested that the sports and activities most commonly associated with traumatic brain injury were as follows (ranked in order of incidence): cycling, football, baseball/softball, basketball, water sports, powered recreational vehicles, soccer, skateboards/scooters, winter sports, and equestrian sports.[4]

The authors of this work report no direct financial interest in the subject matter or any material discussed in this article or with a company making products described.

[a] Department of Neurosurgery, Vanderbilt University Medical Center, 2009 Mallory lane, Franklin, TN 37067, USA; [b] Department of Orthopedic Surgery, Vanderbilt University Medical Center, 2009 Mallory lane, Franklin, TN 37067, USA
* Department of Neurosurgery, Vanderbilt University Medical Center, 2009 Mallory lane, Franklin, TN 37067.
E-mail address: allen.sills@vanderbilt.edu

Prim Care Clin Office Pract 40 (2013) 253–258
http://dx.doi.org/10.1016/j.pop.2013.02.003 **primarycare.theclinics.com**

DEFINITION AND CLASSIFICATION

Concussion is defined as a complex pathophysiologic process that affects the brain and is induced by traumatic biomechanical forces.[5] Concussion is essentially a form of mild traumatic brain injury, although some have objected to the use of the term mild with the view that no type of traumatic brain injury should be viewed as mild.

Concussions are complex injuries that cause changes in neurologic function including balance and cognition as well as a variety of symptoms. Most sports concussions occur without loss of consciousness or overt neurologic signs.[6]

Previously, the presence of certain symptoms was used in an attempt to divide concussions into certain grades of severity based on established guidelines.[7] However, concussions are no longer divided as such, since these grading systems had little clinical usefulness. Instead, concussions are now considered individually and described based on duration and nature of symptoms. Several modifiers have been suggested as reflecting the severity and likely recovery from a concussion.[8] These modifiers include symptoms, neurologic signs, any sequelae such as convulsions, temporal factors in terms of number of events over time and how close the injuries are together, threshold for future injuries, age of the patient, comorbidities of other neurologic conditions, concurrent use of medications, behaviors that are encouraged, repeat injuries, and whether the sport is considered a contact or collision sport as well as the level of play.

In general, athletes who have suffered concussions previously will take longer to recover from their injury because of prolonged symptoms. There is some evidence to suggest that a longer time to recovery is required for each subsequent concussion.[9] Genetics may actually play some role in the risk of concussion. Some neuropathologic studies have indicated an association between ApoE4 promoter genotypes and risk of concussion and a relationship between the tau protein polymorphism and increased risk of concussion.[10]

Age of the athlete also may affect recovery for concussion. Younger athletes may be more vulnerable to injury because of the developing state of their brain and variable rates of their neurologic development. In general, children and adolescents are felt to be more susceptible to concussion than adults, tend to have more symptoms, and have more prolonged recoveries (7–10 days in high school athletes vs 2 to 7 days in college athletes).[11]

BASELINE EVALUATIONS

Concussions frequently present with symptoms such as headaches, fogginess, dizziness, light or noise sensitivity, or with impairments of balance and/or cognitive deficits. Each of these areas can be tracked using symptom scales, specific testing of balance, and neurocognitive testing. All of these functions can be measured at baseline in the noninjured state, and these are all known to be sensitive to significant changes in the first few days following injury. Generally, these factors (and thus most concussions) will normalize over the first 2 weeks.[12–14]

To establish an appropriate baseline for each individual athlete, a history should be obtained, and focused assessment done. The history should focus on previous concussions with regard to duration and nature of symptoms and time loss both from school and from sport. This information helps the provider to better understand the severity of previous injuries. History should also obtain any data about related neurologic conditions such as presence of migraine headaches, seizures, learning disabilities, or other major neurologic illness. Each of these factors has been suggested to favor a prolonged recovery from concussion.

A focused neurologic examination should be done to include basic assessment of major cranial nerves as well as general motor and sensory function. Balance assessment may be done by a variety of methods, the most simple of which is the BESS (balance error scoring system) examination. The BESS examination is an independent measure of a subject's ability to maintain balance when visual cues are removed. It can be performed in any environment and requires only the test subject and a foam pad. This also can be modified without use of foam for quicker assessment.[15]

Neuropsychological testing has traditionally been performed by pencil-and-paper tests; however, due to limited availability of practitioners who can perform these evaluations, there has been marked increase interest in use of computerized cognitive tests that measure the acute effects of concussion.[16,17] Various commercially available products have been developed for performing these neurocognitive studies. The best studied of these tools is the ImPACT test (immediate postconcussion assessment and cognitive testing). This product can be purchased by schools or individual providers and is administered to the patient on a desktop computer. The test takes approximately 20 minutes to take and is scored automatically with a printout of results. The test measures visual and verbal memory, processing speed, and reaction. All of these parameters may be altered in the concussed patient. The idea behind baseline testing is that if each athlete takes this test prior to competition, then there will be an established individual baseline that can be used as comparison against testing done in the concussed athlete. These tests are reproducible but should be administered in a quiet environment with encouragement for maximum effort of the athlete in order to produce the most appropriate data.[18]

POSTINJURY MANAGEMENT

The cornerstone of modern concussion management in all age groups and all sports is physical and cognitive rest. Primarily, rest is used to avoid aggravation of postconcussion symptoms, which can be made worse by either physical or mental exertion in the acute postinjury period. Another driving feature is in an attempt to avoid diffuse cerebral swelling and brain herniation, which can occur in a subset of young athletes who receive a second injury to the brain during the period when they are still recovering from an initial insult.[19] Development of this devastating brain edema typically leaves the patient with severe impairments and is referred to as second impact syndrome.[19]

Current recommendations for managing a sports-related concussion is to rest until symptoms resolve and then begin stepwise increases in activity prior to considering full clearance and return to sport.[8] Attempts are made to avoid stimuli that may aggravate concussion symptoms such as loud noises, bright lights, or even cognitive tasks such as reading or studying, since aggravation of symptoms tends to prolong recovery. The optimal amount of rest has yet to be determined, as this concept has not been well studied from the standpoint of clinical trials or even case series but is based rather on consensus expert opinion.[20]

Repeat cognitive evaluation, either computerized or pencil-and-paper, is done to determine when an athlete has returned to baseline. Some controversy exists about the optimal timing for this repeat evaluation. Given that the general purpose of the evaluation is to ensure a return to baseline function, it is generally agreed that the athlete should be asymptomatic before repeating this test; however, whether the athlete should be retested before beginning a stepwise return to play protocol or as a final step before full clearance remains an area of active debate.

Symptoms of concussion such as headache, balance, and emotional problems will rarely require medical treatment given that most individuals recover in 7 to 10 days.[21]

For the small subset of patients whose deficits persist for more than 10 to 14 days, medical management may need to be considered. For example, if the athlete's persistent symptom is headache, agents that are used for migraine headaches may be tried. Balance problems may be treated with vestibular rehabilitation therapy or occasionally with antiemetics or medications used to treat vertigo.[22] Attention should be paid to emotional issues such as the presence of concurrent depression, since failure to recognize and treat these symptoms will delay the patients overall recovery. Previous work in nonsport traumatic brain injury demonstrated benefit of sertraline in treating depression.[23] Many athletes who have persistent symptoms will require some modification of school work such as extra time to complete assignments or tests; avoidance of noisy areas such as the cafeteria, assemblies, or music class; shorter assignments; and frequent breaks during homework or tests.

Imaging studies are rarely needed, because they will be normal in the overwhelming majority of cases; however, computed tomography or magnetic resonance imaging may be sought if symptoms seem to be escalating after 10 to 14 days, or if focal neurologic deficits such as weakness, numbness, or focal cranial nerve deficits are noted.

Athletes are typically returned to play by stepwise progression of increasing activity that begins with low-impact aerobic activities, then progresses to sport specific noncontact activity and eventually to contact activity.[24] It is generally agreed that athletes who become symptomatic at a certain activity step should rest for 24 hours then return to a lesser level of activity before continuing through the progression. Some leeway is generally given to older athletes (over age 21) for the duration of each of these phases, as it is generally not strictly held that each phase must be 24 hours in the older athlete. However, in high school age and younger athletes, current practice patterns dictate that each return to play step be evaluated for at least a 24-hour period before advancing to the next stage.

No activity should be undertaken until the patient is completely asymptomatic at rest. The first stage then involves light aerobic exercise such as walking or stationary bike. The goal at this stage is to keep the heart rate only mildly elevated and to do only a 20- to 30-minute period of exercise. If there are no symptoms, the athlete can progress the following day to sport-specific training. This involves movements and drills that mimic some of the athlete's movements in his or her sport but again does not reach full-speed activity or involve other players. The following day involves noncontact drills. During this time, the athlete may participate with his or her team in activities that do not cause exposure to contact such as full team warm-ups and other drills. The following day includes a stage of full-contact participation and practice. If the athlete has no symptoms during unrestricted practice, then he or she is ready to return to game action.

LONG-TERM EFFECTS OF CONCUSSION

Increasing reports have been gathered concerning potential for long-term cognitive problems in athletes who have a high exposure to head impacts during career and collision sports.[25] Recent studies have also published findings of pathologic changes in retired athletes, and this has raised questions of potential links between head trauma exposure and these pathologic changes.[26] However, the specificity of these findings, as they relate to cognitive function during life, remains to be elucidated. Also, the specificity of these pathologic changes for sports-related trauma is still unclear, since many older adults who have not been exposed to contact sports will also show similar changes in their brains at autopsy. One other factor that makes correlation of the pathologic findings with clinical behavior difficult is the fact that behavioral changes such as depression, combativeness, and other psychiatric illnesses do have some prevalence in the general population and again may not directly be the result of the pathologic changes that are seen. Additionally, dementia rates in the general population are obviously significant, and thus to correlate late cognitive decline later in life with previous injury exposure is quite difficult. This remains an area of active research.

Currently there are no good data to define a clinical threshold for "how many is too many" with regard to concussions. Clinicians should take into account the fact that short time interval between concussions, duration of symptoms greater than 2 weeks after concussion, and presence of several concussions in adolescent years are all factors that suggest a more significant injury. Extreme caution should be used in allowing these athletes to resume sport activities that are likely to result in additional concussion injury. As with many other medical conditions, the life and occupational goals of the athlete also play a role in determining the acceptable level of risk for continued sport participation.

SUMMARY

Concussions remain a significant sports medicine-related problem. All sports are at risk for athletic brain injury, and proper management depends on early recognition, diagnosis, and treatment. Baseline evaluation of athletes in team sports should be considered, as this will assist in determining when an athlete has returned to baseline. General strategies for postconcussive treatment include avoidance of aggravating stimuli and then a progressive return to play once symptoms have resolved. Continued research is ongoing into potential long-term effects of concussions, but as of yet, causal links between specific numbers of events and severity of concussive events and long-term pathologic and neurodegenerative changes have not been established.

REFERENCES

1. Mehan WP, d'Hemecourt P, Comstock RD. High school concussions in the 2008-2009 academic year: mechanisms, symptoms, and management. Am J Sports Med 2010;38:2405–9.
2. Langlois JA, Rutland-Brown W, Wald MM. The epidemiology and impact of traumatic brain injury: a brief overview. J Head Trauma Rehabil 2006;21:375–8.
3. Bakhos LL, Lockhart GR, Myers R, et al. Emergency department visits for concussion in young child athletes. Pediatrics 2010;126(3):e550–6.
4. American Association of Neurological Surgeons. Patient information: sports-related head injury. National Electronic Injury Surveillance System (NEISS); 2011. Available at: http://www.aans.org/Patient%20Information/Conditions%20and%20Treatments/Sports-Related%20Head%20Injury.aspx. Accessed December 1, 2012.
5. Aubry M, Cantu R, Devorak J, et al. Summary and agreement statement of the First International Conference on Concussion in Sport, Vienna 2001. Recommendations for the improvement of safety and health of athletes who may suffer concussive injuries. Br J Sports Med 2002;36(1):6–10.
6. McCrea M, Guskiewicz KM, Marshall SW, et al. Acute effects and recovery time following concussion in collegiate football players: the NCAA concussion study. JAMA 2003;290:2556–63.
7. Cantu RC. Guidelines for return to contact sports after a cerebral concussion. Phys Sportsmed 1986;14:75–83.

8. McCrory P, Meeuwisse W, Johnston K, et al. Consensus statement on concussion in sport—3rd International Conference on Concussion and sport held in Zurich. J Sci Med Sport 2009;12:340–51.
9. Benson BW, Meeuwisse WH, Rizos J, et al. A prospective study of concussions among National Hockey League players during regular season games: the NHL/NHLPA concussion program. CMAJ 2011;183:905–11.
10. Terrell TR, Bostick RM, Abramson R, et al. APOE, APOE promoter, and tau genotypes and risk for concussion in college athletes. Clin J Sport Med 2008;18:10–7.
11. Sim A, Terryberry-Spohr L, Wilson KR. Prolonged recovery of memory functioning after mild traumatic brain injury in adolescent athletes. J Neurosurg 2008;108:511–6.
12. Collins MW, Grinder SH, Lovell MR, et al. Relationship between concussion and neuropsychological performance in college football players. JAMA 1999;282:964–70.
13. Guskieweicz KM, Ross SE, Marshall SW. Postural stability and neuropsychological deficits after concussion in collegiate athletes. J Athl Train 2001;36:263–73.
14. McCrea M, Kelly JP, Randolph C, et al. Immediate neurocognitive effects of concussion. Neurosurgery 2002;50:1032–40.
15. Finnoff JT, Peterson VJ, Hollaman JH, et al. Intrarater and interrater reliability of the balance error scoring system (BESS). PM R 2009;1:50–4.
16. Lovell MR, Collins MW, Iverson GL, et al. Recovery from mild concussion in high school athletes. J Neurosurg 2003;98:296–301.
17. Iverson GL, Lovell MR, Collins MW. Interpreting change on ImPACT following sport concussion. Clin Neuropsychol 2003;17:460–7.
18. Moser RS, Schatz P, Neidzwski K, et al. Group versus individual administration effects baseline neurocognitive test performance. Am J Sports Med 2011;39:2325–30.
19. Bey T, Ostic KB. Second impact syndrome. West J Emerg Med 2009;10:6–10.
20. McCrory P, Meeuwisse W, Johnston K, et al. Consensus statement on concussion in sport, 3rd International Conference on Concussion Sport held in Zurich, November 2008. Clin J Sport Med 2009;19:185–200.
21. Duhaime AC, Beckwith JG, Maerlender AC, et al. Spectrum of acute clinical characteristics of diagnosed concussions in college athletes wearing instrumented helmets. J Neurosurg 2012;117:1092–9.
22. Gottshall K. Vestibular rehabilitation after mild traumatic brain injury with vestibular pathology. NeuroRehabilitation 2011;29:167–71.
23. Fann JR, Uomoto JN, Katon WJ. Sertraline in the treatment of major depression following mild traumatic brain injury. J Neuropsychiatry Clin Neurosci 2000;12:226–32.
24. McCrory P, Meeuwisse W, Johnston K, et al. Consensus statement on concussion in sport: 3rd International Conference on Concussion in Sport held in Zurich, November 2008. Br J Sports Med 2009;43(Suppl 1):i76–90.
25. McCrory P. Sports concussion and the risk of chronic neurological impairment. Clin J Sport Med 2011;21(1):6–12.
26. McKee AC, Cantu RC, Nowinski CJ, et al. Chronic traumatic encephalopathy in athletes: progressive tauopathy after repetitive head injury. J Neuropathol Exp Neurol 2009;68:709–35.

Treatment of Neck Injuries

Robert Brian Bettencourt, MD, CAQSM[a,*], Michael M. Linder, MD[b,c]

KEYWORDS

• Spine board • Stinger • Spinal stenosis • Cervical cord neuropraxia
• Cervical disc disease • Return to play • Neck injury

KEY POINTS

- Severe cervical spinal injuries are uncommon in contact and collision sports, however, pre-event planning and practice are essential components of sideline medical team preparedness for such occurrences.
- Cervical soft tissue injuries can present complex challenges for athletes and those who care for them.
- Diagnostic imaging techniques, medical treatment, and surgical recommendations in this setting are continuing to evolve.
- Return-to-play guidelines in many instances are incomplete, not standardized, and are the subject of continued debate.
- Most guidance in the literature relies on occasionally conflicting expert opinion, and return to play after central cord neuropraxia in the setting of cervical spinal stenosis is particularly polarizing.
- This conflict can present challenges to medical professionals in forming thoughtful, knowledgeable, and individualized management and return-to-play considerations for the health and safety of athletes.

CERVICAL SPINAL INJURY IN US SPORTS

Every year there are an estimated 11,000 new spinal cord injuries in the United States, with sports participation injuries accounting for 8% of that total. Sports-related injuries are the second most common cause of spinal cord injury (SCI) in people less than 30 years of age, and the fourth most common cause overall. Of all US sports, football is associated with the highest number of catastrophic spinal injuries.

Before 1976, head-first contact during blocking and tackling maneuvers was a commonly used technique. Participants were often taught to engage an opponent

[a] Department of Family Medicine, University of South Alabama College of Medicine, 1504 Springhill Avenue, Room 3414, Mobile, AL 36604, USA; [b] Primary Care Sports Medicine Fellowship Program, Department of Family Medicine, University of South Alabama, 1504 Springhill Avenue, Room 3414, Mobile, AL 36604, USA; [c] Family Medicine Residency Program, Department of Family Medicine, University of South Alabama, 1504 Springhill Avenue, Room 3414, Mobile, AL 36604, USA

* Corresponding author.
E-mail address: Robert.B.Bettencourt@kp.org

Prim Care Clin Office Pract 40 (2013) 259–269
http://dx.doi.org/10.1016/j.pop.2013.02.012 **primarycare.theclinics.com**
0095-4543/13/$ – see front matter

using the crown of the helmet as a primary contact point. Spearing, as it was called, subjected the cervical spine to significant axial loading and substantially heightened the risk of SCI.

The National Collegiate Athletic Association and high school governing bodies banned spearing in 1976. With rule changes, football coaches began modifying their technique teachings. Players were taught to keep their heads up during blocking and tackling, such that initial contact was generally made with the shoulder pads and/or facemask. See what you hit became a common mantra encouraging players to keep their heads up, and avoid head-down engagement during contact.

Over the next decade there was a 70% reduction in the rate of cervical spine injuries and an 82% decrease in cases of traumatic quadriplegia in US football. Even after the institution of these rule and technique changes, there continues to be about 14 catastrophic cervical spinal injuries a year, resulting in a spectrum of permanent neurologic impairment. Because of its popularity in the United States, football tends to garner media attention, but is not the only sport in which neck injuries are a concern. Sports such as cheerleading, gymnastics, ice hockey, lacrosse, and equestrian events also place participants at risk for significant cervical spinal injuries with associated SCI.[1]

TRAUMATIC SCI

SCI is the most feared complication of forces acting on the cervical spine. The spectrum of SCI ranges from transient and temporary to complete and irreparable. Awareness, recognition, and a rapid coordinated response to a possible SCI event is the responsibility of the sideline medical professional. Prompt on-field assessment of potentially catastrophic injuries begins with the primary survey: assessing level of consciousness, airway patency, breathing, and circulation.

Any athlete with an altered level of consciousness or who complains of significant bilateral neurologic complaints or midline neck pain should be treated as having an unstable spinal injury until proved otherwise. When such an injury is suspected, cervical spine stabilization and transfer to a rigid spine board or similar device is of paramount importance to preserve function and prevent further injury.[2–4]

There are 2 currently recommended techniques for initial manual cervical spine immobilization. The head-squeeze technique has the lead rescuer secure the athlete's head or helmet between the palms of the hands with the rescuer's ulnar fingers just below the mastoid process or posterior edge of the helmet.[5] In the trap-squeeze technique, the lead rescuer holds the head or helmet between the forearms while gripping the athlete's trapezius muscles with thumbs placed anteriorly.[4] Both techniques seem to be equally efficacious in the cooperative patient. However, in the confused or combative patient, the trap squeeze may be superior to the head squeeze for cervical spine stabilization.[2]

SPINE BOARDING AND TRANSFER

After on-field stabilization of the cervical spine, athletes are typically transferred and secured to a long spine board or other similar full-body spinal immobilization device (SID) for transfer to an appropriate emergency facility. The key objective is to minimize spinal movement during the transfer process. The designated rescue team is typically composed of 5 to 7 rescuers. This team should review, rehearse, and become comfortable with techniques that best minimize spinal movement.[6]

Several techniques are used to transfer, immobilize, and transport the injured athlete after cervical stabilization. Two common types used for transfer onto spinal immobilization equipment are the log-roll and the lift-and-slide techniques. The log roll involves the rescue either rolling a prone athlete backward into an SID, or rolling the athlete up onto one side, positioning the SID, and then rolling the patient back down. The lift-and-slide technique calls for the rescue team to, in concert, bodily elevate the supine athlete to the extent that a rigid SID can be slid into position and the athlete lowered onto the equipment for immobilization.

In the past there was some disagreement on which technique resulted in safest transfer. In the last few years, several reports have advocated for the lift and slide as the preferred technique for transfer of the supine athlete. The lift-and-slide technique of transfer has been reported to produce less motion at the head and in the cervical spine than the log roll. In a 2009 National Athletic Trainers' Association (NATA) position statement, the organization recommended that the lift-and-slide technique be used for the supine athlete. The investigators also stated that all potential rescuers must be familiar with the log-roll method for the prone athlete with suspected cervical spine injury.[2,6,7]

SPORTING EQUIPMENT CONSIDERATIONS

Effective rescue of the collision sport athlete may be complicated by sporting equipment considerations. During rescue of the athlete with suspected cervical spine injury, stabilization and maintenance of neutral cervical spinal alignment with preservation of the normal cervical lordotic curve allows for the most space around the spinal cord within the cervical spinal column.[3] The combined effect of intact shoulder pads and helmet in the supine position favorably support the maintenance of the normal lordotic curve of the cervical spinal column resulting in the preferred position of neutral spinal alignment. Unless the equipment fits badly and hinders primary rescue operations, removal of the helmet and/or shoulder pads is not recommended. If the helmet has been removed and shoulder pads remain in place, padding should be placed under the occiput to maintain neutral cervical alignment.[2,3,6,8,9]

PHARMACOLOGIC SCI MANAGEMENT

After publication of the NASCIS (National Spinal Cord Injury Study) 2 study in 1990, the use of a high-dose methylprednisolone protocol for the treatment of acute SCI became a standard of care. Soon afterward, several publications and evidence-based reviews questioned the methods and analysis used to show treatment benefit. The American Association of Neurologic Surgeons and the American Academy of Emergency Medicine, among other organizations, published position statements that glucocorticoid administration in acute SCI must not be considered a standard of care, but only a treatment option with unproven benefit.[10,11]

In 2008, the Consortium for Spinal Cord Medicine also stated that, No clinical evidence exists to definitely recommend steroid therapy.[12] In addition, a survey of 305 US neurosurgeons published in *Spine* showed that although 91% used the glucocorticoid protocol in treatment of SCI, only 24% used it out of a belief that it would improve clinical outcome.[13]

Many investigators do not recommend the routine use of steroids in patients with SCI because of concerns for side effects including increased risk of serious infections and gastrointestinal bleeding. However, other investigators argue that there may be a place for the high-dose methyprednisolone protocol. One recent article proposes that exceptions to the unfavorable risk-benefit profile might be considered for patients with C3-level SCI in whom a 1-level improvement in function could make the difference in a ventilator-dependent or independent outcome.[14] Debate about glucocorticoid therapy continues. Perhaps the current state of the argument is still best described by the 2009 NATA position statement: Until additional reliable data are available, the use of high-dose methylprednisolone for acute spinal cord injury remains controversial.[6]

Other interventions designed to reduce inflammation and swelling and improve SCI outcomes have been under study. Hypothermia has shown potential to reduce morbidity in myocardial infarction and brain injury. The 2007 case of a National Football League (NFL) lineman who recovered from significant SCI after being treated acutely with moderate systemic hypothermia as well as conventional medical and surgical intervention garnered widespread media attention. Although there have been some experimental models and clinical studies showing efficacy in SCI, data to support its common institution are currently insufficient. At least 1 large scale trial is pending.[15–17]

Gangliosides are compounds that occur naturally in cell membranes and with greater density in neuronal membranes. A few early studies suggested that gangliosides may promote neural protection and growth. One ganglioside, GM1, was the focus of attention and research.[18] However, a large multicenter trial failed to show clinical benefit from the use of GM1 in SCI.[19] In addition, a recent Cochran Review concluded that there was no substantial evidence to support the use of gangliosides in the treatment of SCI.[20]

CERVICAL CORD NEUROPRAXIA AND TRANSIENT QUADRIPARESIS

Few cervical injuries in sport result in transection of the spinal cord, but sensory and motor loss can still occur. Cervical cord neuropraxia (CCN) is defined as a transient neurologic deficit following spinal cord trauma. Approximately 80% of such injuries involve all four extremities with variable weakness and combined sensory deficits. Clinical characteristics of CCN include tingling or pain and paresthesias in more than one extremity. A common complaint is the so-called burning hands syndrome, with painful paresthesias in both hands. This bilateral presentation represents a central SCI, and must not be confused with the single upper-extremity presentation of a stinger or burner. A spectrum of muscle weakness from full strength to complete quadriplegia may be present in CCN. With the possible exception of burning paresthesia, neck pain is not present at the time of injury.[3,21]

CCN resulting in 4-limb paralysis is known as transient quadriplegia (TQ), and is estimated to occur in 0.2 per 100,000 high school football players and 2 per 100,000 collegiate football players. By definition, neurologic symptoms in TQ are temporary. There is rapid and complete resolution of symptoms from 10 minutes to 48 hours in adults, but symptoms have persisted for up to 5 days in children. Although repeated episodes of neuropraxia may occur in some adults, there are no reported recurrences in the pediatric population.[22,23]

Regardless of symptom resolution, on-field management should be the same as for a suspected catastrophic cervical spine injury with cervical stabilization, transfer to full-body immobilization, and transport to an appropriate medical facility for further evaluation. Initial imaging has typically been cervical spine radiographs, although computed tomography (CT) can more readily diagnose a cervical fracture or dislocation. In suspected TQ or any CCN, magnetic resonance imaging (MRI) imaging should be performed to evaluate the cervical spinal cord for injury or impingement. Although MRI may occasionally show some cord edema, no fractures or frank cord injuries should be seen on imaging in patients with suspected CCN spectrum.[24]

Cervical spinal stenosis (CSS) is a congenital or acquired narrowing of the spinal canal, and is closely associated with CNN and TQ. After Torg defined CSS via a ratio based on radiographic measurements (spinal canal/vertebral body), there was disagreement in the literature about the usefulness of that description.[21] Although a Torg ratio of 0.8 or less identifying significant cervical stenosis was prevalent in patients who had experienced CCN, its low positive predictive value (0.2%) for CCN left it ineffective as a screening tool. Continued research indicated that the Torg ratio might be useful in identifying those adult athletes at risk for recurrent CCN and TQ after an initial event. One separate small retrospective study of 13 pediatric patients with CCN showed that none of the patients studied had CSS. That finding suggested that the Torg ratio defining CSS might not be applicable to the pediatric population.[21–23]

MRI techniques have been used to measure and describe the anatomy and mechanics of CSS, and have surpassed standard radiographic imaging in this regard. The ability of MRI to directly image herniated discs and allow measurement of the spinal column, vertebral discs, and spinal canal and cord make it the preferred method of evaluation. Recent publications place emphasis on quantifying an amount of functional stenosis observed on cervical imaging. The functional reserve of the spinal canal refers to cerebrospinal fluid that is able to flow freely around the spinal cord.[24] Although its clinical usefulness remains to be proved, some investigators are advocating dynamic MRI in flexion and extension to evaluate for functional CSS and possibly to inform return-to-play decision making.[3]

TRANSIENT QUADRIPARESIS AND RETURN TO PLAY

Opinions differ regarding the development of clear guidelines on return-to-play decisions because large-scale studies on such rare events as transient quadriparesis do not exist. Torg and colleagues[25] reported on a collection of 110 athletes who experienced an episode of TQ. Fifty- seven percent of them returned to contact sports, and, although more than half of those (56%) experienced a second episode of TQ, none of them were reported to have suffered a catastrophic or permanent neurologic injury. In one of the earlier studies defining CCN, Torg and colleagues[24] reported a poll of 117 individuals listed on the NFL Registry of Head and Neck as having suffered complete irreversible SCI. Two reported memory of previous transient sensory disturbance, but none recalled any motor paresis or TQ before their catastrophic SCI.[24] A significant amount of research has been devoted to describing CSS and evaluating its relevance to SCI in an attempt to identify athletes at risk. Stenosis of the cervical spinal canal does not predict, but is strongly correlated with, the CCN/TQ injury spectrum in adults but not necessarily in the pediatric population.

There is a paucity of published literature providing data to firmly guide return-to-play decisions after an episode of transient quadriparesis. There has been long-standing debate in the literature as to whether TQ is a risk factor for future spinal cord injury, specifically catastrophic or complete SCI. Some investigators think that a single episode of CCN in the setting of CSS should be an absolute contraindication to return to contact sport. Others hold that an episode of CCN or TQ with associated CSS increases only the likelihood of similar recurrence, and in no way portends worse or permanent injury. To date, research best supports the position that, in the absence of cervical spine instability or CSS, temporary CCN and transient quadriparesis are not associated with a significantly increased risk for permanent or catastrophic SCI. However, investigators vary widely in their opinions on return-to-play criteria after TQ or CCN in the setting of CSS.[21–27]

STINGERS AND BURNERS

Stingers or burners are perhaps the most common peripheral nerve injury in contact sports. Athletes typically present with complaints of unilateral upper extremity burning or paresthesias with associated motor weakness after a contact or collision event. These symptoms occur in the absence of frank cervical pain or limited cervical range of motion (ROM). Any symptoms occurring in a bilateral pattern or including a lower extremity are similarly signs of an SCI and cervical spine precautions must be initiated. Up to 65% of collegiate football players report a stinger-type injury at least once in their playing history, and there has been as much as an 87% recurrence rate reported.

The C5 and C6 nerve distributions are most commonly involved in stingers. In addition to sensory disturbance, concurrent transient weakness may be expected in the biceps, deltoid, or other shoulder abductors; the C5 and C6 nerve roots serve most sensory dermatomes of the upper extremity save the ulnar sides of the arm and little finger. The spectrum of burning, tingling, or lancinating sensory disturbance that tend to define this injury may vary. The symptoms are usually short-lived and resolve spontaneously within a few minutes. Symptoms sometimes persist for 2 or more weeks; however, any athlete with persistent symptoms for greater than 24 to 36 hours should be evaluated for possible SCI.[28]

Stingers seem to result from either traction of the brachial plexus or compression of the cervical nerve root. There is disagreement in the literature as to the exact location, and therefore the predominant mechanism of the nerve injury. A few studies suggest that nerve root compression may be responsible for the preponderance of stinger-type injuries. The debate has been hampered by the failure of imaging and electromyography to accurately identify nerve lesions corresponding with symptoms in affected athletes.

The mechanism for the traction injury is depression of the shoulder ipsilateral to the injury with concomitant lateral flexion of the neck to the contralateral side. During this motion the brachial plexus is stretched, which may lead to nerve damage. This type of traction injury seems to occur more commonly in young athletes with less experience and weak neck and shoulder musculature without a history of cervical spine injury and who tend to lack radiographic evidence of cervical spondylosis.[24]

Stingers also occur secondary to forceful hyperextention of the neck with head rotation to the ipsilateral side during contact. This action narrows the neural foramina leading to an increased risk of compression and injury at the cervical nerve root. There is continued debate in the literature, but this extension-compression may be the most common causative mechanism resulting in the stinger presentation.[28] Several investigators have described its association with older college-aged and professional athletes, especially those with preexisting cervical disc disease, cervical stenosis, or other related conditions.[22]

Most players have resolution of symptoms within a few minutes, with normal sensation and full strength. Athletes with pain-free cervical ROM and complete resolution of stinger symptoms within 15 minutes from onset may be returned to play in the same game. For those with longer lasting symptoms, return to play may be allowed once symptoms have abated and brachial stretch and axial loading tests are not provocative.

In some cases, symptoms can persist for days or weeks. It is thought that the duration may be related to the degree of axonal or nerve root injury but, again, electromyography has so far yielded inconsistent results. However, myelographic imaging such as MRI, possibly accompanied by electrodiagnostic studies, is suggested in patients with symptoms lasting longer than 2 weeks.

Athletes who have experienced a stinger should have their contact technique reviewed for at-risk head positioning during contact. Proper shoulder pad and helmet fitting should be ensured. Participation in a year-round neck strengthening program may also be helpful. Cervical collars (Cowboy, Bullock, and KerrCollars) or neck rolls have been used to limit neck ROM in football players with the intent of decreasing stinger recurrence. Use of these is controversial, with some investigators advocating their use for limiting neck ROM. Other investigators argue that limiting extension may produce the unwanted effect of placing the player's head in a more flexed position, thereby potentially increasing the risk of severe spinal injury. There is currently no good evidence that cervical collars or neck rolls protect against stingers. There is also no strong evidence that recurrent stingers increase the risk of more serious injury, but some investigators propose that a third stinger during a season should prompt consideration for removal of the athlete from play.[21,28,29]

CERVICAL SPRAIN AND STRAIN

Cervical strains and sprains are common entities in contact sports and there is often overlap with elements of both from one event. They characteristically present as localized neck pain with the absence of radiation or neurologic deficit. Mildly limited ROM may be present. Almost all complaints of neck injury occurring in contact sport require the physician to rule out serious cervical spinal injury with a thorough physical examination and imaging as indicated.

A strain involves injury to cervical muscle or musculotendinous junctions. Strains generally occur as a result of a force applied to the head or neck during muscle contraction. The contraction becomes eccentric in nature leading to microscopic or gross tissue shearing. The healing process for these injuries has been described to occur in 3 phases. The destructive phase involves hematoma formation and initiation of the inflammatory response, and this is followed by the repair phase, characterized by phagocytosis of necrotic tissue, myofiber regeneration, and fibrous tissue formation. The third phase, the remodeling phase, involves the remodeling and maturation of muscle and scar tissue.[30]

Acute cervical sprains are seen frequently in collision sports. Athletes often complain of a jammed neck with localized cervical pain and a limited cervical ROM. When acute structural injury is not suspected, the clinical examination should focus on ROM. A restricted ROM precludes immediate return to play. If an athlete is unable or unwilling to perform an ROM examination, a more significant injury should be ruled out.

In adults, a cervical radiographic finding between adjacent vertebral bodies demonstrating greater than 3.5 mm horizontal displacement, or greater than 11 degrees of angulation, is indicative of instability. Such findings require specialist consultation and are a contraindication to contact or collision sport participation.[31] However, in the pediatric population there is often a hypermobility of segments C2 to C4 on imaging, known as pseudosubluxation. Recognition of this entity may reduce the incidence of overdiagnosis and unnecessary treatment.[21,31,32]

The initial treatment of a cervical sprain or strain is similar, and should be tailored to the severity of the injury. Rest, ice, nonsteroidal antiinflammatory drugs (NSAIDs), and soft-collar neck support, as needed, are appropriate interventions. The postinjury period generally involves radiographic evaluation of the cervical spine. Soft-collar support may be discontinued after muscle spasm has subsided, followed by ROM and isometric strengthening exercises. Return to play is allowable once all symptoms of the sprain or strain have resolved and pain-free ROM with full strength has returned.

DISC DISEASE/HERNIATION

Cervical disc disease is an uncommon cause of neck, shoulder, and arm pain in young people. However, it does occur with increased frequency in those who participate in collision sports. Vertebral discs can be thought of as having a gelatinous center, the nucleus pulposis (NP), enclosed within a fibrous sheath, the annulus. These shock absorbers are intercalated between vertebrae throughout the spinal column. Significant deformation of cervical discs can cause symptomatic impingement most commonly affecting the C4 to C7 nerve roots. An acute disc herniation is also capable of causing direct spinal cord compression, resulting in varying degrees of transient or even permanent paralysis. Cervical disc disease is described as occurring in 2 forms: soft disc disease or hard disc disease.

The term hard disc disease refers to a chronic degenerative process producing a spectrum of spondylotic cervical changes. It is the more common of the two forms and tends to occur in adult athletes and the adult population. The changes involved include the bony vertebral structures with marginal osteophyte formation and often facet arthropathy. There is associated desiccation of the NP and decreased elasticity of the disc annulus, which can contribute to annular bulging or frank herniation of annular contents. The symptoms of hard disc disease tend to emerge over time as waxing and waning stiffness and pain that may be exacerbated by contact or collision events.

Soft disc disease describes an acute herniation of the gelatinous nucleus pulposus through the annulus of a cervical disc. This annular rupture with extrusion is usually the result of a collision or contact event producing acute neck pain and paraspinal muscle spasms. The NP commonly extrudes in a posterior-lateral direction, where it can cause foraminal nerve root impingement. Depending on the cervical level, a spectrum of neurologic symptoms may manifest.

A disc herniation usually affects the nerve root exiting at that segment. Therefore, a herniated C4 to C5 disc can compress the C5 nerve root, producing pain radiating from neck to deltoid, weakness of shoulder adduction, lateral shoulder paresthesia, and a decreased biceps reflex. C5 to C6 herniation may impinge on the C6 nerve root, producing weakness of the biceps and wrist extensors with pain radiating into the radial half of the hand. Seventh nerve root compression correlates with loss of reflex and weakness of the triceps, as well as weakness of wrist flexors and finger extensors. Pain may radiate from the neck down the posterior arm into the forearm and hand. Impingement of cervical nerve 8 can affect strength in the finger flexors and intrinsic muscles of the hand, with pain and paresthesias radiating to the ulnar forearm, hand, and fingers.[33]

MRI is an important tool in the evaluation and diagnosis of herniated discs. It can provide excellent delineation of discs, nerves, and surrounding soft tissue structures. However, imaging alone should not be substituted for a thorough clinical examination. Imaging must be correlated with clinical findings, because more than 30% to 40% of asymptomatic adults have some degree of disc protrusion on MRI.

In the absence of myelopathy on imaging or progressive neurologic deficits, conservative measures are the cornerstone of management. Rest, activity modification, NSAIDs, and muscle relaxants to treat paraspinal muscle spasm are frequently recommended therapies.[31] Narcotic analgesia may be necessary if pain is not well controlled. Although it is commonly used during conservative treatment, a recent evidence-based review found insufficient evidence to adequately address the usefulness of physical therapy in this setting.[34]

For patients not responding to conservative measures, cervical epidural steroid injections have frequently been used. CT or fluoroscopic-guided transforaminal epidural steroid injections may provide relief for up to 60% of patients, and 25% of patients with clear surgical indications may obtain at least short-term pain relief negating the need for surgery.[34]

SURGERY

Symptoms of cervical compression with myelopathy on imaging and significant or progressive neurologic symptoms may call for acute surgical intervention. Many surgical techniques have been used to decompress the spinal cord and roots using anterior or posterior approaches. Overall clinical outcomes for single-level cervical disc surgery are commonly reported as satisfactory in 90% to 95% of cases in the general population. Decisions on surgery should be individualized. Many experts currently advocate return to play in collision sport for asymptomatic athletes after a single-level anterior cervical discectomy and fusion (ACDF).[26] Traditional recommendations have been to reserve surgery for patients failing conservative measures after from 4 to 12 weeks. However, given the high percentage of good outcomes, many investigators recommend early surgical intervention rather than other medical treatments.[34]

A recent study of NFL athletes made a case for surgical intervention in these professionals. Performance-based outcomes of athletes undergoing cervical disc surgery, usually ACDF, were compared with those opting for conservative treatment. Seventy-two percent of those opting for surgical intervention successfully returned to play, whereas only 46% of those treated with conservative measures alone returned to play successfully.[35]

It is not clear how the study of NFL players can inform the decision-making process for young athletes. The study was retrospective and nonrandomized. It did not evaluate for concomitant CSS and did not detail the type or grade of disc disease among the two groups. Professional athletes who have spent more time involved in collision sport could be expected to have a higher degree of cervical spondylosis than high school or college-aged athletes. However, the results of the NFL study will likely influence management decisions with regard to the elite athlete.

SUMMARY

Spinal cord injuries are uncommon in sports. Planning and practice for their occurrence, however, remains an essential component of Sideline Medical Team preparedness. Evaluation of cervical nerve injury, cervical cord injury, and cervical disc disease can be complex. Medical management, diagnostic imaging techniques and surgical recommendations in this setting continue to evolve. Most published guidance offers occasionally opposed expert opinion with sport participation after Cervical Cord Neuropraxia in the setting of Cervical Spinal Stenosis appearing particularly polarizing. Such conflicts can present challenges to clinicians in forming management and Return to Play decisions for the health of their athletes.

REFERENCES

1. Banerjee R. Catastrophic cervical spine injuries in the collision sport athlete, part 1: epidemiology, functional anatomy, and diagnosis. Am J Sports Med 2004;32(4): 1077–87.
2. Boissy P, Shrier I, Brière S, et al. Effectiveness of cervical spine stabilization techniques. Clin J Sport Med 2011;21(2):80–8.
3. Bailes JE, Petschauer M, Guskiewics KM, et al. Management of cervical spine injuries in athletes. J Athl Train 2007;42:126–34.
4. Kleiner D, Almquist J, Bailes JE. Prehospital care of the spine- injured athlete. Dallas (TX): Inter-Association Task Force for Appropriate Care of the Spine-Injured Athlete; 2001.

5. National Association of EMTs. Prehospital trauma life support. 6th edition. Philadelphia: Mosby; 2007. p. 222–69.
6. Swartz E, Boden B, Courson R, et al. National Athletic Trainers' Association position statement: acute management of the cervical spine-injured athlete. J Athl Train 2009;44(3):306–31.
7. Waniger K. Cervical spine injury management in the helmeted athlete. Curr Sports Med Rep 2011;10:45–9.
8. Decoster LC, Burns MF. Maintaining neutral sagittal cervical alignment after football helmet removal during emergency spine injury management. Spine (Phila Pa 1976) 2012;37(8):654–9.
9. Bracken M, Shepard M, Collins WF, et al. A randomized, controlled trial of methylprednisolone or naloxone in the treatment of acute spinal-cord injury- results of the second National Acute Spinal Cord Injury Study. N Engl J Med 1990;322: 1405–11.
10. Hurlbert R. Methylprednisolone for acute spinal cord injury: an inappropriate standard of care. J Neurosurg 2000;93(Suppl):1.
11. Sayer FT, Kronvall E, Nilsson OG. Methylprednisolone treatment in acute spinal cord injury: the myth challenged through a structured analysis of published literature. Spine J 2006;6(3):335.
12. Consortium for Spinal Cord Medicine. Early acute management in adults with spinal cord injury: a clinical practice guideline for health-care professionals. J Spinal Cord Med 2008;31(4):403–79.
13. Eck JC, Nachtgill D, Humphreys SC, et al. Questionnaire survey of spine surgeons on the use of methylprednisolone for acute spinal injury. Spine 2006; 31(9):E250.
14. Markandaya M, Stein D, Menaker J. Acute treatment options for spinal cord injury. Curr Treat Options Neurol 2012. [Epub ahead of print].
15. Dietrich WD, Cappuccino A, Cappuccino H. Systemic hypothermia for the treatment of acute cervical spinal cord injury in sports. Curr Sports Med Rep 2011; 10(1):50–4.
16. Dietrich WD. Therapeutic hypothermia for acute severe spinal cord injury: ready to start large clinical trials? Crit Care Med 2012;40(2):691–2.
17. Maybhate A, Hu C, Bazley FA, et al. Potential long-term benefits of acute hypothermia after spinal cord injury: assessments with somatosensory-evoked potentials. Crit Care Med 2012;40:573–9.
18. Michael LJ. Pharmacologic therapy after acute cervical spinal cord injury. Neurosurgery 2002;50(Suppl 3):S63–72.
19. Geisler FH, Coleman WP. The Sygen multicenter spinal cord injury study. Spine 2001;26(Suppl 24):s87–98.
20. Chinnock P, Roberts I. Gangliosides for acute spinal cord injury. Cochrane Database Syst Rev 2005;(2):CD004444.
21. Torg JS. Cervical spine injuries and the return to football. Sports Health 2009; 1:376.
22. Chao S, Pacella MJ, Torg JS. The pathomechanics, pathophysiology and prevention of cervical spinal cord and brachial plexus injuries in athletics. Sports Med 2010;40(1):59–75.
23. Clark AJ, August K, Sun PP. Cervical spinal stenosis and sports-related cervical cord neuropraxia. Neurosurg Focus 2011;31(5):E7.
24. Concannon L, Harrast M, Herring S. Radiating upper limb pain in the contact sport athlete: an update on transient quadriparesis and stingers. Curr Sports Med Rep 2012;11(1):28–34.

25. Torg JS, Pavlov H, Genaurio SE, et al. Neuropraxia of the cervical spinal cord with transient quadriplegia. J Bone Joint Surg Am 1986;68:1354–70.
26. Dailey A, Harrop JS, France JC. High-energy contact sports and cervical spine neuropraxia injuries: what are the criteria for return to participation? Spine 2010;35(Suppl 21):S193–201.
27. Davis G, Ugokwe K, Roger EP, et al. Clinics in neurology and neurosurgery of sport: asymptomatic cervical canal stenosis and transient quadriparesis. Br J Sports Med 2009;43:1154–8.
28. Mayer JE, Cho SK, Qureshi SA, et al. Cervical spine injury in athletes. Current Orthopedic Practice 2012;23(3):181–7.
29. Standaert C, Herring S. Expert opinion and controversies in musculoskeletal and sports medicine: stingers. Arch Phys Med Rehabil 2009;90:402–6.
30. Zmurko MG, Tannoury TY, Tannoury CA, et al. Cervical sprains, disc herniations, minor fractures, and other cervical injuries in the athlete. Clin Sports Med 2003; 22:513–21.
31. Chang D, Bosco J. Cervical spine injuries in the athlete. Bull NYU Hosp Jt Dis 2006;64(3–4):119–29.
32. Proctor M, Cantu R. Head and neck injuries in young athletes. Clin Sports Med 2000;19(4):693–715.
33. Sherping SC. Cervical disc disease in the athlete. Clin Sports Med 2002;21(1): 37–47.
34. Bono C, Ghiselli G, Gilbert T, et al. An evidence-based guideline for the diagnosis and treatment of cervical radiculopathy from degenerative disorders. Spine J 2011;11:64–72.
35. Hsu W. Outcomes following nonoperative and operative treatment for cervical disc herniations in National Football League Athletes. Spine 2011;36(10):800–5.

Back Pain in Adults

Jonathan A. Becker, MD[a,b,*], Jessica R. Stumbo, MD[a,b,c]

KEYWORDS

• Back pain • Lumbar spine • Disk herniation • Imaging • Therapeutics
• Pharmacotherapy

KEY POINTS

- Back pain is common with most experiencing full relief of symptoms with minimal intervention within 4 to 6 weeks.
- The initial patient history and examination should focus on identifying any "red flags" that lead the clinician to suspect more severe pathology, such as cancer, infection, fracture, or cauda equina syndrome.
- For most patients, there is no indication for imaging of the lumbar spine and obtaining early studies does not improve outcomes.
- Radiographs are the initial imaging modality of choice, but rarely yield a definitive diagnosis.
- In nearly all complicated cases of back pain, MRI is the most useful imaging modality.
- NSAIDs are commonly used as a first-line therapy for back pain, but carry significant gastrointestinal, renal, and cardiovascular side effects.
- Despite their frequent use for more severe cases of back pain, there is only variable evidence regarding the effectiveness of opioids and systemic corticosteroids.
- Physical therapy is recommended when pain persists for more than 2 to 3 weeks. There is no standard protocol and the evidence supporting specific modalities is limited.
- Epidural steroid injections have been shown to provide a moderate short-term benefit for those with back and leg pain.
- Back surgery is indicated for the minority of patients, but provides the greatest benefit for those with sciatica, pseuoclaudication, or spondylolisthesis.

INTRODUCTION AND EPIDEMIOLOGY

Low back pain is a common problem accounting for a staggering use of the health care system with direct and indirect costs exceeding $100 billion per year in the United States.[1] To illustrate, low back pain is the second most common reason for a physician visit, it accounts for 2% to 3% of all physician visits, and 25% of all adults in the United States report at least 1 day of pain over a 3-month period.

Disclosures: None.
[a] Primary Care Sports Medicine Fellowship, Jewish Hospital and University of Louisville, Louisville, KY, USA; [b] Department of Family and Geriatric Medicine, University of Louisville, Louisville, KY, USA; [c] Centers for Primary Care, 215 Central Avenue, Suite 205, Louisville, KY 40208, USA
* Corresponding author. Department of Family and Geriatric Medicine, 201 Abraham Flexner Way, Suite 690, Louisville, KY 40202.
E-mail address: jon.becker@louisville.edu

Prim Care Clin Office Pract 40 (2013) 271–288
http://dx.doi.org/10.1016/j.pop.2013.02.002 primarycare.theclinics.com
0095-4543/13/$ – see front matter

For most, this is a self-limited condition with 90% experiencing full relief of symptoms with minimal intervention.[2] However, nearly one-third experience pain in excess of 6 months[3] and one-fourth experience a recurrence within 1 year.[1] The prevalence of low back pain has been increasing since 1990 with patients more likely to seek care, require multiple visits, and report chronic pain. Those with chronic pain are more likely to become less physically active and report higher levels of disability.[4]

As in the general population, low back pain is common in athletes. Although overall prevalence is unknown, published rates in competitive athletes range from 1% to 30%.[5] In young and healthy populations, participation in sports seems to be a risk factor for back pain with athletes having a higher incidence compared with those who are sedentary. However, in former elite athletes, there seems to be a lower lifelong incidence.[5,6]

There are specific activities that carry a higher prevalence of low back pain, especially those that involve repetitive hyperextension, such as gymnastics, diving, volleyball, golf, or football (offensive line). Throwing athletes, such as quarterbacks and pitchers, also seem to be at higher risk for back issues. Most of these cases are self-limited and do not cause any alteration in activity. However, low back pain is the most common reason for lost time in a competitive athlete.[5,6]

HISTORY

Regardless of the level of activity of the patient, the history should focus on identifying any "red flags" for a severe pathology. Low back pain is such a common problem that an accurate history may be the only reliable way to determine if the patient's pain is from a benign cause rather than one necessitating rapid diagnosis and treatment. These causes include cancer, cauda equina syndrome, infection, and fracture. A patient's low back pain is not attributable to a spinal abnormality or disease state in 85% of cases so a rigorous work-up is not indicated unless there are clues in the history or physical examination. Even in the presence of a "red flag," only a minority of patients have significant pathology.[3,6–8]

The evaluation of all patients presenting with low back pain starts with a detailed history. At the minimum, it should include the onset, duration, location, and frequency of the pain. Attention should be paid to any clues of a neurologic deficit, radicular pain, spinal stenosis, or an inflammatory condition. Any history of a back injury, use of prior treatments, and their efficacy is also important to review. Perhaps more than in other conditions, a thorough psychosocial history should be taken with emphasis on substance abuse, injury litigation, workmen's compensation, job dissatisfaction, or psychiatric issues.

The history is crucial to finding any underlying "red flags" for more severe processes, such as cancer, vertebral fracture, cauda equina syndrome, or infection. The following should yield concern for neoplasm: any prior history of cancer or metastases; pain unrelieved by rest or when supine; systemic symptoms, such as fever, night sweats, or weight loss; advanced age (>50 years old); and greater than 6 weeks of pain. Those with a history of trauma, osteoporosis (or anything that affects bone health), substance abuse, long-term corticosteroid use, and the elderly are at higher risk for a vertebral fracture. Cauda equina syndrome should be considered if there are bowel or bladder symptoms; sudden onset of pain; or any progressive loss of neurologic function, such as loss of sensation or weakness. Spinal infection may present in the setting of prior lumbar surgery; unrelenting pain not relieved with rest; fever; immunosuppression; long-term corticosteroid use; intravenous drug use; or recent infection (eg, urinary tract, tuberculosis).

Other clues in the history may prompt further investigation for specific causes. The combination of back and leg pain, symptoms worse with sitting, the presence of numbness or tingling are all typical of radicular pain from a herniated disk or sciatica. Spinal stenosis may present with leg pain that is in excess of back pain, pain exacerbated by standing or walking, or pain relieved by sitting or flexing the spine. Morning stiffness is the hallmark of an inflammatory condition. Patients may also present with constant pain, concomitant gastrointestinal or dermatologic problems, or the presence of other autoimmune diseases.

When treating athletes, it is crucial to obtain specific information regarding their sports or activities. Age, gender, and level of fitness are all useful pieces of information, but any changes in training patterns should also be noted. Review any changes in their training, such as technique, volume, or intensity. Also be sure to note how their symptoms have affected their ability to participate or their performance. The nature of their activity may also play a role in their pain if it involves hyperextension, throwing, twisting, or running. If the athlete has any condition that affects bone health, it places them at a unique risk for stress fractures. These include any aspects of the female athlete triad, deficiencies in calcium and vitamin D intake, any personal or family history of osteoporosis, or prior corticosteroid use.[6]

PHYSICAL EXAMINATION

Before a cause has been determined for low back pain, the physical examination should include at least the following elements:

- Inspection of the lumbar spine
  - Assess for kyphosis, lordosis, or scoliosis
  - Rashes, wounds, signs of trauma or infection
  - Hair patches, sacral dimple, nevi, cafe au lait spots
- Range of motion
  - Lumbar flexion stresses the anterior spine (disk, vertebrae)
  - Lumbar extension stresses the posterior spine (pars, facets)
- Gait evaluation
  - Limping
  - Foot drop
  - Tandem gait
  - Trendelenburg gait
- Palpation of the spine and paraspinal areas
- Straight leg raise testing for those with leg pain[9]
  - Done with the patient supine, examiner passively raises the leg
  - Recreates radicular pain between 10 and 60 degrees
  - When present, a sensitive, but not specific sign
  - Crossed straight leg raising (testing the unaffected leg) carries a higher sensitivity
- Lower extremity neurovascular examination
  - Strength, sensation, and reflex testing (**Table 1**)
  - Focus on L4-S1 nerve roots because this accounts for nearly all disk pathology[3,9]
  - Diminished reflexes may be normal with advanced age
  - Spinal stenosis may have a similar presentation as vascular disease

Significant vertebral tenderness, limited range of motion, fever, or open wounds may be indicative of infection. Fractures also present with limited range of motion and marked vertebral tenderness. Progressive neurologic deficits, such as marked weakness, sensory deficits, loss of anal sphincter tone, or saddle anesthesia, yield a concern for cauda equina syndrome. Lymphadenopathy or other abnormal physical

Table 1
Correlation of physical examination findings with corresponding nerve roots

Nerve Root	Reflex	Strength	Sensory
L4 (L3-L4 disk space)	Patella	Ankle dorsiflexion (tibialis anterior); heel walk	Medial side of the lower leg (medial malleolus)
L5 (L4-L5 disk space)	None	Dorsiflexion of the great toe (extensor hallucis longus)	Lateral aspect of the lower leg and dorsum of the foot
S1 (L5-S1 disk space)	Achilles	Plantar flexion and eversion (peroneus longus and brevis); toe walk (gastrocnemius)	Lateral and plantar side of the foot; lateral malleolus

examination findings related to potential sites of cancer may be present with neoplasm or malignancy.[6,7,9,10]

IMAGING

For most patients with low back pain, imaging is not warranted and does not improve outcomes.[3,7,11] During the first 4 to 6 weeks of symptoms, the American College of Physicians advises that imaging be delayed unless there are signs or symptoms of a serious underlying "red flag" condition. They, along with the American College of Radiology, have developed criteria for early imaging (**Table 2**).

When imaging the lumbar spine, radiographs are generally the initial test of choice. Although they typically do not provide definitive diagnosis, they can be useful to rule out fractures in the setting of "minor" red flags, such as low-velocity trauma or advanced age. Radiographs may also reveal signs of osteoporosis. For most, magnetic resonance imaging (MRI) is the test of choice for complicated low back conditions. These include pain for greater than 4 to 6 weeks, the presence of any historical "red flags," concern for spinal stenosis, radicular symptoms, or neurologic findings. MRI has the advantage of provide details of the bony anatomy and the soft tissues.[3,10]

Table 2
Indications for early imaging of the lumbar spine

American College of Physicians Practice Guideline: Indications for Early Imaging in Low Back Pain	American College of Radiology Appropriateness Criteria for Imaging
Progressive neurologic findings	Symptoms >6 wk
Constitutional symptoms	Trauma
Age >50 y old	Age >70 y old (or trauma at >50 y old)
Trauma	Weight loss
History of malignancy	Fever (unexplained)
Osteoporosis	Cancer
Risk factors for infection (steroid use, immunosuppression, intravenous drug use)	Long-term steroid use or osteoporosis Intravenous drug use Immunosuppression Progressive neurologic deficit Disabling symptoms Prior surgery

Data from Chou R, Qaseem A, Owens DK, et al. Diagnostic imaging for low back pain: Advice for high-value health care from the American College of Physicians. Ann Intern Med 2011;154:181–9; and American College of Radiology. ACR Appropriateness Criteria. Low back pain. http://www.acr.org/~/media/ACR/Documents/AppCriteria/Diagnostic/LowBackPain.pdf. Accessed July 9, 2012.

Computerized tomography (CT) is useful for patients who cannot undergo MRI, those with surgical hardware, or if there is a need for precise bony anatomy. Myelography, diskography, and bone scan are reserved for when specific conditions are suspected. Bone scan with single photon emission CT (SPECT) imaging provides the sensitivity of a bone scan along with three-dimensional resolution. This makes SPECT a particularly attractive option for the diagnosis of stress fracture. Unlike traditional bone scan, SPECT scans take images from multiple angles and the data can be manipulated to display the anatomy in thin slices much like CT or MRI. Fire scan is an emerging technology that digitally combines CT in tandem to bone scan with SPECT images. It has the unique ability to provide sensitivity of bone scan with bony detail of CT scan. It is purported to have a unique ability to identify areas of bone turnover in great detail, particularly in facet disease.[12]

Athletes carry a higher suspicion of stress fracture than the general population. In light of that, bone scan with SPECT imaging is frequently used early in the evaluation of back in athletes. However, even in those cases where there is high suspicion for bony abnormality, it has been recommended that MRI remain the preferred modality. MRI identifies the subtle changes of bony injury while also providing further detail regarding other structures, such as intervertebral disks. Further modalities could then be used if the diagnosis remains in question.[13]

DIFFERENTIAL DIAGNOSIS

Tables 3–9 illustrate the differential diagnosis.[3,6,10,14–18]

Table 3
Common causes of low back pain

Diagnosis	Key Historical and Physical Examination Findings	Diagnostic Studies
Lumbar strain	• Acute onset, possibly an injury • Symptoms worse with activity, relieved with rest • Paraspinal spasm or tenderness	• Only to exclude alternative diagnoses
Disk herniation	• Pain often worse with sitting • Symptoms radiate to lower extremities, typically below the knees • Follows dermatomal pattern • Positive straight leg raise	• MRI if symptoms >4 wk • Electromyography and nerve conduction studies if diagnosis in question
Degenerative disk disease	• Pain worse with flexion or sitting • Chronic pain	• Radiographs • MRI
Facet disease	• Pain worse with extension • Worse with standing or walking	• Radiographs • MRI
Spondylolisthesis	• Leg pain may be greater than back pain • Worse with extension, relieved by flexion • Pain worse with activity	• Radiographs • MRI
Spinal stenosis	• Pain relived by sitting or flexion • Lower-extremity paresthesias, possibly bilateral • Neurogenic claudication (pseudoclaudication) • Elderly	• MRI • CT may be useful to delineate bony anatomy • Vascular studies to rule out claudication

Table 4
Causes of low back pain warranting emergent treatment

Diagnosis	Key Historical and Physical Examination Findings	Diagnostic Studies
Neoplastic: • Myeloma • Spinal cord tumor • Metastases	• Systemic symptoms: fever, weight loss, fatigue • Pain when lying down or night pain • History of cancer	• Radiographs • MRI
Cauda equina syndrome	• Saddle anesthesia • Progressive motor or sensory changes • Urinary retention • Bowel or bladder incontinence • Loss of rectal tone	• MRI
Infection • Osteomyelitis • Diskitis • Epidural abscess	• Fever • Loss of range of motion • History of intravenous drug abuse • Severe pain • Recent surgery or infection • Immunosuppression	• MRI • Complete blood count • Blood culture • Sedimentation rate • C-reactive protein
Fracture	• History of trauma • Low bone mineral density/osteoporosis • Corticosteroid use • Vertebral tenderness • Elderly	• Radiographs • Additional imaging if diagnosis in question

Table 5
Inflammatory causes of low back pain

Diagnosis	Key Historical and Physical Examination Findings	Diagnostic Studies
Ankylosing spondylitis	• Younger population • Predominantly males • Morning stiffness • Pain relieved by activity • Night pain	• Radiographs • Sedimentation rate • C-reactive protein • HLA-B27
Reactive arthritis	• Aseptic arthritis triggered by an extra-articular infection • History of recent gastrointestinal or genitourinary infection • Lower extremities most commonly involved • Classic triad: uveitis, arthritis, urethritis	• Sedimentation rate • C-reactive protein • HLA-B27 (30%–50%) • Imaging to exclude alternative diagnosis
Psoriatic arthritis	• Asymmetric and distal joint involvement • Frequent sacroiliac joint involvement • History of psoriasis with skin and nail changes	• Radiographs
Inflammatory bowel disease	• Systemic manifestation of inflammatory bowel disease • Does not have to correlate with inflammatory bowel disease flare	• Used to exclude alternative explanation for pain
Transverse myelitis	• Develops over 24 h • Typically thoracic spine involvement • Symptoms usually bilateral and occur below level of the lesion • Presents with weakness and sensory deficits or paralysis	• MRI • Cerebrospinal fluid analysis

Table 6
Vascular causes of low back pain

Diagnosis	Key Historical and Physical Examination Findings	Diagnostic Studies
Spinal cord vascular malformation	• Men > women • Typically >50 y old • Progressive radicular symptoms • Psuedoclaudication as in spinal stenosis	• MRI with angiography
Spinal cord infarction	• Rapid onset, often in setting of hypotension or aortic pathology • Pain caused by ischemia • Neurologic deficit ranges from weakness to paresis • Correlates with level of impairment (most common is T8) • History of vascular disorder (eg, vascu litis, hypercoagulable state) • History of diabetes mellitus	• MRI (may be normal for up to 24 h)
Epidural hematoma	• Most often a complication of a procedure (epidural injection or surgery) • Rarely spontaneous • Back or radicular symptoms • Progresses to motor and sensory deficits, possible bowel or bladder involvement	• MRI

Table 7
Metabolic causes of low back pain

Diagnosis	Key Historical and Physical Examination Findings	Diagnostic Studies
Paget disease	• Aching pain that persists into the night • Bony changes and overgrowth lead to pain and spinal stenosis • Cord compression may lead to ischemia	• Radiographs • Alkaline phosphatase • Tests for increased bone turnover • MRI to exclude alternative cause for symptoms
Osteoporosis	• Any comorbidity affecting bone health • History of low bone mineral density • Family history of osteoporosis	• Imaging to rule out fractures • Bone density (DEXA) scan

Table 8
Miscellaneous causes of low back pain

Diagnosis	Key Historical and Physical Examination Findings	Diagnostic Studies
Episacroiliac lipoma ("back mouse")	• Low back pain described as moving to different locations • Rubbery, mobile mass deep subcutaneous tissue	• Done to rule out alternative diagnoses
Zoster	• Vesicular rash • Dermatomal pattern	• Confirmation with polymerase chain reaction testing or culture
Lyme disease (or other tick-borne illness)	• History of tick bite • Travel to endemic area • Characteristic rash ("target lesion")	• EIA Western blot
Statin-induced myopathy	• Use of statin medications	• Elevated creatinine kinase level

Table 9
Extraspinal causes of low back pain

Diagnosis	Key Historical and Physical Examination Findings	Diagnostic Studies
Aortic dissection or aneurysm	• Pulsatile abdominal mass • Hypertension (or hypotension if ruptured)	• Radiographs may reveal abnormality, but CT scan diagnostic
Kidney stone	• History of stones • Hematuria • Pain radiates to groin	• Red blood cells in urine • Radiographs or CT scan
Pyelonephritis	• Fever, systemic symptoms • Costovertebral angle tenderness	• White blood cells or casts in urine
Retroperitoneal hematoma or abscess	• Recent trauma • Anticoagulant use • Fever, immune deficiency • Retroperitoneal tenderness	• CT scan or ultrasound
Psoas abscess	• Psoas sign • Fever, immune deficiency	• CT scan or ultrasound
Splenic rupture or infarct	• Trauma • Viral infection (mononucleosis) • Hemoglobinopathy	• CT scan or ultrasound
Sickle cell crisis	• History of sickle cell disease (or trait)	

TREATMENT OPTIONS

Most acute episodes of low back pain resolve with conservative therapy within 4 to 6 weeks. However, 5% to 10% of patients develop chronic symptoms (pain lasting greater than 3 months) for which a uniformly effective treatment regimen is lacking. Decisions are complicated by lack of high-quality randomized controlled trials. The goals of treatment should be to educate patients, decrease pain, improve function, and minimize side effects associated with chosen treatment modalities.

Medications

There are a variety of different classes of medications that can be used in the management of low back pain. A main goal of therapy is to use the lowest effective dose for the shortest period of time necessary.

Nonsteroidal anti-inflammatory drugs

Various nonsteroidal anti-inflammatory drugs (NSAIDs) are used in back pain.[3,10,19–26] A recent large Cochrane review[24] supported the use of NSAIDs as first-line management in the treatment of acute and chronic low back pain without sciatica. This review included 65 randomized controlled studies and found statistically significant results in favor of NSAIDs over placebo for improved functional status, number of patients recovered, and decrease in pain intensity from baseline. The 2008 Cochrane review also examined the effectiveness of NSAIDs and found moderate evidence that NSAIDs are equally effective as paracetamol/acetaminophen for pain relief and global improvement.

A higher rate of side effects with all NSAIDs is noted when compared with acetaminophen/paracetamol. This is true for nonselective NSAIDs and the cyclooxygenase-2

(COX-2) selective drugs. The Cochrane review from 2008 concluded that NSAIDs were associated with an increased risk of side effects compared with paracetamol with a relative risk of 1.76 (95% confidence interval, 1.12–2.76; N = 309).

Nephrotoxicity is a concern with all NSAIDs, especially in the elderly and those with underlying renovascular disease. Gastrointestinal adverse events including dyspepsia, ulcer disease, and bleeding are also known side effects. In select populations including those with a history of NSAID-induced peptic ulcer disease, coadministration of a proton pump inhibitor with an NSAID had similar efficacy when compared with COX-2 therapy in terms of arthritic pain control and had less dyspepsia than the COX-2 treatment group (15% vs 5.7%).[25]

The risk of adverse cardiovascular events varies with the NSAIDs. Rofecoxib, a COX-2, was removed from the market because of increased cardiovascular events. A meta-analysis published in 2006[26] found an increase in vascular events in not only the COX-2 medications but also the nonselective NSAIDs, specifically ibuprofen and diclofenac. A 42% relative increase in vascular events compared with placebo was found with use of COX-2 inhibitors. Traditional NSAIDs had a vascular event rate similar to COX-2 medications. Of note, naproxen seemed to have less of a risk of vascular events in this meta-analysis compared with placebo and ibuprofen and diclofenac. Caution is advised when prescribing all NSAIDs especially to those with underlying cardiovascular disease or risk factors for cardiovascular disease.

If a patient does not respond to one NSAID it is worthwhile to try another NSAID of a different class before abandoning NSAIDs as a potential treatment option.

Acetaminophen

Acetaminophen is effective for pain relief and is an option for first-line management of low back pain. It is associated with fewer side effects when compared with NSAIDs. The main concern associated with its use is hepatotoxicity especially in patients with underlying liver disease or alcohol use. Asymptomatic elevations in aminotransferase levels can also occur even in healthy patients especially in doses greater than 4 g per day.[3,10,19–24]

Tramadol

Tramadol acts as a weak opioid receptor agonist and inhibits the reuptake of serotonin and norepinephrine. A 2007 Cochrane review found tramadol to be more effective than placebo for pain control in low back pain. Other studies have demonstrated short-term improvements in pain and function but no long-term studies exist. Most common side effects are headache and nausea. Use with caution in patients with a history of narcotic addiction because of its action at the opioid receptor.[3,10,19–23,27]

Opioids

Too few high-quality studies exist with regards to efficacy of opioids in the management of low back pain. Therefore, use is based on clinical judgment. They are typically not considered a first-line management option. In this author's opinion opioids may be considered a treatment option in patients with severe pain that is not effectively controlled by NSAIDs, acetaminophen, or other conservative management options. Pain that interferes with sleep may also warrant consideration for opioid use. Side effects include nausea, constipation, sedation, confusion, addiction, and dependence.[10,21,27–29]

Systemic corticosteroids

These are not recommended for treatment of isolated low back pain because of lack of evidence showing efficacy.[10,20] There is variable evidence regarding use in acute low back pain with radicular symptoms, but they may be of benefit.[3,22] Patients should be educated about potential adverse effects when these medications are used including agitation, irritability, insomnia, and poor glycemic control in those with diabetes mellitus.

Topical analgesics

These agents provide the advantage of avoiding systemic toxicities, but have the limitation of providing treatment to a localized area. Side effects include skin irritation or allergic reaction. Topical analgesics can be used alone or in conjunction with other therapies including oral medications.[30–33]

Capsaicin, a derivative of cayenne peppers, has shown positive but weak evidence in the treatment of neuropathic and musculoskeletal pain.[30,31] Its proposed mechanism of action is depletion of substance P from the sensory afferent nerve fibers. It must be applied multiple times a day for several weeks to get the full benefit. Topical capsaicin is well tolerated by most, but some experience an intolerable burning sensation. A 2006 Cochrane review[31] reported improvement on the visual analog scale at Days 3 and 14 with regards to acute low back pain and treatment with a topical cream containing capsicum. Similar findings were found for chronic low back pain using a capsicum-containing plaster.

Lidocaine 5% patch is another topical option, but there is no documented evidence regarding effectiveness for the treatment of acute or chronic low back pain. The Food and Drug Administration (FDA) has approved it for the treatment of the pain associated with postherpetic neuralgia. It has also shown potential use for myofascial pain[32,33]; however, more studies are needed. Lidocaine patches are generally well tolerated.

Muscle relaxants

These are effective for short-term symptomatic relief of low back pain especially when combined with NSAID therapy. There is mixed evidence to support long-term use in chronic low back pain. There is a high rate of side effects including dizziness and sedation.[3,21,29,34]

Antidepressants

Conflicting conclusions exist regarding the efficacy of antidepressants in the treatment of chronic low back pain and they should not be considered first-line therapy. A 2003 systemic review of seven randomized controlled trials[35] concluded that tricyclic antidepressants but not selective serotonin reuptake inhibitors provided moderate symptom reduction for patients with chronic low back pain. However, a 2008 Cochrane review[36] stated antidepressants were no more effective than placebo in the treatment of chronic low back pain.

Amitriptyline, a tricyclic antidepressant, is useful in patients with neurogenic pain. Its role in the treatment of back pain is not well defined, but its sedative qualities make it a good option for nighttime use in patients with sleep disturbances.[10,21,35–37]

Depression screening is recommended in patients with chronic low back pain because these two conditions frequently coexist. In 2010, duloxetine was FDA approved for the treatment of chronic musculoskeletal pain including low back pain.[38]

Herbal therapy

Long-term safety data do not exist but short-term studies show herbal preparations, such as devil's claw, white willow bark, and cayenne, may have a role in the treatment of chronic low back pain.[31]

Others

Anticonvulsants including gabapentin are sometimes used for chronic low back pain complicated by radiculopathy and show possible benefits in some trials. At this time, this is not an FDA-approved indication.[39]

Benzodiazepines are commonly used for muscle relaxation in severe cases. This class of drugs can be associated with abuse, addiction, and tolerance. Therefore, they should be used cautiously.[3,10,21,29,40]

Bed Rest

Activity modification is advocated for the treatment of acute low back pain rather than bed rest and immobilization. Bed rest may be recommended for 1 to 2 days if there is severe pain, but patients should be educated that longer periods of bed rest can be associated with a delayed recovery, joint stiffness, and muscle wasting. Provide patient reassurance and education that it is safe to get out of bed and perform activities as tolerated.[3,19,22,41,42]

Physical Therapy

Referral for a course of physical therapy is typically recommended if symptoms persist for more than 2 to 3 weeks. No standard protocol exists. The variety of interventions and modalities used make comparing studies difficult. Individualized regimens that include therapist supervision, stretching, and strengthening tend to be associated with the best outcomes. The McKenzie method, spine stabilization exercises, and home exercise program all display benefits. Traction therapy is "probably not effective" as a single treatment for low back pain according to the 2010 Cochrane review.[3,10,20,22,29,43]

Topical Cold Versus Heat Therapy

Heat therapy seems to be beneficial in reducing pain associated with acute low back pain. Additional pain relief and improved function are achieved when combined with exercise. Minimal evidence exists for the use of cold therapy in acute low back pain.[3,10,29,44,45]

Transcutaneous Electrical Nerve Stimulation

Based on a 2010 review, current evidence does not support the use of transcutaneous electrical nerve stimulation unit in the management of chronic low back pain. As of 2012, Medicare no longer provides coverage for a transcutaneous electrical nerve stimulation unit for this purpose.[10,46,47]

Lumbar Corsets

Evidence for efficacy is unclear regarding use of lumbar corsets in the management of acute and chronic low back pain. Studies show a possible benefit if a lumbar corset is combined with additional spinal support, such as a heat-moldable plastic insert.[3,10,48]

Injection Therapy

The rates of epidural steroid injections and facet injections rose 271% and 231%, respectively, between 1994 and 2001 in the Medicare population.[49]

Epidural steroid injections

Numerous studies have failed to yield a definitive answer regarding the efficacy of epidural steroid injections with published ranges of efficacy between 18% and

90%.[21,22,49–53] The wide range of published efficacy reflects the lack of standardization in injection technique, patient heterogeneity, and the differences in the methodology of the studies analyzing the data. Moderate short-term benefit in patients with chronic low back pain with radiculopathy has been shown.[50] Injections should always be used in conjunction with a multidisciplinary treatment plan.

In a recent study of National Football League players,[52] epidural steroid injections were found to be safe and effective in the treatment of symptomatic acute lumbar disk herniations and allowed a quick return to play. Loss of practice and game time is of high concern in all athletes but especially so in the professional athlete. Therefore, interventions that provide a more rapid return to play are always being sought. In this study, 17 players who had 27 acute disk herniations that were confirmed on MRI from 2003 to 2010 underwent epidural steroid injections. The outcomes were promising because the success rate for returning the athletes to play was 89% with an average loss of 2.8 practices (range, 0–12). Only three players failed conservative treatment and went on to surgery. Risk factors for failed conservative management in this study were disk sequestration noted on MRI and weakness on physical examination. In patients without radicular symptoms no benefit with epidural steroid injections has been shown.

Facet injections and medial branch nerve blocks

Conflicting evidence exists for the efficacy of intra-articular corticosteroid facet injections and medial branch nerve blocks on short- and long-term pain control for facet-related back pain. However, they may be of benefit.[10,22,51,54,55]

Prolotherapy

Prolotherapy is an injection therapy that is thought to aide in the healing of chronic degenerative soft tissue conditions potentially by triggering an acute inflammatory response.[22,56–58] A variety of injected solutions including dextrose, sodium morrhuate, and phenol have been used. No standardized protocol exists.

A Cochrane review[58] published in 2007 found that prolotherapy alone is not effective in the treatment of chronic low back pain. However, when combined with other interventions it may be of benefit. More studies are needed.

Complementary and Alternative Medicine

This broad group of therapies is a popular addition to traditional medical management for acute and chronic low back pain.[19,20,22,59,60] A total of 45% of individuals with back pain see a chiropractor, 24% use massage therapy, and 11% receive acupuncture. Most patients often fail to disclose use of these treatment options to their health care provider.

More high-quality studies are needed to further elucidate the evidence for these treatment options when used alone or in combination with standard medical treatment. Various modalities exist including acupuncture, mobilization/manipulation, and massage that seem to show promise in the treatment of select individuals with acute and chronic low back pain. The safety profile for most complementary and alternative therapies is acceptable.

Stem Cell Therapy

Autologous mesenchymal stem cell therapy for chronic low back pain caused by degenerative disk disease has shown benefit in animal studies and is now being examined as a treatment option in humans.[61] In a pilot study published in 2011, 10 patients with degenerative disk disease with a preserved external annulus fibrosis who had failed conservative therapy (physical and medical options) underwent mesenchymal stem cell and showed statistically significant improvements in lumbar pain levels and level of disability. Although more research is needed, stem cell therapy is another nonsurgical option on the horizon in the treatment of chronic low back pain.

SPECIAL CONSIDERATIONS FOR ATHLETES

Back pain is the most common reason for time away from sports.[5,6,13,20,22,42] Rates vary among sports and data regarding prevalence compared with the general population are inconsistent. Combined with the lack of high-quality randomized studies, it is difficult to make general recommendations. Nonetheless, some inferences can be made:

- Treatment algorithms for athletes should be similar to the general population.
- Relative rest or time off from sports may be appropriate, but there is no role for bed rest in the treatment of low back pain.
- Earlier imaging does not improve outcomes. Radiographs rarely provide definitive diagnosis. Despite a higher rate of stress fracture than the general population, MRI remains the advanced imaging modality of choice for most athletes.
- Injury-specific and postsurgical return to play guidelines lack standardization.
- Despite the variability in protocols and lack of high-quality data, physical therapy or an exercise program that focuses on spine stabilization and core strengthening are programs with encouraging outcomes.

REFERRAL AND SURGICAL INDICATIONS

Back surgery is indicated for only a minority of patients with low back pain.[10,19,21,62–70] However, the rates of low back surgery in the United Sates are increasing. Patients with persistent pain, despite conservative management or progressive neurologic deficits, should be referred for a surgical evaluation especially in cases of herniated disk, spinal stenosis, and spondylolisthesis. The National Institutes of Health–supported Spine Patient Outcomes Research Trial (SPORT) was designed to evaluate the surgical and nonsurgical treatment of intervertebral disk herniations, degenerative spondylolisthesis, and lumbar spinal stenosis. The SPORT studies were randomized, prospective, multicenter trials that included an observational cohort arm.

Intervertebral Disk Herniation

SPORT participants had to meet strict inclusion criteria, which included symptoms for at least 6 weeks, imaging that supported clinical findings, and neurologic signs.[62–65] The surgical procedure was open discectomy.

Nonsurgical and surgical groups showed improvement. In the intent-to-treat analysis all measures favored surgery; however, this difference was not statistically significant regarding the primary outcome measures (self-reported improvements in impairment and health-related quality of life) but was statistically significant for secondary outcome measures (patient satisfaction, self-rated progress, and improvements in sciatica symptoms). When the randomized group and the cohort group are analyzed together, the as-treated analysis shows a statistically significant improvement in all measured outcomes for the surgery group compared with the nonsurgical patients. Improvements after surgery were maintained at greater than 4 years follow-up. Characteristics that increased the treatment effect of surgery were being married, absence of joint problems, and worsening symptoms from baseline.

Degenerative Spondylolisthesis

The surgical procedure was a posterior laminectomy with or without bilateral single level fusion with or without instrumentation.[66] Inclusion criteria included symptoms for at least 12 weeks and imaging confirmation of degenerative spondylolisthesis.

In a combined as-treated analysis of the randomized group and the cohort group, surgery was favored and demonstrated statistically significant improvements in all primary and secondary outcome measures including pain, improvements in disability and function, and patient satisfaction.

Lumbar Spinal Stenosis

The surgical procedure was a posterior decompressive laminectomy.[63,67,68] All patients had symptoms for at least 12 weeks, had neurogenic claudication or radicular leg symptoms, and imaging showing lumbar spinal stenosis at one or more levels.

Similar to the findings with disk herniation and spondylolisthesis, when a combined analysis is done including the randomized and cohort groups, surgery for symptomatic lumbar spinal fusion was favored in all primary and secondary outcome measures including improvements in pain and function and patient satisfaction when compared with nonsurgical treatment. The improvements were also maintained at the 4-year follow-up.

A systemic review[68] published in 2003 also showed surgery was more effective than continued conservative treatments for patients with symptomatic lumbar spinal stenosis who had underwent at least 3 to 6 months of conservative management. The improvements were seen in pain, function, and quality of life, but not walking ability.

Disk Replacement and Spinal Fusion

Disk degeneration is a common part of the aging process and frequently deemed to be the source of nonspecific chronic low back pain. After patients have failed a trial of conservative management, they are referred to surgery to remove the degenerative disk.

Traditional surgical procedures involve removing the disk and doing a fusion of the inferior and superior vertebrae. New techniques involve disk replacement with a plastic or metal artificial implant.

A recent Cochrane review[69] examined seven randomized controlled trials. Six of the trials compared disk replacement with spinal fusion and one compared disk replacement with nonsurgical treatment. The conclusion of the Cochrane review was that based on the short-term studies that are available, disk replacement is at least equivalent but not superior when compared with fusion with respect to pain control, disability levels, and improved quality of life. In patients with nonspecific chronic low back pain who have failed adequate trials of at least 2 years of nonsurgical interventions, surgery can be considered an option.[70]

ACKNOWLEDGMENTS

The authors thank Dr Melvin Law of Premiere Orthopedics in Nashville, Tennessee, for contributing to and expertly reviewing this article.

REFERENCES

1. Deyo RA, Mirza SK, Martin BI. Back pain prevalence and visit rates: estimates from U.S. national surveys, 2002. Spine 2006;31:2724–7.

2. Croft PR, Macfarlane GJ, Papageorgiou AC, et al. Outcome of low back pain in general practice: a prospective study. BMJ 1998;316:1356–9.
3. Casazza BA. Diagnosis and treatment of acute low back pain. Am Fam Physician 2012;85:343–50.
4. Freburger JK, Holmes GM, Agans RP, et al. The rising prevalence of chronic low back pain. Arch Intern Med 2009;169:251–8.
5. Bono CM. Current concepts review: low back pain in athletes. J Bone Joint Surg Am 2004;86:392–6.
6. Daniels JM, Pontius G, El-Amin S, et al. Evaluation of low back pain in athletes. Sports Health 2011;3:336–45.
7. Chou R, Fu R, Carrino JA, et al. Imaging strategies for low back pain: systemic review and meta-analysis. Lancet 2009;373:463–72.
8. Bhangle SD, Sapru S, Panush RS. Back pain made simple: an approach based on principles and evidence. Cleve Clin J Med 2009;76:393–9.
9. Cochrane Collaboration. Physical examination for lumbar radiculopathy due to disc herniation in patients with low back pain. New York: John Wiley & Sons Ltd; 2010.
10. Chou R, Qaseem A, Snow V, et al. Diagnosis and treatment of low back pain: a joint clinical practice guideline from the American College of Physicians and the American Pain Society. Ann Intern Med 2007;147:478–91.
11. Chou R, Qaseem A, Owens DK, et al. Diagnostic imaging for low back pain: advice for high-value health care from the American College of Physicians. Ann Intern Med 2011;154:181–9.
12. Willick SE, Kendall RW, Roberts ST, et al. An emerging imaging technology to assist in the localization of axial spine pain. PM&R 2009;1:89–92.
13. Ganiyusufoglu AK, Onat L, Karatoprak O, et al. Diagnostic accuracy of magnetic resonance imaging versus computed tomography in stress fractures of the lumbar spine. Clin Radiol 2010;65:902–7.
14. Healy PJ, Helliwell PS. Classification of the spondyloarthropathies. Curr Opin Rheumatol 2005;17:395–9.
15. Kaplin AI, Krishnan C, Deshpande DM, et al. Diagnosis and management of acute myelopathies. Neurologist 2005;11:2–18.
16. Cheshire WP, Santos CC, Massey EW, et al. Spinal cord infarction: etiology and outcome. Neurology 1996;47:321–30.
17. Wang VY, Chou D, Chin C. Spine and spinal cord emergencies: vascular and infectious causes. Neuroimaging Clin N Am 2010;20:639–50.
18. Hadjipavlou AG, Gaitanis LN, Katonis PG, et al. Paget's disease of the spine and its management. Eur Spine J 2001;10:370–84.
19. Deyo RA, Weinstein JN. Low back pain. N Engl J Med 2001;344:363–70.
20. Petering RC, Webb C. Treatment options for low back pain in athletes. Sports Health 2011;3:550–5.
21. Last AR, Hulbert K. Chronic low back pain: evaluation and management. Am Fam Physician 2009;79:1067–74.
22. Shen FH, Samartzis D, Andersson GB. Nonsurgical management of acute and chronic low back pain. J Am Acad Orthop Surg 2006;14:477–87.
23. Carragee EJ. Persistent low back pain. N Engl J Med 2005;352:1891–8.
24. Roelofs PD, Deyo RA, Koes BW, et al. Non-steroidal anti-inflammatory drugs for low back pain. Cochrane Database Syst Rev 2008;(1):CD000396. http://dx.doi.org/10.1002/14651858.CD000396.pub3.
25. Lai KC, Chu KM, Hui WM, et al. Celecoxib compared with lansoprazole and naproxen to prevent gastrointestinal ulcer complications. Am J Med 2005;118:1271–8.

26. Kearney PM, Baigent C, Godwin J, et al. Do selective cyclo-oxygenase-2 inhibitors and traditional non-steroidal anti-inflammatory drugs increase the risk of atherothrombosis? Meta-analysis of randomized trials. BMJ 2006;332:1302.
27. Deshpande A, Furlan AD, Mailis-Gagnon A, et al. Opioids for chronic low-back pain. Cochrane Database Syst Rev 2007;(3):CD004959. http://dx.doi.org/10.1002/14651858.CD004959.pub3.
28. Martell BA, O'Connor PG, Kerns RD, et al. Systematic review: opioid treatment for chronic back pain: prevalence, efficacy, and association with addiction. Ann Intern Med 2007;146:116–27.
29. Kinkade S. Evaluation and treatment of acute low back pain. Am Fam Physician 2007;75:1182–8.
30. Mason L, Moore RA, Derry S, et al. Systemic review of topical capsaicin for the treatment of chronic pain. BMJ 2004. http://dx.doi.org/10.1136/bmj.38042.506748.EE.
31. Gagnier JJ, van Tulder MW, Berman BM, et al. Herbal medicine for low back pain. Cochrane Database Syst Rev 2007;(2):CD004504. http://dx.doi.org/10.1002/14651858.CD004504.pub3.
32. Kroenke K, Krebs EE, Bair MJ. Pharmacotherapy of chronic pain: a synthesis of recommendations from systemic reviews. Gen Hosp Psychiatry 2009;31:206–19.
33. Dalpiaz AS, Lordon SP, Lipman AG. Topical lidocaine patch therapy for myofascial pain. J Pain Palliat Care Pharmacother 2004;18:15–34.
34. Van Tulder MW, Touray T, Furlan AD, et al. Muscle relaxants for nonspecific low back pain: a systemic review within the framework of the Cochrane collaboration. Spine 2003;28:1978–92.
35. Staiger TO, Gaster B, Sullivan MD, et al. Systemic review of antidepressants in the treatment of chronic low back pain. Spine 2003;28:2540–5.
36. Urquhart DM, Hoving JL, Assendelft WJ, et al. Antidepressants for non-specific low back pain. Cochrane Database Syst Rev 2008;(1):CD001703. http://dx.doi.org/10.1002/14651858.CD001703.pub3.
37. Machado LA, Kamper SJ, Herbert RD, et al. Analgesic effects of treatments for non-specific low back pain: a meta-analysis of placebo-controlled randomized trials. Rheumatology 2009;48:520–7.
38. Skljarevski V, Desaiah D, Liu-Seifert H, et al. Efficacy and safety of Duloxetine in patients with chronic low back pain. Spine 2010;35:E578–85.
39. Yildirima K, Denizb O, Guresera G, et al. Gabapentin monotherapy in patients with chronic radiculopathy: the efficacy and impact on life quality. J Back Musculoskelet Rehabil 2009;22:17–20.
40. Chou R, Huffman LH. American Pain Society guideline on the evaluation and management of low back pain. Glenview (IL): American Pain Society; 2007.
41. Vroomen P, de Krom M, Wilmink JT, et al. Lack of effectiveness of bed rest for sciatica. N Engl J Med 1999;340:418–23.
42. Malvivaara A, Hakkinen U, Aro T, et al. The treatment of acute low back pain: bed rest, exercises, or ordinary activity? N Engl J Med 1995;332:351–5.
43. Clarke JA, van Tulder MW, Blomberg SE, et al. Traction for low-back pain with or without sciatica. Cochrane Database Syst Rev 2007;(2):CD003010. http://dx.doi.org/10.1002/14651858.CD003010.pub4.
44. French SD, Cameron M, Walker BF, et al. A Cochrane review of superficial heat or cold for low back pain. Spine 2006;31:998–1006.
45. Kettenmann B, Wille C, Lurie-Luke E, et al. Impact of continuous low level heatwrap therapy in acute low back pain patients: subjective and objective measurements. Clin J Pain 2007;23:663–8.

46. Khadilkar A, Odebiyi DO, Brosseau L, et al. Transcutaneous electrical nerve stimulation (TENS) versus placebo for chronic low-back pain. Cochrane Database Syst Rev 2008;(4):CD003008. http://dx.doi.org/10.1002/14651858.CD003008.pub3.
47. Jacques L, Jensen TS, Rollins J, et al. Decision memo for transcutaneous electrical nerve stimulation for chronic low back pain (CAG-00429N). In: Centers for Medicare and Medicaid Services. 2012. Available at: http://www.cms.gov/medicare-coverage-database/details/nca-decision-memo.aspx?NCAId=256&ver=1&NcaName=Transcutaneous+Electrical+Nerve+Stimulation+for+Chronic+Low+Back+Pain&bc=ACAAAAAAIBAA&. Accessed July 15, 2012.
48. Million R, Nilsen KH, Jayson MI, et al. Evaluation of low back pain and assessment of lumbar corsets with and without back supports. Ann Rheum Dis 1981;40:449–54.
49. Friedly J, Chan L, Deyo R. Increases in lumbosacral injections in the medicare population 1994 to 2001. Spine 2007;32:1754–60.
50. Benoist M, Boulu P, Hayem G. Epidural steroid injections in the management of low back pain with radiculopathy: an update of their efficacy and safety. Eur Spine J 2012;21:204–13.
51. Staal JB, de Bie R, de Vet HC, et al. Injection therapy for subacute and chronic low-back pain. Cochrane Database Syst Rev 2008;(3):CD001824. http://dx.doi.org/10.1002/14651858.CD001824.pub3.
52. Krych AJ, Richman D, Drakos M, et al. Epidural steroid injection for lumbar disc herniation in NFL athletes. Med Sci Sports Exerc 2012;44:193–8.
53. Cohen SP. Epidural steroid injections for low back pain. BMJ 2011;343:d5310.
54. Boswell MV, Colson JD, Sehgal N, et al. A systemic review of therapeutic facet joint interventions in chronic spinal pain. Pain Physician 2007;10:229–53.
55. Peterson C, Hodler J. Evidence-based radiology (part 1): is there sufficient research to support the use of therapeutic injections for the spine and sacroiliac joints? Skeletal Radiol 2010;39:5–9.
56. Watson JD, Shay BL. Treatment of chronic low back pain: a 1-year or greater follow-up. J Altern Complement Med 2010;16:951–8.
57. Rabago D, Slattengren A, Zgierska A. Prolotherapy in primary care practice. Prim Care Clin Office Pract 2010;37:65–80.
58. Dagenais S, Yelland MJ, Del Mar C, et al. Prolotherapy injections for chronic low-back pain. Cochrane Database Syst Rev 2007;(2):CD004059. http://dx.doi.org/10.1002/14651858.CD004059.pub3.
59. Furlan A, Yazdi F, Tsertsvadze A, et al. Complementary and alternative therapies for back pain II. Evidence Report/Technology Assessment No. 194. Prepared by the University of Ottawa Evidence-based Practice Center under Contract No. 290-2007-10059-I (EPCIII). AHRQ Publication No. 10(11)-E007. Rockville (MD): Agency for Healthcare Research and Quality; 2010.
60. Gay R. Back pain: complementary and alternative medicine module. Am Col Physicians/PIER. 2012. Available at: http://pier.acponline.org/physicians/alternative/camdz417/camdz417.html. Accessed July 15, 2012.
61. Orozco L, Soler R, Morera C, et al. Intervertebral disc repair by autologous mesenchymal bone marrow cells: a pilot study. Transplantation 2011;92:822–8.
62. Pearson A, Lurie J, Tosteson T, et al. Who should have surgery for intervertebral disc herniation? Spine 2012;37:140–9.
63. Asghar FA, Hilibrand AS. The impact of the Spine Patient Outcomes Research Trial (SPORT) on orthopaedic practice. J Am Acad Orthop Surg 2012;20:160–6.

64. Weinstein JN, Lurie JD, Tosteson TD, et al. Surgical versus non-operative treatment for lumbar disc herniations: four-year results for the Spine Patient Outcomes Research Trial (SPORT). Spine 2008;33:2789–800.
65. Tosteson AN, Tosteson TD, Lurie JD. Comparative effectiveness evidence from the spine patient outcomes research trial: surgical versus nonsurgical care for spinal stenosis, degenerative spondylolisthesis, and intervertebral disc herniation. Spine 2011;36:2061–8.
66. Weinstein JN, Lurie JD, Tosteson TD, et al. Surgical compared with nonoperative treatment for lumbar degenerative spondylolisthesis: four-year results in the Spine Patient Outcomes Research Trial (SPORT) randomized and observational cohorts. J Bone Joint Surg Am 2009;91:1295–304.
67. Weinstein JN, Tosteson TD, Lurie JD. Surgical versus non-operative treatment forlumbar spinal stenosis four-year results of the Spine Patient Outcomes Research Trial. Spine 2010;35:1329–38.
68. Kovacs FM, Urrutia G, Alarcon JD. Surgery versus conservative treatment for symptomatic lumbar spinal stenosis: a systemic review of randomized controlled trials. Spine 2011;36:E1335–51.
69. Jacobs W, Van der Gaag NA, Tuschel A, et al. Total disc replacement for chronic back pain in the presence of disc degeneration. Cochrane Database Syst Rev 2012;(9):CD008326. http://dx.doi.org/10.1002/14651858.CD008326.pub2.
70. Airaksinen O, Brox JI, Cedraschi C, et al. Chapter 4. European guidelines for the management of chronic nonspecific low back pain. Eur Spine J 2006;15(Suppl 2):S192–300.

Lumbar Injuries of the Pediatric Population

Brian S. Harvey, DO[a,*], Gabriel Brooks, PT, DPT, MSPT, MTCH[b],
Albert Hergenroeder, MD[c]

KEYWORDS

- Pediatric low back pain • Muscular strains • Ligamentous sprains
- Facet arthropathy • Sacroiliac joint dysfunction • Spondylolysis • Scoliosis
- Sheurmann's kyphosis

KEY POINTS

- Athletes with poor flexibility of the hamstrings and lumbar and decreased core strength with poor lifting technique, with a dramatic increase in exercise frequency or intensity, or who experience repetitive lifting or twisting are at risk for lumbar strains, sprains and spasm along with sacroiliac joint dysfunction.
- Spondylolysis is an important cause of low back pain (LBP) in adolescents. Although there is no gold standard for imaging, MRI is growing as the acceptable imaging modality in the pediatric patients due to the low ionizing radiation factor and abilities to detect soft tissue abnormalities and detect early stress reaction within the pars intarticularis. Treatment should include complete rest, physical therapy (once pain-free), and a slow return to play (once asymptomatic).
- Fever, unexplained weight loss, night sweats, unrelenting or worsening pain, morning stiffness, and night pain are all indicators of underlying pathology and require further evaluation.

INTRODUCTION

Back pain is estimated to be second in office visits only to the common cold. It is estimated that the United States spends approximately $90 billion[1] on LBP per year. Surveys of Finnish and Dutch adolescents indicate a prevalence of back pain between 7% and 17%.[2,3] Of the 6% of patients, mean age 9.7 years, presenting to a primary care pediatric practice with a musculoskeletal problems, 6.5% were for back pain.[4] Back pain increases through adolescence into young adulthood, with 30% to 50% of 15 year olds to 20 year olds experiencing at least 1 episode of back pain in their lifetime.[5] The frequency and severity of lumbar pain in young athletes demands an

[a] Salina Regional Health Center, Salina, KS, USA; [b] Physical Medicine and Rehabilitation, Adolescent and Sport Medicine Clinic, Texas Children's Hospital, Houston, TX, USA; [c] Adolescent Medicine and Sports Medicine Section, Department of Pediatrics, Baylor College of Medicine, Houston, TX, USA
* Corresponding author.
E-mail address: BHarvey14@hotmail.com

Prim Care Clin Office Pract 40 (2013) 289–311
http://dx.doi.org/10.1016/j.pop.2013.02.011 **primarycare.theclinics.com**

in-depth understanding of spinal anatomy and function to manage patients with LBP, whether acute, chronic, or caused by systemic disease. This article focuses on the diagnosis and treatment of LBP in the pediatric population, starting with mechanical LBP, proceeding to other causes of LBP, and ending with red flags (indicators of more serious underlying disease) associated with LBP. This article focuses on the updates, advancements, and controversies of pediatric LBP in the field of primary care sports medicine.

MECHANICAL LOW BACK PAIN

Epidemiology

Recent studies report that only 12% to 26% of pediatric patients with back pain have a diagnosable cause.[5] Many of these, in the authors' experience, can be attributed to mechanical LBP associated with lumbar instability. Mechanical back pain (defined as back pain with negative imaging) accounts for approximately 53% of overall pediatric LBP[6] and has been documented in up to 26% of pediatric patients presenting to the primary care sports medicine office.[7] The mean age of onset of symptoms was 13 years. The medians for point, period, and lifetime LBP prevalence were, respectively, 14%, 24%, and 39%.[8] Sports participation seems to influence the prevalence of mechanic LBP and has been reported as high as 50.7% in gymnastics.[9]

Lumbar Instability

Anatomy and spinal mechanics

There have been advances in improving the understanding of the role of key muscles in stabilizing the lumbar spine and pelvis and the consequences of failure to do so.[10–14] Improvements in imaging techniques, including in diagnostic musculoskeletal ultrasound, have led to advancements in identifying and treating acute and chronic spinal dysfunction.[15] Practitioners should understand that the core comprises the musculature of greatest importance in stabilizing the spine and pelvis, and dysfunction of the named muscles should be identified and addressed in patients with low back complaints. Those muscles are the

1. Transversus abdominus
2. Lumbar multifidus
3. Internal and external obliques
4. Gluteus maximus
5. Gluteus medius
6. Pelvic floor (including levator ani)

This section focuses on mechanical lumbar pain associated with lumbar instability, without identified other primary causes, which are discussed later.

Lumbar vertebral segment mechanics

Understanding the lumbar spine's expected segmental movement aids in the diagnosis of mechanical dysfunction. Mechanical dysfunction can be defined as abnormal motion range or quality within the lumbar spine. Normal motion should take place smoothly and symmetrically regardless of the speed at which it is performed. There should be no signs of sharp angulations, fulcrum points, or accelerations throughout the ranges of motion. Failure of the normal muscle performance in the lumbar spine leads to deviations from these normal characteristics, which are clues to underlying dysfunction.[16,17]

Pathophysiology

Lumbar spine functional instability is literally the failure of the muscles to control the spinal segment in the neutral zone. The neutral zone is a region of intervertebral motion around the neutral posture where little resistance is offered by the passive spinal column. The neutral zone is a clinically important measure of spinal stability function. It may increase with injury to the spinal column or with weakness of the muscles, which in turn may result in spinal instability or a low back problem. It may decrease and may be brought within the physiologic limits, by osteophyte formation, surgical fixation/fusion, and muscle strengthening.[18] It can be thought of as the normal physiologic range of spinal segment component motions within which there is no compromise of the osseous, soft tissue, or neural tissues. This condition results from a progressive misuse or disuse of the muscular corseting mechanism. Progressive muscular dysfunction then allows the vertebral segment to exceed the normal ranges of motion and this failure to control movement within a normal range allows strain deformation of the ligaments that govern the spinal segment. With plastic deformation of these stabilizing ligaments, a continued increase in motion can occur, compromising nerve roots and other pain-sensitive structures.[19–24]

Presentation

Patients present with chronic lumbar pain, defined as duration of greater than 3 months during sport and during sustained, unsupported positions, such as standing and sitting.[25] Typically symptoms are improved with changing positions frequently. The pain is better in the morning, worse at end of day when muscles are more fatigued, and relieved with rest in supine lying. The symptoms may include generalized LBP that does not pass the gluteal fold and is of the achy variety; this complaint is characteristic of early stages of this disease, whereas catching sensations, sharp pain, and locking are late stage characteristics.[16,18]

Physical examination

A biomechanical examination is essential in diagnosing lumbar spine dysfunction because functional instability is a movement disorder and is not well demonstrated on static examination.

Observation Examiners should inspect for hypertrophic banding across 1 or both sides of the lumbar spine, which is consistent with instability.

Palpation The areas of the affected segments are tender to palpation.

Active range of motion There are 6 cardinal plane spine movements—forward flexion, extension, left/right lateral flexion, and left/right rotation. Movement is typically abnormal in quality rather than limited in range. Trick movements, hyperextended segments, and accelerations through the range of motion involving the dysfunctional segment are typical of functional instability.

Muscle performance Gross functional stabilization should be tested in full load bearing and partial load bearing in both gravity-resisted and assisted maneuvers. This can be accomplished in 3 movements:

- Single-leg squat: deviations into trunk side bending (Trendelenburg sign), rotation, and lower-extremity functional valgus indicate failure of the lumbopelvic core stabilizing muscles (**Fig. 1**).
- Quadruped lumbar stabilization with arm and leg displacement: side bending, rotation, or hyperextension of the spine from neutral indicates failure of the lumbopelvic core stabilizing muscles.

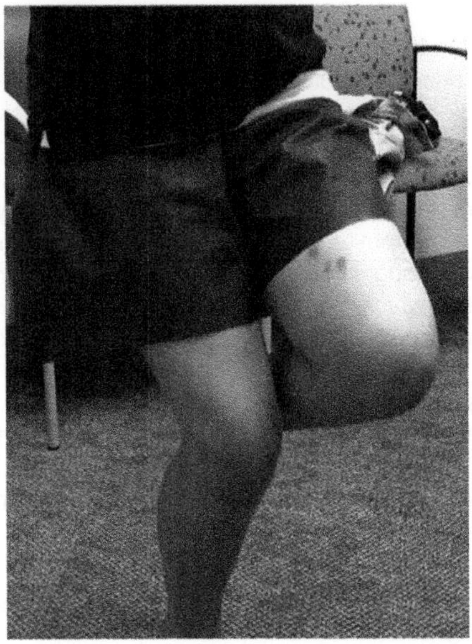

Fig. 1. Functional valgus of the lower extremity in single-leg squat testing.

- Supine lumbar stabilization with hip flexion: transverse plane deviations from neutral or spinal backward bending indicate failure of the lumbopelvic core stabilizing muscles.

Radiologic evaluation

Plain film imaging in cases of lumbar segmental functional instability likely is noncontributory unless the instability has progressed to spondylolysis as a result of fatigue failure of the pars interarticularis. Diagnostic ultrasound in a dynamic examination may help identify muscular atrophy of the transversus abdominus and or multifidus, thereby demonstrating failure of the primary stabilization mechanism, and is a finding consistent with chronic LBP.[15] If the primary care provider has access or specialized training in diagnostic musculoskeletal ultrasound, this radiologic imaging technique may be useful in identifying deficits in the core musculature.

Treatment

Mechanical LBP should be approached with a prescription for spinal stabilization exercises.[26] There has been controversy in the type of exercise that best improves LBP. The authors advocate spinal stabilization exercises targeting the deep spinal musculature over the more superficial muscles, such as the rectus abdominus or erector spinae.[10,19–24,27] Spinal stabilization exercise regimens and superficial spine strengthening programs are advocated to improve lumbar instability.[28]

Back pain in adolescents can be associated with stress and depression,[2] and these maladies should be considered in patients who do not improve with a seemingly adequate rehabilitation program.

Supervised exercise programs are advocated for the rehabilitation of LBP,[29] but there is conflicting information regarding the use of supervised group exercise programs versus individually supervised programs. There is evidence that supervised spinal stabilization programs are superior to education alone and superior to a nonsupervised exercise programs in respects to pain, disability, and improvements in general health status.[26,30]

Contusion

Pathophysiology

A contusion results from a direct blow to the musculature surrounding the lumbar spine causing bleeding into the muscle fibers. Athletes involved in contact or collision sports are at the greatest risk for lumbar contusions; however, contusions can occur in all sports and recreational activities.

Presentation and physical examination

Patients present with pain that may be progressive. It is less likely for patients to have discoloration and/or swelling. Depending on the extent of the injury, patients have decreased range of motion due to pain and spasm. As a result of the direct blow, bleeding into the surrounding tissue disrupts the normal lumbar mechanics. The altered mechanics may generate pain because patients are overusing the surrounding, uninjured musculature for spinal stability and stabilization, leading to an altered posture or gait.

Radiologic evaluation

Radiographic evaluations in contusions of the lumbar spine are typically unnecessary, unless there is concern for underlying fracture or retroperitoneal or peritoneal soft tissue injury.

Treatment

Initial treatment consists of rest, ice, and analgesic medication. Once the pain is controlled, warmth and gentle message may be used; some patients improve with ice, although they are a minority in the authors' experience. Physical therapy is used for pain control and to help restabilize the lumbar spine, improve flexibility of the surrounding musculature, and provide an increase in strength and endurance of the lumbar spine musculature to prevent future injury.

Muscular Strains and Ligamentous Sprains

Pathophysiology

Muscular strain or ligamentous sprains occur after an acute twist, sudden forward flexion, or extension from a poorly performed lifting action or with a seemingly minor action after a long exercise period in which muscles are exhausted (eg, after a long day of working in the garden or bent over riding a bicycle). The movement overloads the supporting muscles/ligaments, causing trauma to those structures. A muscular strain can vary in severity, from fiber disruption to complete muscular tear. Sprain of the lumbar spine occurs when 1 or more the stabilizing ligaments are disrupted or torn, most likely the interspinous process ligament.[31] Athletes with poor flexibility of the hamstrings and lumbar extensor muscles, decreased core strength with poor lifting technique, a rapid increase in exercise frequency or intensity, or who experience repetitive lifting or twisting are at risk for strains and sprains.

Presentation and physical examination

The pain is often sharp, sudden, and debilitating (as opposed to the more chronic nature of lumbar instability). Patients may experience pain with rotation, flexion, and extension as well as with Valsalva maneuvers, such as coughing or sneezing. Patients may have difficulty with simple activities of daily living. Lumbar sprains and strains are often difficult to differentiate from disk herniation, although disk herniation in the pediatric population is rare, accounting for only 0.9% to 2% of adolescent back pain in North America.[5,32] Muscular strains and ligament sprain typically do not cause sciatica in adolescents, unless spasm leads to narrowing of the neuroforamen and nerve root compression.

Radiologic evaluation

Lumbar strains/sprains or patients with facet syndrome may require plain film analysis and/or MRI analysis depending on the complaints and physical examination. Patients with midline tenderness, sciatica, or radicular symptoms or patients who have any concern for spondylolysis should have further imaging.

Treatment

Initial management includes pain control with ice and analgesic medications. A 5-day course of prednisone has been useful in the authors' experience if patients are experiencing pain that limits activities of daily living. Prednisone and analgesia allow physical therapy to be initiated more effectively. Initiation of painless exercises as soon as possible is beneficial whereas bed rest for any length of time is detrimental to the patient's recovery. Typically, complete resolution of symptoms in strains and sprains occurs in 4 to 6 weeks. Patients are allowed to return to play once they are pain-free and functionally rehabilitated.

Facet Arthropathy

Pathophysiology

Facet arthropathy, or facet syndrome, is a posterior element process resulting from inflammation of a facet joint. In young athletes, facet syndrome occurs from repetitive spinal movement, in particular increased rotational or hyperextension forces disrupting the facet joint capsule/ligaments, leading to inflammation. This is in contrast to the adult population, where facet syndrome is linked to degenerative disk disease, which places an increased shearing load on the facet joints, with resultant periosteal and synovial irritation, arthritis, and joint capsule deterioration.

Presentation and physical examination

Facet syndrome may be difficult to differentiate from spondylolysis in young athletes. Facet syndrome is a diagnosis of exclusion. Patients are likely to have pain with palpation over the paraspinous area and, similar to spondylolysis, there is pain with standing hyperextension. Patients may be painful with rotation away from the affected side (Farfan maneuver), placing increased stress on the affected facet joint.[33]

Radiologic evaluation

Because facet syndrome is considered a diagnosis of exclusion, pediatric patients may often undergo either a single-photon emission CT (SPECT) scan with limited CT scan or an MRI effectively ruling out spondylolysis.

Treatment

The initial treatment includes rest and avoidance of aggravating movements, ice directly over the lateral posterior elements, and analgesic medication. In adult studies, intra-articular injections may provide long-term relief, in 18 to 63% of patients.[34,35] The authors do not advocated the use of intra-articular injections in the pediatric population. Radiofrequency denervation is controversial in the adult population and no reports were found in the pediatric population. Once the pain is well controlled, focusing on core strength, flexibility, and endurance during physical therapy, like the treatment of mechanical LBP (discussed previously), is the key to recovery and prevention of future injury.[33,36,37]

Sacroiliac Joint Dysfunction

Although LBP is multifactorial and it is occasionally difficult to determine the exact tissue at fault, inclusion of the SI joints (SIJs) in the lumbar examination is warranted because they have been observed as the primary cause of symptoms in 10% to 27% of adult patients with LBP or buttocks pain.[38–45]

In children, the exact incidence of SI pathology is unknown, but in one pediatric neurosurgery clinic,[46] SI pain was the primary pain generator in approximately one-third of children referred for LBP. The SIJ may develop malalignment from either acute or repetitive insult, but in the majority, no inciting event is identified.[46] Girls and women may be more at risk for SIJ injury than boys and men due to

- Broader and flatter pelvic architecture in girls and women than boys and men[46–50]
- Cyclic hormonal-released collagen relaxation about the pelvis[51]
- Differences in center of mass distribution and mechanical loading of the pelvis[52]

Young athletes are more at risk for SI injury and malalignment than adults due to

- Lack of neuromusculoskeletal coordination (possibly associated with axial growth disturbance of afferent input and mechanoreceptors)
- Lack of muscular strength/power
- Joint hypermobility
- Developmental loss of muscular extensibility and resultant shunting of force to axial spine[46]

Anatomy

The SIJ is a diarthrodial joint that serves as a force transducer from the legs to the spine.[47] It is well governed by ligamentous constraints (**Figs. 2** and **3**) and achieves the remainder of the joint's stability from the muscular corseting about the pelvis.

Pathomechanics

The sacrum functions best in its role as a force transducer when muscular strength and flexibility are well balanced. The directional loads on the joint, however, are frequently asymmetric, leading to aberrant loading, strain, and pain in the SIJ.[47] The imbalances occur via disuse atrophy of the gluteals and lower abdominals and hyper-activation of the iliopsoas or hamstrings. When the SIJ is effectively unlocked in this manner, it is no longer able to properly distribute force from legs to spine, and failure of stabilizing structures leads the joint to positional fault and pain.[53,54]

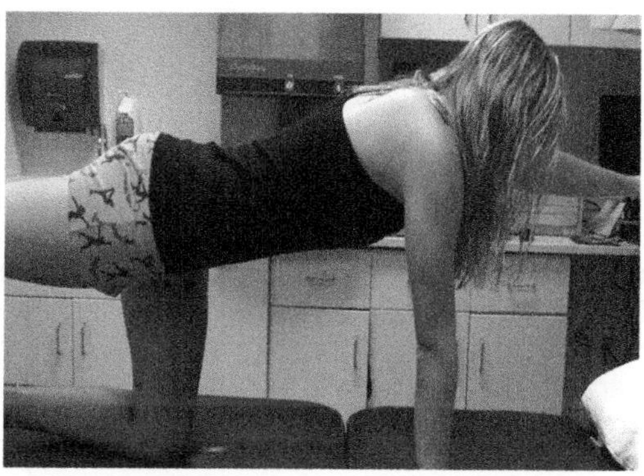

Fig. 2. Stability testing in quadruped.

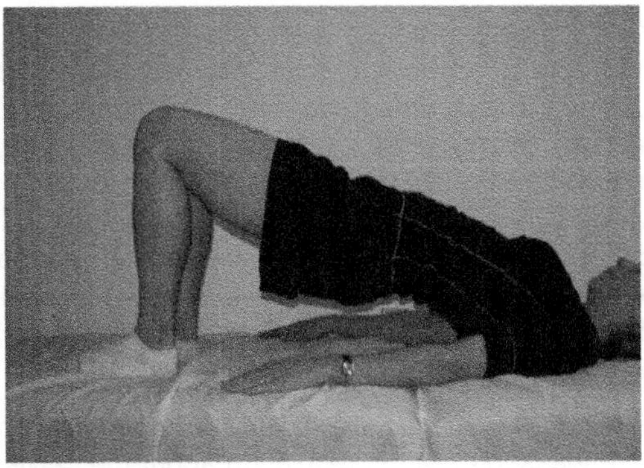

Fig. 3. Stability testing in supine.

Clinical presentation

Pain that originates in the SIJ is commonly perceived in the low back, posterior pelvis, and gluteal region, although pain is often referred into the lower and upper lumbar regions, groin, or lower limbs. Pain of SIJ origin may mimic lumbar disk injury with radiculitis and it is further complicated when a disk bulge has been identified on MRI. In the absence of a straight leg test and the absence of neurologic signs, however, such as decreased motor strength, sensory alterations, or asymmetric deep tendon reflexes with positive pain provocation tests for SIJ dysfunction, the SIJ should be considered a primary source of the pain.[44]

Physical examination

Because SIJ pain is difficult to distinguish from other forms of LBP and because individual tests have weak sensitivity and specificity, a combined battery of tests is often used to help ascertain a proper diagnosis.[55–58] The most sensitive (89%), although nonspecific, finding on physical examination is tenderness in the sacral sulcus, the soft tissue just medial to the posterior superior iliac spine.[51] Full biomechanical testing of the pelvis may require referral to a specialist.

Radiologic evaluation

Radiologic imaging contributes little in the diagnosis of SIJ dysfunction unless red flag symptoms, such as rapidly progressive pain, loss of bowel or bladder function, fever, ankylosing spondylitis, and lumbar disk herniation, are present.[43]

Definitive diagnosis

The only definitive way to diagnose SI joint pathology is via an SI joint block done under fluoroscopy, where a 75% reduction of symptoms is considered diagnostic.[51]

Treatment

Nonoperative treatment of sacroiliac joint dysfunction Treatment of SIJ pain includes supervised physical therapy consisting of joint manipulation, pelvic muscular stabilization exercises, and addressing the underlying mechanical causes, such as muscular weakness in controlling lumbosacral shear forces, lumbopelvic movement dyscoordination, and posture and gait disturbances.[47,59–64] One study[46] reported that bedside hip flexion and extension against an examiner's resistance (affording realignment of the SI joint) resulted in complete and immediate resolution of symptoms in 53% of cases (N = 48) and marked improvement in 80%.

Passive supports Belts, braces, and binders may be used to provide temporary mechanical SIJ stabilization and proprioceptive input to patients.[47] The belt is properly positioned when placed directly superior to the greater trochanters and as such it can significantly limit SIJ motion and thereby decrease pain.[65,66]

Adjunctive treatment modalities Based on the methodologic limitations in the published literature, there are insufficient data to endorse the use of back schools, low-level laser therapy, patient education, massage, traction, superficial heat/cold, and lumbar supports for chronic lumbosacral or LBP in pediatric patients.

Resistant cases of sacroiliac joint dysfunction Conservative physical therapy may be augmented by fluoroscopically guided SIJ infiltration of anesthetic or corticosteroid.[43,47] Fluoroscopic guided intra-articular SIJ infiltrations with local anesthetic and corticosteroids hold the highest evidence rating.[43] Anesthetic blocks are the diagnostic gold standard but must be interpreted with caution, because false-positive results as well as false-negative results occur frequently.[67]

The authors have little experience in pediatric patients with the use of corticosteroid injections, anesthetic blocks, and radiofrequency treatments.

Operative treatment of sacroiliac joint dysfunction Surgery should be considered a last-line management strategy because most cases can be ameliorated with other more conservative efforts. When conservative treatments fail, arthrodesis of the SIJ for chronic, nontraumatic, painful dysfunction may be considered.[68] Complications include infection, radicular irritation, and pseudoarthrosis. Clinical judgment should be used if lumbar spine pathology coexists with SIJ dysfunction. In the authors' experience, surgery is rarely indicated in the pediatric population with SI joint dysfunction.

SPONDYLOLYSIS

Epidemiology

Spondylolysis is a defect, congenital or acquired and bilateral or unilateral, within the pars interarticularis. Acquired spondylolysis in young athletes is secondary to repetitive hyperextension, rotation, or flexion of the lumbar spine. The most common site is L5, representing 82% to 95% of the cases, although spondylolysis can occur at any spinal level.[69–76] Congenital spondylolysis occurs in 4% of the general population.[77] Spondylolysis (both congenital and acquired) has been reported to occur in 5.2% of 12 year olds[7,77,78] and approximately 6% to 8% in the general population. Increased rates are seen, however, in subsets of athletes.[70–76] Sports in which spondylolysis is more frequently reported include overhead athletics (eg, baseball, tennis, and field throwing), gymnastics, cricket, rowing, and dance.[78] The prevalence remains approximately 6% into adulthood but is an uncommon cause of LBP in the adult population. Among adolescent patients referred to a sports medicine physician, 47 of 100 were diagnosed with symptomatic spondylolysis compared with only 5 out of 100 adult patients.[7] Not all patients with spondylolysis are symptomatic. In a 25-year prospective study by Fredrickson and colleagues[77] of 500 children, the incidence of spondylolysis in asymptomatic 6-year-old patients was 4.4%, 5.2% in 12 year olds, and 5.6% in 16 year olds. After 25 years, only 4 patients with asymptomatic spondylolysis developed back pain, with 3 of the 4 resolving with conservative management and 1 patient having radicular symptoms resolving with diskectomy and laminectomy.[77]

Pathophysiology

The pathogenesis, although debatable, is likely to be genetic predisposition combined with repetitive stress and shearing forces of the inferior articular process of the segment above and superior articular process of the segment below leading to stress reaction and eventual fracture of the pars intartiuclaris (**Fig. 4**).[73]

Presentation

The typical adolescent presentation of spondylolyisis is LBP that is worsened with activity and relieved with rest. Neurologic changes, including weakness, numbness, and tingling and loss of bowel and bladder control are rare in isolated spondylolyisis without the presence of spondylolisthesis. Any focal neurologic or systemic finding (eg, fever, chills, and weight loss) should lead physicians to another diagnosis.

Physical Examination

Although nondiagnostic, some common physical examination findings include

- Exaggerated lordosis in combination with tight/spasm hamstrings
- Decreased range of motion in the lumbar vertebrae secondary to pain
- Pain with extension
- Pain with standing single-leg hyperextension
- Pain with palpation over the region of the pars localized to the affected segment or regionally if guarding and muscular spasm is present
- Negative neurologic examination, included the straight leg raise

Imaging Modalities

Radiography

When spondylolysis is considered in the differential diagnosis, anteroposterior, lateral, and bilateral 45° oblique views are the initial imaging tests of choice. A 5th collimated lateral view of the lumbosaral junction can improve sensitivity in detecting the pars defect. When using all 5 views to evaluate for spondylolysis, 96.5% of fractures through the pars iterarticularis were detected, with the majority found on the

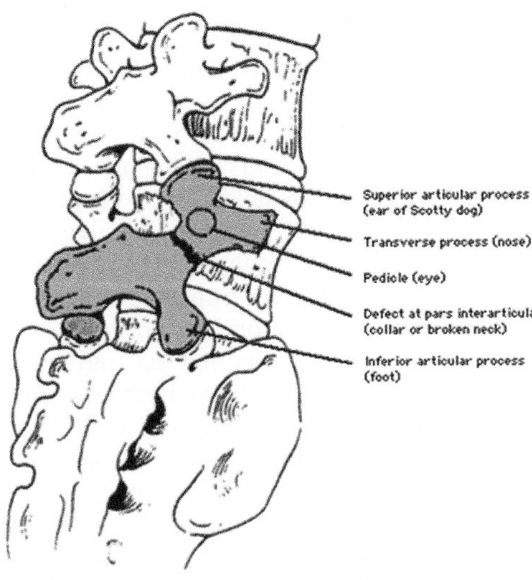

Fig. 4. Schematic representation of fracture through the pars interarticularis. (*From* Smith AJ, Hu SS. Management of spondylolysis and spondylolisthesis in the pediatric and adolescent population. Orthrop Clin North Am 1999;30:487; copyright 1999 W. B. Saunders; with permission.)

collimated view.[73] Due to the plane in which the pars fracture is located, 20% of spondylolysis defects are seen only on the oblique views.[79] With the majority of pars fractures occurring in the coronal plane, however, the collimated lateral view of the lumbosacral junction is determined to be the best view to identify spondolylysis defects, identifying up to 84% of defects.[80]

Keys to looking at plain radiographs

1. A fracture through the pars interarticularis is referred to as the Scottie dog sign.[69]
2. In general, acute fractures often have a narrow and irregular appearance whereas chronic fractures have a larger gap and smooth edges.
3. The contralateral pedicle can have a sclerotic appearance due to overload or represent healing callus formation from an old spondylolysis injury.

When a pars interarticularis fracture is present, the sensitivity of plain radiographs appear excellent; however, pars defects without complete fracture or fractures that lie outside the plane captured by radiograph are radiographically occult.[80,81] Due to the possibility of having an incomplete fracture, radiograph alone is not sufficient in ruling out spondylolysis and further studies are needed. The imaging modality of choice is under debate. Despite the need for further imaging, there are no evidence-based guidelines on which imaging modalities are used after plain radiography.

Radionucleotide imaging

SPECT is a useful tool in aiding the diagnosis of spondylolysis and has been shown more sensitive than plain radiographs in the diagnosis of pars interarticularis defects. SPECT scans show increased uptake in metabolically active lesions within the bone and, as such, are able to delineate an active spondylolysis (**Fig. 5**).

If patients have a positive SPECT scan, the next step is to obtain a CT scan to define the extent and healing potential for the fracture. A negative SPECT scan does not, however, effectively rule out inactive or chronic spondylolytic lesions, particularly if patients have a history and physical examination consistent with spondylolysis. These lesions, however, are often asymptomatic, and other diagnosis should be considered and pursued.[69]

Limitations to SPECT

- The radiation dose is approximately 5 mSv; however, the need for CT scan to further depict the fracture adds another 10 mSv to 20 mSv. A 6-view radiograph of the lumbar spine is equal to 1.5 mSv.[73] A simple chest radiograph is 0.1 mSv.

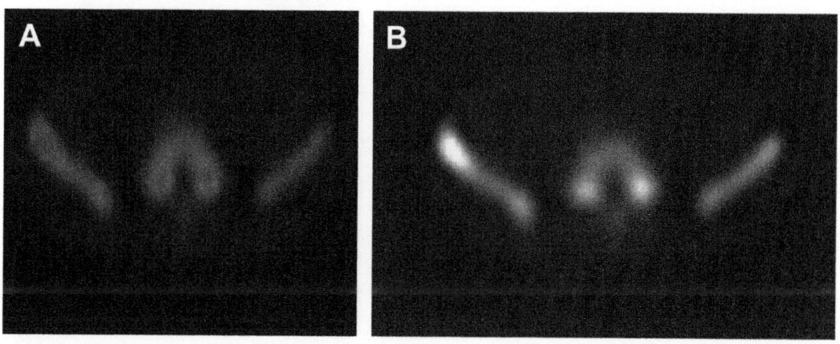

Fig. 5. (*A, B*) SPECT scans showing increased uptake in the bilateral pars interarticularis.

- SPECT cannot delineate actively healing lesions or acutely progressing lesions, because both have uptake on the SPECT scan.
- SPECT scans are not specific and cannot differentiate spondylolysis from osteomyelitis, tumors, facet arthritis, or other metabolically active lesions.

CT

A thin-cut CT scan is recommended if a patient has a positive SPECT scan to further identify the defect. CT is often considered the modality of choice to further identify the pars intarticularis fracture, with improved bone anatomy detail, and is most accurate in identifying partial fractures. CT cans further identify other lesions that are positive on the SPECT scan (eg, osteoid osteoma), bone cysts, and osteomyelitis. As with SPECT scanning, CT uses a large radiation dose, does not have the ability to differentiate acute or chronic lesions, and cannot accurately identify soft tissue pathology (**Fig. 6**).[73]

Limitations to CT

- CT cannot accurately differentiate acute or chronic lesions.
- CT cannot accurately identify nerve root compression.
- CT has a large radiation dose.

MRI

MRI is the authors' diagnostic test of choice in evaluation of spondylolysis. MRI has the ability to identify acute stress reaction within the pars and identify other soft tissue pathology and does not have a radiation dose associated with its protocol. There are several advantages to using MRI: MRI is improving in its technical precision, decreasing the slice size to 2 mm to 3 mm, and improving its image quality with larger magnet size.[82] MRI can detect complete fractures as well as early stress reactions, manifested as bone edema (**Figs. 7** and **8**). MRI has no radiation dose.[69] MRI can accurately define nerve root compression and depict the size and patency of the neural foramen. MRI is also able to accurately define a herniated disk, diskitis, and other soft tissue tumors.

Limitations to MRI

- Inability to adequately define cortical disruption without complete pars fracture
- Inability to pick up occult osteoid osteomas

The authors propose an algorithm for the diagnosis of spondylolysis (**Fig. 9**).

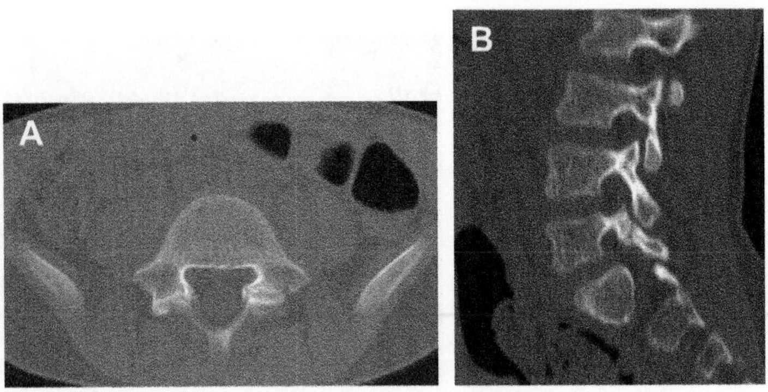

Fig. 6. Axial (*A*) and sagittal (*B*) cuts showing pars intarticularis fracture.

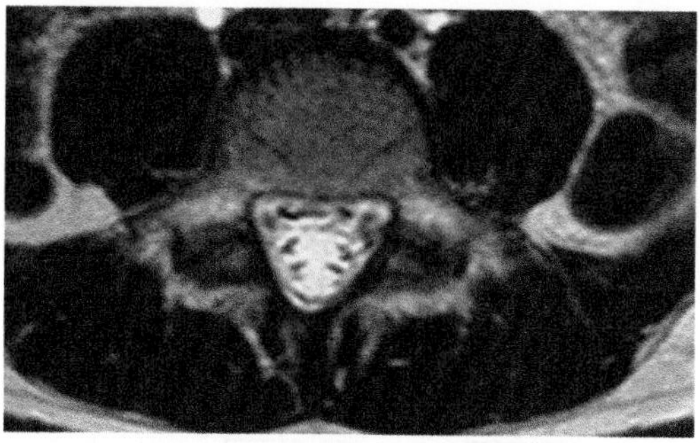

Fig. 7. Axial T2 MRI showing increasing uptake in the bilateral pars interarticularis.

Treatment

Conservative management

The goal of treatment of patients with spondylolysis is for patients to be pain-free with activities of daily living, reducing the possibility of progression to spondylolisthesis, having a bone or fibrous union along the fracture, and having patients be rehabilitated in an appropriate way as to help prevent future injuries to the low back. Initial management of spondylolysis is rest and removal from all physical activity that would load the posterior elements of the spine.

Bracing There are differing opinions with regards to bracing. Success in conservative management without bracing is no different from conservative management with bracing, either method being effective in approximately 80% of patients.[72,83] Advocates of bracing suggest using a thoracolumbosacral orthotic (TLSO) brace, such as a BOB, corset style brace for 3 to 6 months for up to 20 hours per day to facilitate stabilization of the affected lumbar segment and promote healing of the fracture. The brace is designed to decrease lordosis and extension while unloading the posterior elements and stress across the pars interarticularis.

There are no guidelines based on randomized controlled trials for what type of brace to use (soft corset, Boston, or TLSO), how long to brace (3 to 6 months or until

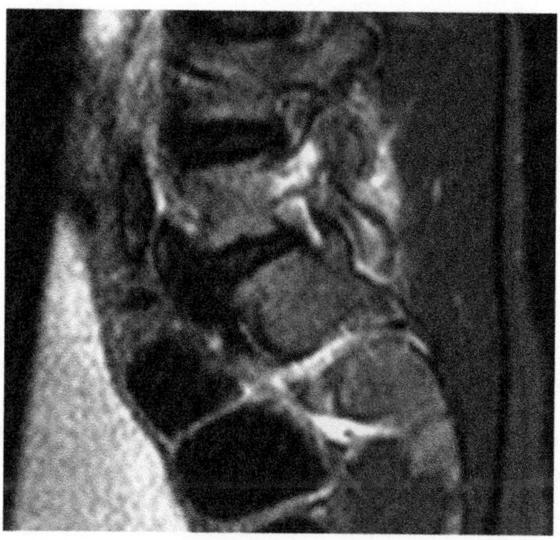

Fig. 8. MRI sagittal stir sequence showing fracture and edema in the pars interarticularis.

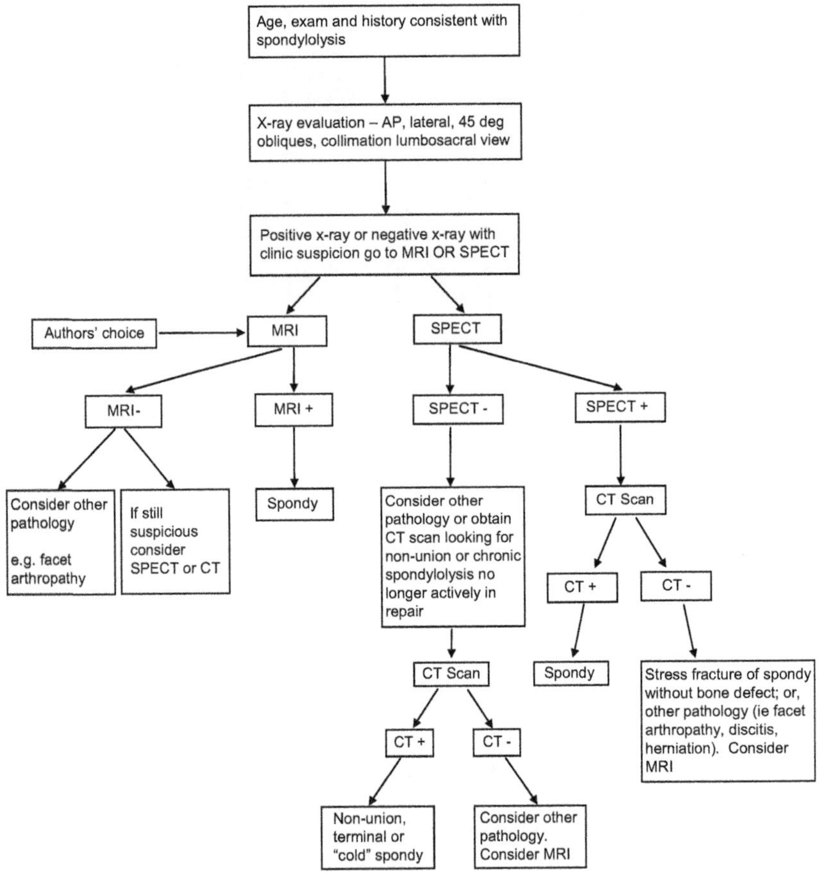

Fig. 9. Algorithm for the diagnosis of spondylolysis. AP, anterioposterior; Spondy, spondylolysis; +, positive; −, negative.

asymptomatic), or a weaning protocol out of the brace before returning to their sporting activity.

A common bracing protocol, and one that the authors use, includes the Boston overlapping brace with 0° of extension for up to 23 hours per day. After 4 to 6 weeks, or once asymptomatic, patients may be allowed to return to sport while in their brace and avoiding hyperextension maneuvers. A physical therapy protocol should be initiated early to target flexibility and strength[84]; 78% of symptomatic spondylolysis patients demonstrated good or excellent results with full return to sports in 4 to 6 months.[84]

Electrical stimulation Another treatment of spondylolysis may be external electrical stimulation, particularly for chronic, painful nonunion lesions.[85,86] Further research is needed to confirm if this therapy is objectively helpful and when it is best to use electrical stimulation. As such, there are no evidence-based guidelines supporting electrical stimulation use in the acute or chronic nonunion setting.

Physical therapy Once pain-free, patients are allowed to initiate a physical therapy program that includes lumbar stabilization (in particular, the multifidus), core stabilization (including the transverse abdominus), and improving flexibility of the surrounding musculature (particularly of the hamstrings and hip flexors).[87] After completing physical therapy, there should be a gradual, graded return to play, starting with functional and sport-specific drills, progressing to practice, and lastly returning to full competitive sport, as long as patients remain pain-free.

Prognosis and expected outcomes In a large meta-analysis of 15 observational studies, nonoperative success rates varied from 66% to 100%. The success rate was approximately 84%.[72] In the same meta-analysis, the success rate for those who followed a bracing protocol was 89% whereas for those who used restricted activity without a brace it was 86% and the difference was not statistically significant.[72] After a period of relative rest, physical therapy, and sport-specific rehabilitation, athletes can be expected to be back into sport within 5 to 7 months.[78]

Follow-up imaging Follow-up imaging is not necessary in late adolescent, unilateral early-stage defects that respond clinically to conservative treatment.[78] Radiograph healing in acute stress reaction on MRI and early-stage defects on CT have been shown to correlate with the resolution of clinical symptoms and, as such, repeat imaging costs time, money and extra radiation.[88,89] If there is a spondylolisthesis greater than 30% at presentation, a pars defect in a young patient at diagnosis who has yet to go through a growth spurt, or bilateral pars defect, repeat diagnostic imaging is warranted.

If patients are not responding to traditional conservative management, repeat imaging may be needed to re-evaluate the diagnosis or document the extent of healing that has occurred with conservative management.

If patients have no signs of spondylolisthesis at diagnosis and are pain-free with conservative therapy, the authors may repeat lateral radiographs when patients have finished growth to document a baseline. The authors do not follow an uncomplicated spondylolysis radiographically, however.[75] In the authors' opinion, if patients have completed a targeted course of physical therapy and continue to remain asymptomatic, it is unnecessary to obtain repeat a CT, MRI, or SPECT scan.

Surgical treatment options Although beyond the scope of this article, there are surgical options available for the treatment of spondylolysis. Surgery is reserved for those who fail conservative management (approximately 10%–15%) with continued pain despite restriction of physical activity for 6 to 9 months, skeletally immature children with a grade 3 or higher spondylolisthesis, a progressive spondylolisthesis, or patients with progressive, focal neurologic signs.[73]

Treatment resistance The treatment of spondylolysis can sometimes be difficult, particularly due to relying on patients to have complete rest and perform adequate rehabilitation on their own or under parental supervision. Complete rest can often be difficult; however, with education of athletes and parents, this can be achieved with or without a brace. One of the main drawbacks to wearing a brace is noncompliance. Approximately 85% of the patients, however, wore the brace at least 80% of the recommended 23 hours per day.[83] Brace wear may enhance treatment compliance, reminding patients to restrict and modify their activities. Another challenge is keeping patients out of activity once they are asymptomatic. Many athletes do not understand the importance of relative rest once they are asymptomatic. Returning to play in the brace after patients were asymptomatic in 4 to 6 weeks is an option for some athletes.[83] The success rate with this approach did not vary from previous studies that excluded all sport participation for 3 to 6 months. Another challenge to treatment is a required home exercise program to gain and maintain strength and flexibility gained within the PT session.

Spondylolisthesis

The progression of spondylolysis to spondylolisthesis in the pediatric population is greatest in skeletally immature adolescents who are less than 16 years of age. Spondylolisthesis is forward movement of the vertebral body in relation to the vertebra below due to an insufficient pars interarticularis. Spondylolisthesis is higher in bilateral pars defects, with the majority of spondylolisthesis found with L5 slipping forward on S1. They are classified according to the degree of slip in relation to the vertebral body below.

- Grade 1: up to 25% of the vertebra is displaced in relation to the vertebra below
- Grade 2: 25% to 50% of the vertebra is displaced in relation to the vertebra below
- Grade 3: 50% to 75% of the vertebra is displaced in relation to the vertebra below
- Grade 4: greater than 75% of the vertebra is displaced in relation to the vertebra below

As with spondylolysis, treatment of grades 1 and 2 spondylolisthesis includes rest, physical therapy, and potentially the use of a TLSO brace. Athletes with grade 3 or 4 slips should avoid contact sports and, if progressive, a referral for surgical correction is warranted. Progression of a grade 1 spondylolisthesis or less than 30% slippage is rare, if recognized and treated early. Skeletally immature patients, however, with greater than 30% slippage should be followed every 6 to 12 months by physical examination and, if warranted, radiography, to assess the progression of spondylolysis to spondylolisthesis.[76,83,90]

Pediatric Low Back Pain Red Flags

Back pain in the pediatric population is a common complaint presenting to general practitioners and sports medicine physicians. The differential diagnoses include trauma, infection, rheumatologic conditions, neoplasm, musculoskeletal conditions, and pain of nonorganic causes. A complete history and physical examination in combination with imaging and laboratory evaluation may be warranted to rule out systemic causes.[91] The history should include location, onset, duration, and quality of pain and an assessment of a mechanism of injury.[92] Although rare, major trauma or high-impact injuries should raise the index of suspicion for fracture in the lumbar spine. Systemic and constitutional signs should suggest an infectious, rheumatologic, or neoplastic cause. A history of fever, chills, weight loss, and night sweats or pain that is unrelenting, wakes a patient up from sleep, or does not improve despite rest suggests a systemic or progressive process.[1]

Infectious

Infections of the lumbar spine, including epidural or paraspinal abscess, diskitis, and osteomyelitis, may present to a primary care sports office as back pain. The index of suspicion should be raised in patients presenting with atypical musculoskeletal pain, ill-appearing patients, and/or febrile patients. Young children may refuse to walk or sit, develop a limp, or refuse to pick anything up from the floor.[1,93] This compensatory mechanism, in an attempt to reduce spinal motion, may be the only presenting symptom. Neurologic complaints are rare; however, adolescents may complain of weakness in the lower extremities or have reduced reflexes on examination. Paraspinal splinting with muscular spasm and decreased range of motion, localized point tenderness with percussion, and abdominal pain may be symptoms of a spinal infection. Other nonspinal infections can present with LBP, including pyelonephritis, pneumonia, pelvic inflammatory disease, and pyomyositis of the surrounding musculature or myalgias related to viral infections.[94]

Neoplasm

Tumors of the lumbar spine account for 0.5% of the primary musculoskeletal tumors occurring in the spine of pediatric patients.[95] Back pain that is unrelenting despite rest is the most common presenting complaint in patients with a tumor in the lumbar spine.[91] Other systemic symptoms include weight loss; malaise; fever; atraumatic LBP; pain that awakens patients at night; pain that is not affected by activity or reduced with rest; progressive symptoms over time; neurologic complaints, including loss of bowel; and bladder control and weakness.

Rheumatologic

Spondyloarthropathies are a subset of rheumatologic conditions, including spondylitis, sacroilitis, and asymmetric peripheral arthritis, accounting for up to 10% to 20% of childhood arthritis.[96] Spondyloarthropathies include differentiated subtypes: ankylosing spondylitis, reactive arthritis, psoriatic arthritis, and arthritis associated with systemic diseases, such as an enteropathic arthopathy associated with inflammatory bowel disease. There is an undifferentiated subtype, including seronegative enthesopathy and arthropathy and juvenile spondyloarthropathy. Each diagnosis has differentiating symptoms on history; however, in general, patients classically present with morning stiffness in the lower back or buttock, typically longer than 30 minutes, which improves throughout the day.[96] The pain may wake them up at night and progressively worsens over time. A family history of a first-degree relative with a rheumatologic condition is another risk factor. Other systems may be involved if related to a systemic disorder or the type of arthritis, including the gastrointestinal tract, eyes, skin, genitourinary system, or other joint involvement. Juvenile spondyloarthropathy presenting as back pain is uncommon and peripheral arthritis often precedes the onset back pain.[96] Physical examination should highlight the presence of conjunctiva involvement, mucus membrane involvement, rashes, urethritis, cervicitis, peripheral joint effusion, and decreased range of motion of the lumbar spine if active disease is present.

Scoliosis

Scoliosis is a 3-D deformity defined as curvature greater than 10°. Adolescent idiopathic scoliosis is the most common, presenting as a right thoracic or left lumbar curvature. Scoliosis should not cause pain and does not increase the risk for LBP. A history of pain requires a more aggressive evaluation, rather than assuming the scoliosis is causing the pain. One study showed, however, that 32% patients with scoliosis had pain and only 9% were found to have a cause other than idiopathic scoliosis.[1]

Sheurmann kyphosis

Scheuermann kyphosis is the most common cause of structural kyphosis and is found in up to 20% to 30% of the general population.[94] It is defined as hyperkyphosis of the thoracic or thoracolumbar spine with radiologic evidence of anterior wedging of more than 5° in 3 or more consecutive thoracic vertebra, resulting in a thoracic kyphotic curve of greater than 35°.[91] This is a mechanical and permanent kyphosis, not a functional or dynamic kyphosis related to posture. Scheuermann kyphosis can cause pain, disfigurement, and complications similar to scoliosis. Those patients with Scheuermann kyphosis may have an increased risk for spondylolysis or spondylolisthesis due to their altered mechanics and underlying anatomy. Typically, patients with

Scheuermann kyphosis respond to conservative management with surgery and bracing used only for those with severe deformity.[93] Poorly formed vertebral bodies with multiple herniations of the lumbar disk through a weak endplate may form Schmorl nodes, which can be found incidentally or cause LBP. A possible lumbar variant exists, consisting of Schmorl node in multiple consecutive lumbar vertebras, which has been theorized to cause pain and possible disruption of normal spinal mechanics. Athletes with this variant are typically found to have hypolordotic and hypokyphotic appearance to their thoracolumbar junction. Neurologic symptoms are rare in Scheuermann kyphosis.

Fracture

Unlike the compression fractures found in adults, a large force, high velocity, or large impact, such as a motor vehicle accident or large collision in contact sports, is typically needed to cause a lumbar fracture in healthy pediatric patients.[97] Physical examination could show bruising, swelling, decreased range of motion, surrounding muscular spasm, and other musculoskeletal injuries. Depending on the location of the fracture, patients may have neurologic symptoms, including loss of bowel and bladder, reflex changes, sensation and temperature changes, or weakness indicative of a medical emergency.

Spinal stenosis

Although uncommon in the pediatric population, spinal stenosis can present with lower extremity parasthesias worse with prolonged standing and relieved by sitting.[98,99] Lying supine worsens the pain. Because spinal stenosis is a chronic process, it presents more commonly in the adult population as the spine degenerates due to age, rather than congenitally in the pediatric population.

Cauda equina

Cauda equina is a medical emergency and is an entity that should be recognized immediately by primary care providers. Progressive neurologic symptoms, including weakness in the lower extremities, decreased reflexes in the lower extremities, loss of bowel or bladder, and saddle paresthesias, should warrant emergent evaluation. Cauda equina have multiple causes, ranging from traumatic fractures, dramatic local inflammation and swelling, and mass effect from a tumor to an epidural bleed into the surround tissue.

SUMMARY

Primary musculoskeletal etiologies, such as stress fractures, strains, facet arthropathy, and SI joint dysfunction, are more common causes of pediatric pain than systemic diseases, both in the office setting and the emergency room. Systemic features, young age, and atypical pain should clue physicians to causes other than a primary musculoskeletal cause and prompt an intensive search for other conditions.

REFERENCES

1. Bernstein R, Cozen H. Evaluation of back pain in children and adolescents. Am Fam Physician 2007;76:1669–76.
2. Diepenmaat AC, van der Wal MF, de Vet HC, et al. Neck/shoulder, low back and arm pain in relations to computer use, physical activity and depression among Dutch adolescents. Pediatrics 2006;117:412–6.

3. Hakala P, Rimpela A, Salminen JJ, et al. Back, neck and shoulder pain in Finnish adolescents: national cross sectional surveys. BMJ 2002;325:743–5.
4. De Inocencio J. Musculoskeletal pain in primary care: analysis of 1000 consecutive general pediatric clinic visits. Pediatrics 1998;102:e63.
5. Gurd D. Back pain in the young athlete. Sports Med Arthrosc 2011;19:7–16.
6. Auerbach JD, Ahn J, Zgonis MH, et al. Streamlining the evaluation of low back pain in children. Clin Orthop Relat Res 2008;466:1971–7.
7. Micheli L, Wood R. Back pain in young athletes: significant differences from adults in causes and patterns. Arch Pediatr Adolesc Med 1995;149: 15–8.
8. Calvo-Muñoz I, Gómez-Conesa A, Sánchez-Meca J. Prevalence of low back pain during childhood and adolescence: a systematic review. Rev Esp Salud Publica 2012;86:331–6.
9. Purnell M, Shirley D, Nicholson L, et al. Acrobatic gymnastics injury: occurrence, site and training risk factors. Phys Ther Sport 2010;11:40–6.
10. Franca FR, Burke TN, Hanada ES, et al. Segmental stabilization and muscular strengthening in chronic low back pain—a comparative study. Clinics (Sao Paulo) 2010;65:1013–7.
11. Hides JA, Boughen CL, Stanton WR, et al. A magnetic resonance imaging investigation of the transversus abdominus muscle during drawing in of the abdominal wall in elite Australian football league players with and without low back pain. J Orthop Sports Phys Ther 2010;40:4–10.
12. Bouche KG, Vanovermeire O, Stevens VK, et al. Computed tomographic analysis of the quality of trunk muscles in asymptomatic and symptomatic lumbar discectomy patients. BMC Musculoskelet Disord 2011;12:65.
13. Pel JJ, Spoor CW, Pool-Goudzwaard AL, et al. Biomechanical analysis of reducing sacroiliac joint shear load by optimization of pelvic muscle and ligament forces. Ann Biomed Eng 2008;36:415–24.
14. Kumar SP. Efficacy of segmental stabilization exercise for lumbar segmental instability in patients with mechanical low back pain: a randomized placebo controlled crossover study. N Am J Med Sci 2011;3:456–61.
15. Teyhen DS, Childs JD, Stokes MJ, et al. Abdominal and lumbar multifidus muscle size and symmetry at rest and during contracted states. Normative reference ranges. J Ultrasound Med 2012;31:1099–110.
16. Panjabi MM. Clinical spinal instability and low back pain. J Electromyogr Kinesiol 2003;13:371–9.
17. Ahmadi A, Maroufi N, Behtash H, et al. Kinematic analysis of dynamic lumbar motion in patients with lumbar segmental instability using digital videofluoroscopy. Eur Spine J 2009;18:1677–85.
18. Panjabi MM. The stabilizing system of the spine. Part II. Neutral zone and instability hypothesis. J Spinal Disord 1992;5:390–7.
19. Hodges PW, Richardson CA. Inefficient muscular stabilization of the lumbar spine associated with low back pain. A motor control evaluation of transversus abdominis. Spine (Phila Pa 1976) 1996;21:2640–50.
20. Hides JA, Stokes MJ, Saide M, et al. Evidence of lumbar multifidus muscle wasting ipsilateral to symptoms in patients with acute/subacute low back pain. Spine (Phila Pa 1976) 1994;19:165–72.
21. Hodges P, Kaigle Holm A, Holm S, et al. Intervertebral stiffness of the spine is increased by evoked contraction of transversus abdominis and the diaphragm: in vivo porcine studies. Spine (Phila Pa 1976) 2003;28: 2594–601.

22. Wilke HJ, Wolf S, Claes LE, et al. Stability increase of the lumbar spine with different muscle groups. A biomechanical in vitro study. Spine (Phila Pa 1976) 1995;20:192–8.
23. Solomonow M, Zhou BH, Harris M, et al. The ligamento-muscular stabilizing system of the spine. Spine (Phila Pa 1976) 1998;23:2552–62.
24. Kaigle AM, Holm SH, Hansson TH. Experimental instability in the lumbar spine. Spine (Phila Pa 1976) 1995;20:421–30.
25. Stanton TR, Latimer J, Maher CG, et al. How do we define the condition 'recurrent low back pain'? A systematic review. Eur Spine J 2010;19:533–9.
26. Kulig K, Beneck GJ, Selkowitz DM, et al. An intensive, progressive exercise program reduces disability and improves functional performance in patients after single-level lumbar microdiskectomy. Phys Ther 2009;89:1145–57.
27. Macintosh JE, Bogduk N. The biomechanics of the lumbar multifidus. Clin Biomech 1986;1:205–13.
28. Ferreira ML, Ferreira PH, Latimer J, et al. Comparison of general exercise, motor control exercise and spinal manipulative therapy for chronic low back pain: a randomized trial. Pain 2007;131:31–7.
29. Henchoz Y, Kai-Lik So A. Exercise and nonspecific low back pain: a literature review. Joint Bone Spine 2008;75:533–9.
30. Bronfort G, Maiers MJ, Evans RL, et al. Supervised exercise, spinal manipulation, and home exercise for chronic low back pain: a randomized clinical trial. Spine J 2011;11:585–98.
31. Bono CM. Low back pain in athletes. J Bone Joint Surg Am 2004;86:382–96.
32. Lauerman W, Shaffer B, DeLee JC, et al, editors. Orthopaedic sports medicine: principles and practices, vol. 1. 2nd edition. Sports injuries to the thoracolombar spine in children and adolescents. Philadelphia: WB Saunders; 2003. p. 1562–75.
33. Khan N, Husain S, Haak M. Thoracolumbar injuries in the athlete. Sports Med Arthrosc 2008;16:16–25.
34. Cohen SP, Raja SN. Pathogenesis, diagnosis, and treatment of lumbar zygapophysial (facet) joint pain. Anesthesiology 2007;106:591–614.
35. Staal JB, de Bie R, de Vet HC, et al. Injection therapy for subacute and chronic low-back pain. Cochrane Database Syst Rev 2008;(3):CD001824.
36. Varlotta GP, Lefkowitz TR, Schweitzer M, et al. The lumbar facet joint: a review of current knowledge: part I: anatomy, biomechanics, and grading. Skeletal Radiol 2011;40:13–23.
37. Varlotta GP, Lefkowitz TR, Schweitzer M, et al. The lumbar facet joint: a review of current knowledge: part II: diagnosis and management. Skeletal Radiol 2011;40: 149–57.
38. Boswell MV, Trescot AM, Datta S, et al. Interventional techniques: evidence-based practice guidelines in the management of chronic spinal pain. Pain Physician 2007;10:7–111.
39. Cohen SP. Sacroiliac joint pain: a comprehensive review of anatomy, diagnosis and treatment. Anesth Analg 2005;101:1440–53.
40. Manchikanti L, Singh V, Pampati V, et al. Evaluation of the relative contributions of various structures in chronic low back pain. Pain Physician 2001;4: 308–16.
41. Maigne JY, Aivakiklis A, Pfefer F. Results of sacroiliac joint double block and value of sacroiliac pain provocation test in 54 patients with low back pain. Spine (Phila Pa 1976) 1996;21:1889–92.
42. Irwin RW, Watson T, Minick RP, et al. Age, body mass index, and gender differences in sacroiliac joint pathology. Am J Phys Med Rehabil 2007;86:37–44.

43. Vanelderen P, Szadek K, Cohen SP, et al. 13. Sacroiliac joint pain. Pain Pract 2010;10:470–8.
44. Weksler N, Velan GJ, Semionov M, et al. The role of sacroiliac joint dysfunction in the genesis of low back pain: the obvious is not always right. Arch Orthop Trauma Surg 2007;127:885–8.
45. Ilaslan H, Arslan A, Koç ON, et al. Sacroiliac joint dysfunction. Turk Neurosurg 2010;20:398–401.
46. Stoev I, Powers AK, Puglisi JA, et al. Sacroiliac joint pain in the pediatric population. J Neurosurg Pediatr 2012;9:602–7.
47. Forst SL, Wheeler MT, Fortin JD, et al. The sacroiliac joint: anatomy, physiology, and clinical significance. Pain Physician 2006;9:61–8.
48. Van de Meent H, Jansen H, Van der Linde H. Study of the human pelvis using CAT-scan: gender differences and anatomy of the ramus ossis ischii. Prosthet Orthot Int 2008;32:385–9.
49. Janssen MM, Drevelle X, Humbert L, et al. Differences in male and female spino-pelvic alignment in asymptomatic young adults: a three dimensional analysis using upright low-dose digital biplanar X-rays. Spine (Phila Pa 1976) 2009;34: E826–32.
50. Seike K, Koda K, Oda K, et al. Gender differences in pelvis anatomy and effects on rectal cancer surgery. Hepatogastroenterology 2009;56:111–5.
51. Dreyfus P, Dreyer SJ, Cole A, et al. Sacroiliac joint pain. J Am Acad Orthop Surg 2004;12:255–65.
52. Abe T, Kearns CF, Fukunaga T. Sex differences in whole body skeletal muscle mass measured by magnetic resonance imaging and its distribution in young Japanese adults. Br J Sports Med 2003;37:436–40.
53. Snijders CJ, Vleeming A, Stoeckart R. Transfer of lumbosacral load to iliac bones and legs. Part I: biomechanics of self-bracing of the sacroiliac joints and its significance for treatment and exercise. Clin Biomech 1993;8:285–94.
54. Forst SL, Wheeler MT, Fortin JD, et al. The Sacroiliac joint: anatomy, physiology, and clinical significance. Pain physician 2006;9:61–8.
55. Hancock MJ, Maher CG, Latimer J, et al. Systematic review of tests to identify the disc, SIJ, or facet joint as the source of low back pain. Eur Spine J 2007;16:1539–50.
56. Szadek KM, Van der wurff P, Van tulder MW, et al. Diagnostic validity of criteria for sacroiliac joint pain: a systematic review. J Pain 2009;10:354–68.
57. Freburger JK, Riddle DL. Using published evidence to guide the examination of the sacroiliac joint region. Phys Ther 2001;81:1135–43.
58. Arab AM, Abdollahi I, Joghataei MT, et al. Inter- and intra-examiner reliability of single and composites of selected motion palpation and pain provocation tests for sacroiliac joint. Man Ther 2009;14:213–21.
59. Gilliss AC, Swanson RL II, Janora D, et al. Use of osteopathic manipulative treatment to manage compensated trendelenburg gait caused by sacroiliac somatic dysfunction. J Am Osteopath Assoc 2010;110:81–6.
60. Gyurcsik ZN, András A, Bodnár N, et al. Improvement in pain intensity, spine stiffness, and mobility during a controlled individualized physiotherapy program in ankylosing spondylitis. Rheumatol Int 2012;32:3931–6.
61. Boulay C, Tardieu C, Hecquet J, et al. Three-dimensional study of pelvic asymmetry on anatomical specimens and its clinical perspectives. J Anat 2006;208: 21–33.
62. Scholtes SA, Gombatto SP, Van Dillen LR. Differences in Lumbopelvic motion between people with and people without low back pain during two lower limb movement tests. Clin Biomech (Bristol, Avon) 2009;24:7–12.

63. Shadmehr A, Jafarian Z, Talebian S. Changes in recruitment of pelvic stabilizer muscles in people with and without sacroiliac joint pain during the active straight-leg-raise test. J Back Musculoskeletal Rehabil 2012;25:27–32.
64. Beales DJ, O'Sullivan PB, Briffa NK. The effects of manual pelvic compression on trunk motor control during an active straight leg raise in chronic pelvic girdle pain subjects. Man Ther 2010;15:190–9.
65. Buyruk HM. Effect of pelvic belt application on sacroiliac joint mobility. In: Vleeming A, Snyders CJ, Stoeckart R, editors. Progress in vertebral column research: First International Symposium on the Sacroiliac Joint: its role in posture and locomotion. Rotterdam (The Netherlands): ECO; 1991. p. 94–5.
66. Vleeming A, Buyruk HM, Stoeckart R. An integrated therapy for peripartum pelvic instability: a study based on biomechanical effects of pelvic belts. In: Vleeming A, Snyders CJ, Stoeckart R, editors. Progress in vertebral column research: First International Symposium on the Sacroiliac Joint: Its role in posture and locomotion. Rotterdam (The Netherlands): ECO; 1991. p. 86–92.
67. Rupert MP, Lee M, Manchikanti L, et al. Evaluation of sacroiliac joint interventions: a systematic appraisal of the literature. Pain Physician 2009;12:399–418.
68. Keating JG, Dims V, Avillar M. Sacroiliac joint fusion in a chronic low back pain population. The integrated function of the lumbar spine and sacroiliac joint. Part 1. Rotterdam (The Netherlands): ECO; 1995. p. 361–5.
69. Maxfield BA. Sports-related injury of the pediatric spine. Radiol Clin North Am 2010;48:1237–48.
70. Herman P. Spondylolysis and spondylolisthesis in the child and adolescent athlete. Orthop Clin North Am 2003;34:461–7.
71. Kim HJ, Green DW. Spondylolysis in the adolescent athlete. Curr Opin Pediatr 2011;23:68–72.
72. Klein G, Mehlman CT, McCarty M. Nonoperative treatment of spondylolysis and grade 1 spondylolisthesis in children and young adults: a meta-analysis of observational studies. J Pediatr Orthop 2009;29:146–56.
73. Leone A, Cianfoni A, Cerase A, et al. Lumbar spondylolysis: a review. Skeletal Radiol 2011;40:683–700.
74. McCleary MD, Congeni JA. Current concepts in the diagnosis and treatment of spondylolysis in young athletes. Curr Sports Med Rep 2007;6:62–6.
75. Syrmou E, Tsitsopoulos PP, Marinopoulos D, et al. Spondylolysis: a review and reappraisal. Hippokratia 2010;14:17–21.
76. Tsirikos AI, Garrido EG. Spondylolysis and spondylolisthesis in children and adolescents. J Bone Joint Surg Br 2010;92:751–9.
77. Fredrickson BE, Baker D, McHolick WJ, et al. The natural history of spondylolysis and spondylolisthesis. J Bone Joint Surg Am 1984;66:699–707.
78. Standaert CJ, Herring SA. Spondylolysis: a critical review. Br J Sports Med 2000; 34:415–22.
79. Libson E, Bloom RA, Dinari G. symptomatic and asymptomatic spondylolysis and spondylolisthesis in young adults. Int Orthop 1982;6:259–61.
80. Harvey CJ, Richenberg JL, Saifuddin A, et al. Pictorial review: the radiological investigation of lumbar spondylolysis. Clin Radiol 1998;53:723–8.
81. Standaert CJ, Herring SA. Expert opinion and controversies in sports and musculoskeletal medicine: the diagnosis and treatment of spondylolysis and adolescent athletes. Arch Phys Med Rehabil 2007;88:537–40.
82. MacDonald J, D'Hemecourt P. Back pain in the adolescent athlete. Pediatr Ann 2007;36:703–12.

83. d'Hemecourt PA, Zurakowski D, Kriemler S, et al. Spondylolysis: returning the athlete to sports participation with brace treatment. Orthopedics 2002;25:653–7.
84. d'Hemecourt PA, Gerbino PG 2nd, Micheli LJ. Back injuries in the young athlete. Clin Sports Med 2000;19:663–79.
85. Stasinopoulos D. Treatment of spondylolysis with external electrical stimulation in young athletes: a critical literature review. Br J Sports Med 2004;38:352–4.
86. Curtis C, d'Hemecourt P. Diagnosis and management of back pain in adolescents. Adolesc Med State Art Rev 2007;18:140–64, x.
87. O'Sullivan PB, Phyty GD, Twomey LT, et al. Evaluation of specific stabilizing exercises in the treatment of chronic low back pain with radiological diagnosis of spondylolysis and spondylolisthesis. Spine (Phila Pa 1976) 1997;22:2959–67.
88. Cohen E, Stuecker RD. Magnetic resonance imaging in the diagnosis and follow up of impending spondylolysis in children and adolescents: early treatment may prevent pars defects. J Pediatr Orthop B 2005;14:63–7.
89. Sairyo K, Sakai T, Yasui N, et al. Conservative treatment for pediatric lumbar spondylolysis to achieve bone healing using a hard brace: what type and how long? J Neurosurg Spine 2012;16:610–4.
90. Agabegi SS, Fischgrund JS. Contemporary management of isthmic spondylolisthesis: pediatric and adult. Spine J 2010;10:530–43.
91. Glancy G. The diagnosis and treatment of back pain in children and adolescents: an update. Adv Pediatr 2006;53:227–40.
92. Selbst SM, Lavelle JM, Soyupak SK, et al. Back pain children who present to emergency department. Clin Pediatr (Phila) 1999;38:401–6.
93. King HA. Back pain in children. Orthop Clin North Am 1999;30:467–74, ix.
94. Balagué F, Nordin M. Back pain in children and teenagers. Baillieres Clin Rheumatol 1992;6:575–93.
95. Sassmannshausen G, Smith BG. Back pain in the young athlete. Clin Sports Med 2002;21:121–32.
96. Tse SM, Laxer RM. Juvenile spondyloarthropathy. Curr Opin Rheumatol 2003;15:374–9.
97. Muñiz AE, Liner S. Lumbar vertebral fractures in children: gour cases and review of the literature. Pediatr Emerg Care 2011;27:1157–62.
98. Tran de QH, Duong S, Finlayson RJ. Lumbar spinal stenosis: a brief review of the nonsurgical management. Can J Anaesth 2010;57:694–703.
99. Amundsen T, Weber H, Nordal HJ, et al. Lumbar spinal stenosis: conservative or surgical management?: a prospective 10-year study. Spine (Phila Pa 1976) 2000;25:1424–35.

The Athlete's Hip and Groin

Kumar Tammareddi, MD[a], Vincent Morelli, MD[b,*],
Miguel Reyes Jr, MD[c]

KEYWORDS

• Hip • Groin • Athlete • Injury • Pain

KEY POINTS

- A large number of hip and groin injuries have multiple components or coexisting injuries often complicating the diagnosis.
- Current data for hip osteoarthritis suggest conservative measures as primary treatment along with non pharmacological and pharmacological treatments.
- Pain due to hip labral tears may return after treatment with conservative therapy and return to sport; it may require surgical management.
- Conservative therapy for femoroacetabular impingement involves avoiding specific activities and likely needs surgery to enable a return to athletics.
- The success rate for conservative therapy in treating a sports hernia is thought to be low; surgical treatment is usually required.

This article focuses on athletic causes for hip and groin pain, although the area is also commonly affected by various non–sport-related conditions (**Table 1**). A large number of hip and groin injuries have multiple components or coexisting injuries often complicating the diagnosis.[1,2] A complete history and physical, and appropriate diagnostic examinations, are needed to diagnose, treat, speed recovery, and prevent reinjures.

Sports-related injuries of the hip and groin region occur in 5% to 9% of high school athletes.[3–5] In adult soccer players, hip and groin injuries account for 12% to 16% of all injuries,[6] and activities with similar quick cutting movements, accelerations, decelerations, and directional changes also have an increased incidence of such injuries. Because the center of gravity is located within the pelvis, and loads generated through athletic performance are transferred through the hip and groin,[7] it is vital to keep the area healthy and stable.

ANATOMY

The anatomy of the hip and groin region is complex and injuries often involve multiple origins and surrounding structures. A detailed discussion of the anatomy is beyond the

[a] Department of Sports Medicine, Meharry Medical College, 1005 Todd Boulevard, Nashville, TN 37208, USA; [b] Department of Family and Community Medicine, Meharry Medical College, 1005 Dr D.B. Todd Boulevard, Nashville, TN 37208, USA; [c] Department of Radiology, Medical Imaging of Dallas, 102 Decker Court, Irving, TX 75062, USA
* Corresponding author.
E-mail address: morellivincent@yahoo.com

Prim Care Clin Office Pract 40 (2013) 313–333
http://dx.doi.org/10.1016/j.pop.2013.02.005 primarycare.theclinics.com
0095-4543/13/$ – see front matter

Table 1
Differential diagnosis of hip and groin pain

Athletic	Nonathletic
Muscle strains	Septic arthritis
Contusions (ie, hip pointer)	Lumbar spine abnormalities
Hip dislocations and subluxations	Avascular necrosis
Acetabular labral tears	—
Femoral fractures	Spondyloarthropathies
Sports hernia and athletic pubalgia	Tumors
Osteitis pubis	Gastrointestinal disorders
Bursitis	Genitourinary disorders
Snapping hip syndrome	Gynecologic disorders
Osteoarthritis	—
Stress fractures	—
Nerve entrapment	—

scope of this article, so the reader is referred to anatomic texts. This article discusses only clinically significant structures in relation to specific injuries.

RISK FACTORS FOR HIP AND GROIN INJURIES

Risk factors leading to an increased incidence of future groin injuries include hip adductor strength less than 80% of abductor strength (in hockey players),[8] decreased hip range of motion, previous injury,[9] and muscular tightness in soccer players.[10] Established risk factors in the development of osteoarthritis of the hip include age, obesity, and sports such as soccer, track, or running, in which repetitive injury is likely.[11]

ADDUCTOR STRAINS

Adductor strains are the most common groin injury among athletes, accounting for roughly 10% of all injuries in soccer players.[6] As mentioned earlier, decreased range of motion and decreased adductor strength have been associated with an increased incidence of adductor strains and are the primary focus of adductor strain prevention programs.[12–14] Adductor strains usually occur at the musculotendinous junction but may also occur at the bone-tendon junction (enthesopathy). Physical examination elicits tenderness on palpation of the involved muscle and pain on stretching/adduction against resistance.

Imaging

Although rarely needed for diagnosis, ultrasound and magnetic resonance imaging (MRI) may be used in cases in which a definitive diagnosis is required (eg, chronic injuries, those nonresponsive to therapy) or to rule out other causes for groin pain. Ultrasound has a reported sensitivity of up to 84%[15] and MRI (gadolinium-enhanced imaging improves visualization of abnormalities)[16] may be used when ultrasound is nondiagnostic and the clinician remains highly suspicious. MRI has been reported as normal in roughly 40% of patients with chronic adductor enthesopathy.[16]

Treatment

Rest and nonsteroidal antiinflammatory drugs (NSAIDs) may be offered for initial treatment of acute adductor strains (see our article elsewhere in this issue for more specifics on NSAID use). Beyond this, the site of the lesion determines the treatment plan. If the insult is near the bone-tendon junction (enthesopathy), physical therapy should be delayed until acute symptoms have improved. Because these areas are less vascular, some healing is needed before rehabilitation. Gentle stretching and strengthening should then follow over a period of weeks. If the tear is near the more vascular musculotendinous junction or in the muscle belly, early and more aggressive therapy can be instituted.[17] Physical therapy should be designed to improving range of motion, strength, and flexibility. In acute strains, when athletes have regained 70% of strength and a pain-free range of motion (usually 4–8 weeks), they may return to sports. In chronic strains, the recovery time may be as long as 6 months.[18]

Injection Therapy

In chronic or recalcitrant cases, steroid injection (80 mg of triamcinolone acetonide and 3 mL of 0.5% of marcaine) is thought to be a reasonable option by some investigators. Schliders and colleagues[19,20] recently evaluated injection of the bone-tendon junction in both competitive athletes and recreational athletes, and evaluated patients 1 year after the intervention. Competitive athletes with documented enthesopathy on MRI (average duration of symptoms 25 weeks) were unlikely to be helped by injection. To identify patients who might be helped by intervention, the investigators noted that competitive athletes with clinical adductor disorders of short duration (average duration of symptoms 6 weeks) and normal MRI all improved with injection. The investigators do not comment on this group having had milder disease or that many of this group might have improved without intervention. The author's conclusion that, "...injections can be expected to afford at least one year of pain relief in patients who have had a short duration of symptoms..." cannot be drawn from this data as there was no control group.

There is currently no good evidence for the use of steroid injections in adductor enthesopathy.

Surgical Repair

Surgical repair with tenotomy has been shown to improve chronic adductor tears that have not responded to conservative therapy for at least 6 months. In a recent study,[21] 70 patients underwent tenotomy for chronic adductor pain. Seventy-three percent were satisfied with the results of the surgery, but only 54% of athletes were able to return to their previous sport.

Acute complete adductor tears generally require surgical repair.

OSTEOARTHRITIS OF THE HIP

Introduction

Osteoarthritis is the most common arthritic disease in developing countries,[22] with an overall prevalence of 10.9%.[23] One in 4 people in their 60s and more than half in their 80s showed radiographic changes of osteoarthritis.[24] Established risk factors such as age, obesity, occupation, trauma, and genetics all play a role in disease initiation and progression. In athletes, a long history of high-mileage distance running or involvement in power sports should be also be considered as risk factors for the development of hip osteoarthritis.[25,26] Comparing active men from 50 to

70 years of age who had undergone hip replacement surgery with age-matched control individuals, Vingard and colleagues[27] found that those with an increased exposure to sports (in hours) had a 4.5 times greater risk of developing osteoarthritis at the hip.

Histopathology

In osteoarthritis, extracellular matrix synthesis is surpassed by its degradation, causing a net breakdown of cartilage.[28] Inflammatory markers such as interleukin 1, prostaglandin E2, and tumor necrosis factor alpha have been found in osteoarthritic cartilage,[28,29] and because inflammation is one of the causative factors in arthritic pain, efforts to reduce the inflammation are major parts of current treatment. Hyaluronic acid has also been found to be decreased in osteoarthritic joints,[30] supporting the rationale behind supplementation therapy. A full discussion of the pathophysiology and histopathology of osteoarthritis is beyond the scope of this article, but aspects on which current therapies are based are discussed.

Symptoms

Arthritic pain is usually described as dull and achy, with noted joint stiffness and limited range of motion particularly with internal rotation and flexion. A feeling of crepitus and grinding may also be noted as joint surfaces become irregular and narrowed because of osteophyte formation. Groin pain has been noted in 22% to 39% of patients with hip osteoarthritis.[31,32]

Diagnosis/Imaging

There is no gold standard diagnostic test for osteoarthritis, but clinical criteria include reduced internal rotation of 15° or less with an erythrocyte sedimentation rate (ESR) of less than or equal to 45 mm/h, pain on internal rotation, morning hip stiffness lasting 60 minutes or less, and age more than 50 years. Together, these clinical criteria have a sensitivity of 86% and specificity of 75%. Adding radiological examinations looking for osteophytes and joint space narrowing and an ESR of 20 mm/h or less increased the sensitivity and specificity to 89% and 91% respectively.[31]

Plain radiographs of the hip (standing AP pelvis - where normal articular width is 4–5 mm – and frog leg views) should be the initial imaging choice but can be normal in early osteoarthritis. X-rays may, however, detect other abnormalities such as fractures, femoroacetabular impingement (FAI) syndrome, and avascular necrosis of the femoral head.

MRI has been increasingly used for evaluation of osteoarthritis, but, in a recent meta-analysis performed for osteoarthritic changes of the knee, hip, and hand, overall sensitivity was only 61% and specificity was 82%.[33]

Treatment

The optimal treatment of hip osteoarthritis includes both nonpharmacologic and pharmacologic options. Risk factor modification should be taken into account. If the patient is overweight, weight reduction has been proved to reduce symptoms and is a key treatment goal.[34] Regular individualized exercise has also been proved to be effective in relieving symptoms[35] and should be encouraged. Ambulation appliances can also be used to help with pain relief in some cases.

Medications

Zhang and colleagues[36] reviewed the medication used in treatment plans for osteoarthritis published between 1966 and 2004 and came to the following conclusions.

Acetaminophen is an initial medication of choice and is generally safer than NSAIDs. NSAIDs can be used in conjunction with acetaminophen if there is inadequate pain relief from acetaminophen alone. They recommend that nonselective cyclooxygenase (COX) inhibitors should be combined with an H2 blocker, misoprostol, or proton pump inhibitors in patients with increased risk of gastrointestinal bleed. Opioids may be added to acetaminophen and NSAIDs but are not more effective than either when used alone. They conclude that opiates should only be used if there is failure of, or contraindications to, other medications. There is conflicting data on the symptom relieving efficacy of glucosamine/chondroitin in arthritic joints,[37–39] but even the most encouraging data affirms only a small benefit with these compounds. There is no evidence of structure modifying effects.

Steroid injection

Steroid injections have also been used for the treatment of osteoarthritis when conservative and oral therapies have failed. The hip is a difficult joint to inject because of its anatomy, and it is generally recommended that imaging be used to confirm placement of the needle, with ultrasound being favored because of its ease of use, lower cost, and safety.[40] In a randomized, double blind, placebo-controlled clinical trial, Lambert and colleagues[41] injected confirmed osteoarthritic hips under fluoroscopy after failed conservative therapy. Using 40 mg of triamcinolone hexacetonide and 10 mg of bupivacaine or 2 mL saline solution, they found a significant improvement in pain scores, which lasted up to 3 months. However, the treatment group was significantly younger than the placebo group, although time since diagnosis was equivalent.

In conclusion, intra-articular steroid injection for osteoarthritis of the hip lacks strong evidence of efficacy and is supported only by category 1B evidence.[36]

Hyaluronic acid

The exact mechanism by which hyaluronic acid works is unknown. Several effects have been found including enhanced synthesis of extracellular matrix proteins, including chondroitin and keratin sulfate, and prostaglandins. In addition, hyaluronic acid has been found to decrease inflammatory mediators, decrease cartilage degradation, and increase the synthesis of the extracellular matrix.[30] Nociceptor activity may also be attenuated by hyaluronic acid, resulting in decreased pain levels.[42]

There remains controversy for the use of hyaluronic acid in hip osteoarthritis. In one study, 42 patients were treated with either hyaluronic acid or mepivacaine injection. Compared with mepivacaine, hyaluronic acid was shown to improve symptoms, decreasing NSAID intake by 49.4%, whereas mepivacaine alone had a reduction of only 24.6%. However, there was no statistical significance between these groups in the reduction of NSAID use.[43] Other studies have shown slight improvement but less than that of corticosteroid therapy.[44] The use of hyaluronic acid remains controversial and needs further investigation before becoming a recommended therapy before total hip arthroplasty.

Surgery

Those patients who fail conservative therapy and have limited functional capacity may need surgical referral for a total hip arthroplasty. A meta-analysis by Vissers and colleagues[45] reviewed literature to compare the recovery of physical function after total hip arthroplasty. Patients recovered 80% of the physical function of normal healthy individuals within 6 months of their arthroplasty. For pain, the proportion of patients who remain free from pain ranges from 43.2% to 84.1%. Revision rates of the hip ranged from 0.8 to 2.04 per 100 person years.[36]

Summary

Osteoarthritis of the hip often affects older athletes. This can be caused by repetitive wear placed on the hip joint or from trauma in the recent or remote past. General treatment guidelines suggest conservative measures as primary treatment with non-pharmacologic and pharmacologic treatments. Corticosteroid injections may be attempted but there remains category Ib evidence for this treatment at this time. Hyaluronic acid can be tried, but remains controversial. Total hip arthroplasty affords significant pain relief, especially in patients with appreciable pain and disability and in those with advanced radiographic changes.[36]

HIP LABRAL TEARS

Introduction

The hip labrum acts as a shock absorber, joint lubricator, and pressure distributor. Tears of the labrum are responsible for hip and groin pain in as many as 22% to 55% of patients with hip and groin pain.[46,47] Labral tears can occur in athletic trauma from isolated or repetitive injury.[48] Most tears are not associated with any known cause and are thought to be caused by repetitive microtrauma.[46,48] Repetitive pivoting on a loaded femur, as in soccer or golf, have been linked to labral disorders. However, tears can also occur with simple running, sprinting, or any activity that places excessive force on the labrum.

Labral tears are often found in association with chondral injury adjacent to the labral disorder. Chondromalacia, thinning of the cartilage, delamination of the cartilage, chondral flap tears, and full-thickness chondral injury with exposed bone have all been documented alongside labral tears.[48,49] FAI can also predispose athletes to labral disorders.

There are several classifications of labral tears, including histologic, anatomic, etiologic, and those based on magnetic resonance arthrogram (MRA)/arthroscopy findings. However, these classification systems do not help provider prognosis or guide treatment. One current study with the Multicenter Arthroscopic Hip Outcomes Research Network has proposed a classification system and is studying labral tears and their prognostic implications, but data have yet to be published.[50]

Clinical Picture

With labral tears, anterior hip or groin pain is the most common complaint from patients, usually beginning without any inciting event. Patients may also report a variety of mechanical symptoms such as clicking, locking/catching, or giving way. Of these symptoms, clicking seems to be the most consistent with a labral tear.[47,49,51] The pain usually worsens with activity and is often aggravated by walking, pivoting, prolonged sitting, and impact activities such as running.[49]

Imaging

Hip radiographs with cross-table views and anterior/posterior pelvis views can be used to evaluate for OA and FAI, but with isolated labral tears, x-rays are normal.

MRA of the hip is the best noninvasive test to evaluate labral disorders, with a sensitivity of 87% and specificity of 64%. Plain MRI has only 66% sensitivity and 79% specificity.[52] Criteria for tears on an MRA include contrast extending into the labrum or acetabular/labral interface, blunted appearance, and displacement/detachment from underlying bone.[48,53] MRA is more effective in finding anterior labral tears than posterior tears.

Arthroscopy is the gold standard for diagnosis and can be both diagnostic and therapeutic. For diagnosis, it is usually reserved for those with an intra-articular pain that cannot be identified through history, physical, or imaging.[54]

Treatment

Conservative therapy should be tried initially with antiinflammatory medications and a physical therapy protocol for 10 to 12 weeks. This treatment does help with the pain but, once the patient has returned to normal activities, the pain may recur.[51] Injections with steroids may be used with associated degenerative changes but, as stated earlier, such intervention is not supported by strong evidence. In younger patients without degenerative changes, intra-articular injections with steroids may damage chondral surfaces.[55]

Arthroscopic procedures are used when conservative measures fail. When a tear is present, in some cases sutures may be used to secure the tear and frayed edges can be shaved. Arthroscopic repair has varied results depending on associated findings during the repair. Most results of arthroscopic surgery are positive. In one study, 89% of patients had an improved status at 16.5 months after arthroscopic debridement.[56] Another article concludes that, depending on associated findings, nonelite athletes were 93% improved but only 76% were able to return to their sport symptom free. Among elite athletes, 96% were improved, but only 85% were able to successfully return to their sports. Factors that influenced poor outcomes included associated arthritis, FAI, and articular cartilage damage.[57]

Following arthroscopic repair, guided physical therapy should include proper range of motion and fixing faulty gait patterns learned with the previous labral tear. Active straight leg raising and deep hip extension or lunges should be avoided initially.

Golfers can be expected to return to competition in an average of 6 weeks, whereas baseball and soccer players average 12 weeks before return.[58]

FAI SYNDROME

Introduction

FAI syndrome or hip impingement syndrome is defined as the abutment between the femoral head and the acetabular rim.[59] FAI syndrome can be caused by anatomic abnormalities of the femoral head/neck (cam lesion) and/or the acetabulum (pincer lesions).[60] Repeated hip flexion during sports can cause impingement of the labrum on the femoral head and may result in early arthritis of the both the femoral head and acetabular surfaces. The prevalence of FAI is not well documented in the literature and radiographic findings are unhelpful in establishing prevalence rates because such changes are also commonly seen in asymptomatic athletes.[61] Further studies are needed to determine which athletes with radiographic changes of FAI will develop the clinical symptoms of the syndrome.

Pathogenesis

The hip is a ball-and-socket joint and, even with normal morphology, extremes of movement can cause impingement of the labrum and femoral neck.[62] Two major morphologic variations of the hip joint that are associated with FAI are the cam (cam comes from the Dutch word meaning cog) lesion and the pincer lesion (**Fig. 1**).

Cam lesions are more common in athletes. A cam impingement is characterized by a nonspherical femoral head and abnormal angles of the femoral neck in relation to the

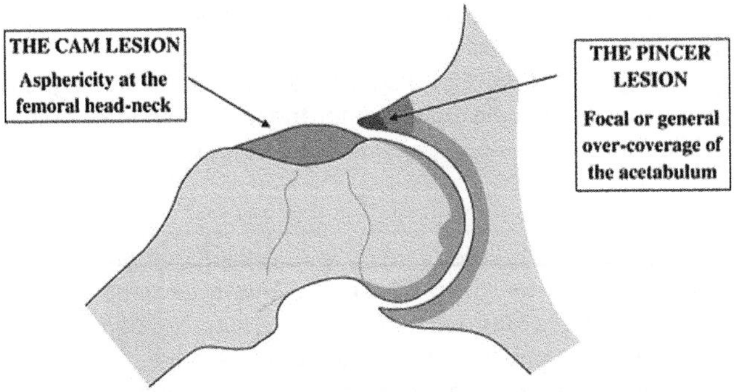

Fig. 1. Cam and pincer lesions. (*From* Chakraverty JK, Snelling NJ. Anterior hip pain – Have you considered femoroacetabular impingement? International Journal of Osteopathic Medicine 2012;15:22–7; with permission.)

head.[63] The pathogenesis of cam deformities is not well understood but the deformity may be caused by developmental disorders such as Legg-Calve-Perthes or slipped capital femoral epiphysis. It may also simply develop during an athlete's growth.[64,65] With the cam lesion's nonspherical femoral head moving within the hip joint during flexion, it contacts the anterosuperior labrum and places shearing forces on the labral surface. Eventual separation of the labrum from the surrounding articular cartilage may result from these repetitive shearing forces. Complaints of pain, stiffness, and decreased range of motion of the hip are common from athletes.[63]

The rim impingement or pincer lesion is located on the acetabular side of the hip joint. This lesion is found mostly in women. A pincer lesion is the result of increased coverage on the femoral head by the anterior portion of the acetabulum.[66] This abnormality can lead to a repetitive crushing of the labrum and can result in a type II labral tear/cystic tear.[67,68]

Diagnosis

FAI syndrome typically presents in active young or middle-aged patients.[69] The onset of painful symptoms may be insidious or may occur after minor trauma. Pain is usually localized to the groin alone (in up to 85%) or to the groin and affected hip (14%).[70,71] Patients may also describe lower extremities locking, catching, or giving way.

Clinical examination is a key element to diagnosis because radiological imaging alone is not sufficient for diagnosis. The impingement test (decreased range of motion and painful limitation in flexion, internal rotation, and adduction of the hip) is the physical examination test of choice, with a sensitivity of 75% and specificity of 43% in identifying those with labral tears.[47,72,73] Much like the McMurry test when seeking meniscal tears, the scour test to detect labral tears is performed by internally and externally rotating the hip in both abduction and adduction to find labral disorders. This test may also discover symptoms related to FAI, including stiffness, locking, catching, or snapping of the hip.[74]

Imaging

Diagnosing FAI requires typical symptoms, physical examination findings, in conjunction with radiographic findings.[75] Radiographic investigations start with radiographs including an anteroposterior (AP) view of the pelvis as well as a cross-table lateral view of the hip. The AP view can reveal deformities of the femoral head including a flattened head-neck junction and a pistol-grip deformity. The alpha angle has been used a measurement to aid in the diagnosis of FAI. The alpha angle is measured on an oblique image through the center of the femoral neck. A circle is used to outline the femoral head, one line is drawn down the long axis of the femoral neck and another line is drawn from the center of the circle to the point where the femoral head is noted beyond the circle (**Fig. 2**).[76] The alpha angle is the angle formed by the intersection of these two lines (see **Fig. 2**; **Fig. 3**). Measurements of the femoral head and neck are taken including the alpha angle and head-neck offset. A head-neck offset of less than 7 mm and an alpha angle of greater than 55° (see **Figs. 2** and **3**).[77]

Rim impingement on an AP pelvis radiograph reveals overcoverage of the femoral head.

MRA is the test of choice for detecting any suspected concomitant labral disorders. A triad of abnormal head-neck morphology, anterosuperior cartilage abnormality, and anterosuperior labral disorders on MRA were found in 88% of patients with FAI.[78]

Treatment

Conservative treatment

Despite the fact that FAI is seemingly an anatomical abnormality causing mechanical problems, conservative treatment (restricted movement of the hip, physical therapy, NSAIDs) may be tried. Some authors have recommended surgical correction as definitive therapy treatment in this malady, but a recent study by Emara and colleagues[71] cast doubt on this 1-size-fits-all approach. In this study of 37 patients with FAI, 33 responded to a trial of conservative treatment with significantly improved Harris Hip Scores and symptoms after 6 months. Twenty-seven of these 33 maintained these benefits at 24 months. However, the conservative regimen included not only diclofenac and physical therapy to increase internal rotation and abduction but also included avoidance of excess physical activity, adaptation of a nonpainful range of motion, and modification of activities of daily living.

Athletes in the study had to avoid running in straight lines and, instead, were instructed to run in a zigzag pattern. Cycling was also avoided, or allowed only with modifications to the normal cycling movement. Although this approach may benefit less active patients, it is not a practical solution for the athletic population.

Surgical treatment

Surgical correction of the mechanical impingement (femoral head abutting against the acetabular rim) is the treatment of choice for FAI that has failed conservative management.[79] Both open and arthroscopic techniques have been described,[62] with the most

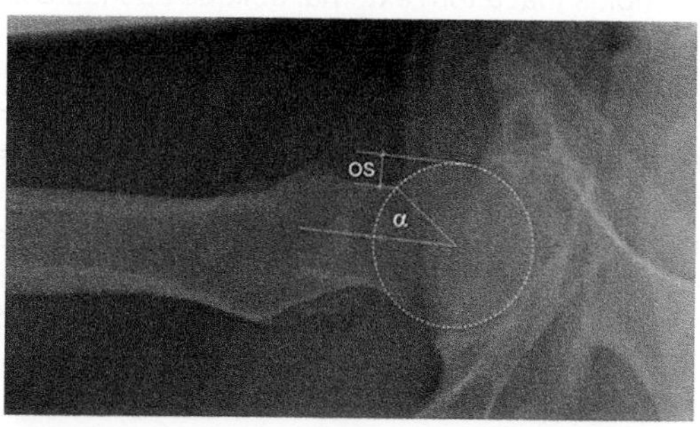

Fig. 2. Cross-table Lateral View: normal alpha angle, less than 55°, head-neck offset of greater than 7 mm. (*From* Hossain M, Andrew JG. Current management of femoroacetabular impingement. Curr Orthop 2008;22(4):306; with permission.)

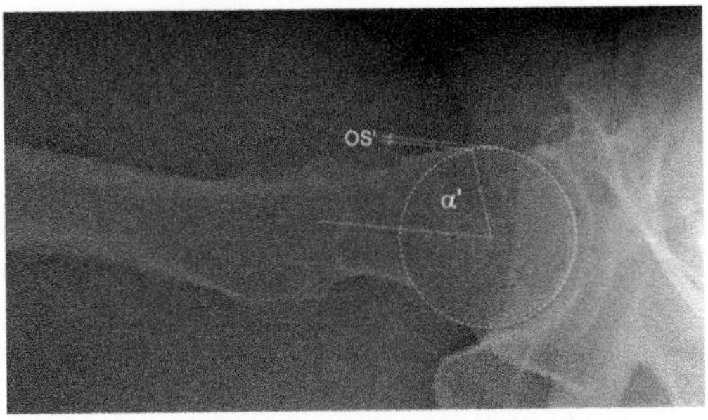

Fig. 3. Cam lesion with alpha angle greater than 55°, head-neck offset of less than 7 mm. (*From* Hossain M, Andrew JG. Current management of femoro-acetabular impingement. Curr Orthop 2008;22(4):307; with permission.)

recent review suggesting that arthroscopic outcomes are equal to or better than open methods, with lower rates of major complications.[80]

Surgical complications, such as heterotrophic ossification (bone growth in extraskeletal soft tissue), can occur and can be seen in open and arthroscopic surgery. Of the 300 cases reviewed by Randelli and colleagues,[81] 5 had heterotopic ossification after arthroscopic surgery. These patients did not have NSAID therapy after surgery. In the patients who were compliant with their NSAID treatment, no heterotopic ossification was noted. NSAID therapy was recommended to patients who underwent arthroscopic and open surgery.

SPORTS HERNIA

Introduction

The sports hernia is not a true hernia but refers to a painful soft tissue injury of the groin and has also been called Gilmore groin, athletic pubalgia, or groin disruption. This article uses the term sports hernia to encompass all three terms and to indicate a soft tissue defect of the posterior abdominal wall and its accompanying pain.

In a sports hernia, the tendons of the oblique muscles (and possibly the adductor tendons) attached to the pubic bone are often torn. These injuries have a reported incidence of 10% to 13% in soccer players and are caused by stress and pivot forces placed on this area.[9,82]

Causes

There are 2 major theories of the causes of sports hernias. One theory, popularized in a study by Gilmore,[83] holds that a torn external oblique aponeurosis causes dilatation of the superficial inguinal ring, leading to a torn conjoined tendon and dehiscence between the inguinal ligament and the torn conjoined tendon. The second school of thought is that athletic pubalgia is secondary to an occult prehernia condition and/or a small, non-detectable hernia caused by a defect in the posterior wall of the inguinal canal or transversalis fascia.[84]

Litwin and colleagues[85] combined these two theories and proposed that a large tear or multiple small tears of the external oblique, rectus abdominis, or muscles forming the conjoint tendon weaken the boundaries of the posterior wall and lead to formation of a hernia.

Clinical Diagnosis

Sports hernias usually present with chronic groin pain that radiates to the inner thigh and is worsened by athletic activity.[86] Inguinal canal tenderness, dilated superficial inguinal ring, pubic tubercle tenderness, and hip adductor origin tenderness are commonly found on physical examination and can be aggravated by sudden movement such as Valsalva, coughing, sneezing, athletic effort, sexual activity, or resisted sit-up or hip adduction.[87] To elicit the pain of sports hernia, the patient should perform a resisted sit-up, with legs extended and with legs flexed, while the examiner palpates the rectus abdominis insertion.[82]

Imaging

The diagnosis of athletic pubalgia is mainly clinical and several studies have shown MRI to have a limited role in assessment of the injury. However, a recent study by Zoga and colleagues[88] found unenhanced MRI to be helpful and to have a sensitivity and specificity of 68% and 100% for rectus abdominis tendon injury and 86% and 89% for adductor tendon injury.

Dynamic ultrasound is less helpful, being highly operator dependent and exhibiting only subtle positive findings.[87]

Treatment

Conservative treatment of a sports hernia should be tried before surgical intervention, although the success rates for this type of therapy are thought to be low when a sports hernia is present.[87,89] Treatment generally includes 6 to 8 weeks of rest followed by hip and adductor strengthening and stretching with a gradual return to sport-specific activities.[90] Treatment may also include nonsteroidal antiinflammatory medications, steroid injections, or platelet-rich plasma injections, although there is little evidence for the efficacy of such interventions. If the athlete is pain free after 10 to 12 weeks, then competitive sports can be attempted.[91]

Surgical correction should only be selected with failure of conservative therapy. Both laparoscopic and open surgical approaches (with or without mesh) to correct the abdominal wall defect have been described. Caudill and colleagues,[87] using mesh-enhanced repairs, found comparable results between laparoscopic and open techniques. Ninety-six percent of those operated on laparoscopically and 92.8% of athletes operated on openly were able to return to sport after surgical intervention. It should be noted that this is a different procedure than usual inguinal hernia repair.

Laparoscopic repair may enable athletes to return to sports faster than open repair. Some studies have reported 87% to 92% of patients returning to training within 4 weeks of their laparoscopic surgery and to full activity within 6 weeks, and no recurrent symptoms at 12.1 months.[92,93] When using open repair, the athlete commonly has to be inactive for the initial 4-week postoperative period[87] and generally has a slower return to full activity (3–6 months).[94–96]

A small prospective study using fibrin glue rather than sutures to secure the mesh has had favorable outcomes with 16 soccer players. All players returned to preinjury levels of sporting activity 31 days (on average) after surgery. The cost of the glue used during surgery was significantly more than suture costs, and this was only a small prospective study. According to the study, sutures may increase operating time and decrease surgeon satisfaction because of an increase in perceived difficulty, and fibrin glue may improve these outcomes.[97] Cost, long-term analysis, and further research are needed to determine whether fibrin glue could replace traditional treatment, but the outcomes of surgeon satisfaction and the difficulty of the operation did improve.

Summary

In conclusion, when treating sports hernia, the primary care physician should inform patients about the various treatment options and discuss the expected results of therapy. It is important to discuss the likely need for surgical intervention with failure of conservative therapy. Open versus laparoscopic correction, and the general time frame for return to full activity, will be determining factors for definitive treatment.

OSTEITIS PUBIS

Introduction

Osteitis pubis, or pubic bone stress injury, is an isolated or repetitive insult to the pubic symphysis and surrounding structures. The trauma can be secondary to vaginal birth, pelvic/perineal surgery, infection, rheumatoid arthritis, or athletic activity.[98–100] In athletes, high-stress forces are transferred through the pelvis, the pubic symphysis, and surrounding structures during kicking, rapid acceleration, deceleration, or sudden directional changes. These forces can cause stress reactions and changes in the normal architecture of the symphysis pubis.[100,101]

Signs and Symptoms

Patients present with pain in the pubic symphysis, proximal adductor pain, or pain in other adjacent structures.[102] Symptoms may also include pain in the lower abdominal muscles, perineal pain, or testicular or scrotal pain.[103] Such overlapping symptoms necessitate ruling out other localized disorders such as sports hernia, FAI, adductor strain, and labral tears.

Physical examination reveals tenderness on direct palpation over the pubic symphysis. Most investigators hold that, if such tenderness is lacking, the diagnosis is less likely.[2] However, Fricker and colleagues[4] noted that only 70% of patients with osteitis pubis had pubis symphysis pain on examination. Other physical examination testing includes pelvic compression testing and flexion, abduction, and external rotation testing, both of which stress the pubic symphysis and reproduce pain in the area.[104]

Imaging

Radiographs are rarely helpful. Sclerosing, irregularity, and widening of the symphysis pubis[105] (initially thought to indicate osteitis pubis) have also been found in up to 76% of asymptomatic young soccer players.[106]

Bone scan can confirm the diagnosis when increased uptake is noted around the symphysis pubis. However, early in the disease, before osteoblast activation, bone scan may be negative. In addition, bone scan does not correlate with the severity of the clinical presentation.[4,107]

MRI is reported to have good diagnostic accuracy in osteitis pubis, but the sensitivity and specificity are not documented in the literature.[108] MRI findings reveal bone marrow edema and signs of stress reaction.

Treatment

The treatment of choice remains conservative therapy, which can include physical therapy, NSAIDs, glucocorticoids, and corticosteroid injections. Experimental conservative therapy is still being developed, but there remains no standardized conservative treatment plan.[109]

Corticosteroids

Corticosteroid injections have shown improvement in the symptoms of osteitis pubis. In a case series, O'Connell and colleagues[105] evaluated 16 high-level athletes with clinically suspected osteitis pubis and a positive MRI or bone scan. The patients were injected with an aqueous suspension of 20 mg of methylprednisolone acetate and 1 mL of 0.5% bupivacaine hydrochloride into the symphyseal cleft. Of the 16 patients, 14 had immediate relief of symptoms and returned to their respective sports activities 48 hours after the procedure. At a 6-month follow-up, 7 of the 16 remained symptom free; 1 patient had 2 more injections (with bupivacaine only), which improved symptoms for an additional 2 weeks; 7 had persistent pain; and 1 was referred to surgery for painful joint disruption. All patients reported some improvement of their pain level.

Another small study of 8 patients by Holt and colleagues[110] used a combination of lidocaine, bupivacaine, and dexamethasone for athletes with osteitis pubis who had failed 16 weeks of conservative treatment. Of the 8 athletes injected, 3 returned to full participation within 3 weeks, 4 required a second injection to alleviate their symptoms and 1 had persistent pain after 2 injections.

However, optimistic expectations with steroid injections should be avoided because the study mentioned earlier had only a small number of patients, did not state the length of time for which symptoms were present, and had no control/placebo-injection comparison group. We could find no other trials of steroid injections in osteitis pubis.

Curettage

Curettage of the pubic symphysis cartilage may be of benefit when nonoperative measures have failed. One such study treated patients in whom a variety of conservative measures had failed over a mean of 13.22 months. First, a corticosteroid/anesthetic was injected into the area of the os pubis. Patients who experienced immediate pain relief from steroid/anesthetic injection then had curettage of the fibrocartilage disc and hyaline endplates of the pubic bodies. Of the 23 patients in the study, 9 reported feeling much better, 9 reported feeling better than before curettage, 3 had symptoms similar to before the procedure, and 2 had increased severity of their symptoms at a mean of 24.31 months (12.5–59.6 months). Seven of the patients were unable to return to full activity. Of those who did return fully, the average time to recovery was 5.63 months.[111] However, this study lacked a control group.

Other smaller studies have been performed with positive results[112] but, because there are a limited number of studies, no firm conclusions can be drawn about the efficacy of this procedure.

Wedge resection surgery

As with curettage, wedge resection in athletes is explored in a limited number of studies[113–115] and no single surgical technique has been proved to be most effective. One study recommends observation, physiotherapy, NSAIDs, and up to 3 pubic symphysis steroid injections over at least 9 months before suggesting surgery.[102] When conservative measures fail, the surgical option can be discussed with the patient. Surgery involves wedge resection of the symphysis pubis with or without a plate arthrodesis. Wedge resection after 6 months of conservative therapy in 10 patients showed a 70% satisfaction rate but also yielded 20% instability at a follow-up of 92 months. After 92 months, 7 patients had no pain, 1 patient had the pain return, another patient had sacroiliac joint pain and clicking of the pubic symphysis, and the remaining patient had instability that required arthrodesis at 79 months but then remained pain free 18 months after arthodesis.[114]

In a study by Williams and colleagues,[115] 7 rugby players with a diagnosis of osteitis pubis had surgical correction with plate arthrodesis. All 7 had resolution of symptoms at 52.4 months without pubic symphysis instability. Patients resumed light training on average at 3.7 months after surgery and a return to competitive fitness 6.6 months after surgery.

Summary

Osteitis pubis is usually seen in athletes involved in sports with high-stress forces transferred through the pelvis, the pubic symphysis, and surrounding structures during kicking, rapid acceleration, deceleration, or sudden directional changes. There is usually pubic symphysis pain noted on direct palpation, but this may not be present in all individuals. Diagnosis can be difficult because radiographs are often unhelpful. MRI may show marrow edema and bone scans may reveal a reactive area around the pubic symphysis. Conservative treatment is still first line, but an effective standardized physical therapy regimen has yet to be developed. Steroid injections and curettage have shown limited benefit. Wedge resection may improve symptoms in select patients but can lead to pelvic instability.

OBTURATOR NERVE IMPINGEMENT

Introduction

The obturator nerve originates from the ventral rami of spinal nerves L2, L3, and L4. These roots combine to form a common trunk that then descends through the psoas muscle, over the pelvic brim, and into the lesser pelvis. Here it transverses through the obturator canal and enters the thigh through the obturator foramen before dividing into anterior and posterior branches. The anterior branches supply the adductor longus, gracilis, and adductor brevis muscles and supplies sensory fibers to the skin of the medial aspect of the midthigh. The posterior division innervates the obturator externus and supplies part of the adductor magnus and a sensory branch to the articular capsule, cruciate ligaments, and synovial membrane of the knee.[116] The adductor magnus and longus are also partially innervated by the sciatic and femoral nerves, thus obturator denervation may cause only a subtle weakness in this muscle group. The adductor brevis remains the only muscle solely supplied by the obturator nerve and, as such, is best suited for specific electromyography (EMG) diagnosis of obturator entrapment.[117]

Clinical Picture

Obturator entrapment, although reportedly not as common as other groin injuries, can also present as a deep ache near the adductor origin that is worsened with exercise and often subsides with rest. Pain may radiate down to the knee because of the innervation of the posterior obturator fibers.

On physical examination there may be a subtle weakness in the adductor muscles. The pectineus stretch may cause pain and is performed with the patient actively externally rotating and abducting the hip. Pain may also be reproduced with internal rotation of the hip against resistance. Both tests are intended to stretch the nerve and cause pain.[117]

Imaging

Plain radiographs are typically normal in obturator entrapment.

MRI may reveal atrophy, especially of the adductor brevis and longus, but is unable to detect any abnormality of the nerve in the thigh or tunnel.[118]

An electromyogram completed by an experienced neurologist (with special focus on the adductor brevis) can be helpful in detecting entrapment. EMG studies may find demyelination if the patient has had symptoms present for more than 2 weeks. If there is no indication of demyelination at initial testing and clinical suspicion remains high, a repeat test can be obtained at 4 to 6 weeks.[119]

Applying a local anesthetic block with lidocaine or bupivacaine to the obturator nerve at the obturator foramen under fluoroscopic guidance can provide further evidence of entrapment if there is significant relief of pain/reproduction of the adductor weakness after injection.[120] Once diagnosed, surgical treatment may be warranted.[116]

Treatment

In a study by Bradshaw and colleagues,[118] patients who failed conservative measures had surgery to release the entrapment of the obturator nerve. They concluded that conservative treatment has limited success and, if denervation is noted on EMG, surgery is the preferred treatment plan. Their results suggest that sports can be resumed in as little as 3 to 6 weeks.

Bradshaw and colleagues'[118] surgical technique was an open one but, in 2007, Rigaud and colleagues[121] reported a laparoscopic procedure that involved surgical neurolysis and incision of the obturator canal. These investigators stated that this minimally invasive technique afforded easier dissection.

SUMMARY

Obturator nerve entrapment is not as common as other hip and groin injuries in athletes. Pain may radiate from the groin down to the knee and weakness in the adductor muscles can be seen on physical examination. Imaging has a limited role, and an electromyogram should be obtained by an experienced neurologist for diagnosis. An anesthetic block with pain relief can also confirm the diagnosis. Conservative therapy has limited success and, if denervation is noted on EMG, surgery is the next option.

REFERENCES

1. Lovell G. The diagnosis of chronic groin pain in athletes: a review of 189 cases. Aust J Sci Med Sport 1995;27(3):76–9.
2. Westlin N. Groin pain in athletes from southern Sweden. Sports Med Arthrosc Rev 1997;5:280–4.
3. Koch RA, Jackson DW. Pubic symphysitis in runners. A report of two cases. Am J Sports Med 1981;9(1):62–3.
4. Fricker PA, Taunton JE, Ammann W. Osteitis pubis in athletes. Infection, inflammation or injury? Sports Med 1991;12(4):266–79.
5. DeLee JC, Farney WC. Incidence of injury in Texas high school football. Am J Sports Med 1992;20:575–80.
6. Werner J, Hägglund M, Waldén M, et al. UEFA injury study: a prospective study of hip and groin injuries in professional football over seven consecutive seasons. Br J Sports Med 2009;43(13):1036–40.
7. Anderson K, Strickland SM, Warren R. Hip and groin injuries in athletes. Am J Sports Med 2001;29(4):521–33.
8. Tyler TF, Nicholas SJ, Campbell RJ, et al. The association of hip strength and flexibility with the incidence of adductor muscle strains in professional ice hockey players. Am J Sports Med 2001;29(2):124–8.
9. Arnason A, Sigurdsson SB, Gudmundsson A, et al. Risk factors for injuries in football. Am J Sports Med 2004;32(Suppl 1):5S–16S.

10. Ekstrand J, Gillquist J. The avoidability of soccer injuries. Int J Sports Med 1983; 4:124–8.
11. Vingard E, Alfredsson L, Malchau H. Osteoarthrosis of the hip in women and its relationship to physical load from sports activities. Am J Sports Med 1998;26(1): 78–82.
12. Niemuth PE, Johnson RJ, Myers MJ, et al. Hip muscle weakness and overuse injuries in recreational runners. Clin J Sport Med 2005;15(1):14–21.
13. Ibrahim A, Murrell GA, Knapman PJ. Adductor strain and hip range of movement in male professional soccer players. J Orthop Surg (Hong Kong) 2007; 15(1):46–9.
14. Tyler TF, Nicholas SJ, Campbell RJ, et al. The effectiveness of a preseason exercise program to prevent adductor muscle strains in professional ice hockey players. Am J Sports Med 2002;30(5):680–3.
15. Megliola A, Eutropi F, Scorzelli A, et al. Ultrasound and magnetic resonance imaging in sports-related muscle injuries. Radiol Med 2006;111(6):836–45.
16. Robinson P, Barron DA, Parsons W, et al. Adductor-related groin pain in athletes: correlation of MR imaging with clinical findings. Skeletal Radiol 2004;33:451–7.
17. Fricker PA. Management of groin pain in athletes. Br J Sports Med 1997;31(2): 97–101.
18. Holmich P, Uhrskou P, Ulnits L, et al. Effectiveness of active physical training as treatment for long-standing adductor-related groin pain in athletes: randomised trial. Lancet 1999;353(9151):439–43.
19. Schilders E, Bismil Q, Robinson P, et al. Adductor-related groin pain in competitive athletes. Role of adductor enthesis, magnetic resonance imaging, and entheseal pubic cleft injections. J Bone Joint Surg Am 2007;89:2173–8.
20. Schilders E, Talbot JC, Robinson P, et al. Adductor-related groin pain in recreational athletes: role of the adductor enthesis, magnetic resonance imaging, and entheseal pubic cleft injections. J Bone Joint Surg Am 2009; 91(10):2455–60.
21. Atkinson HD, Johal P, Falworth MS, et al. Adductor tenotomy: its role in the management of sports-related chronic groin pain. Arch Orthop Trauma Surg 2010;130(8):965–70.
22. Das SK, Farooqi A. Osteoarthritis. Best Pract Res Clin Rheumatol 2008;22(4): 657–75.
23. Pereira D, Peleteiro B, Araújo J, et al. The effect of osteoarthritis definition on prevalence and incidence estimates: a systematic review. Osteoarthritis Cartilage 2011;19(11):1270–85.
24. Felson DT. The epidemiology of knee osteoarthritis: results from the Framingham Osteoarthritis Study. Semin Arthritis Rheum 1990;20(3 Suppl 1):42–50.
25. Marti B, Knobloch M, Tschopp A, et al. Is excessive running predictive of degenerative hip disease? Controlled study of former elite athletes. BMJ 1989; 299(6691):91–3.
26. Kujala UM, Kaprio J, Sarna S. Osteoarthritis of weight bearing joints of lower limbs in former elite male athletes. BMJ 1994;308(6923):231–4.
27. Vingard E, Alfredsson L, Goldie I, et al. Sports and osteoarthritis of the hip: an epidemiologic study. Am J Sports Med 1993;21(2):195–200.
28. Sarzi-Puttini P, Cimmino MA, Scarpa R, et al. Osteoarthritis: an overview of the disease and its treatment strategies. Semin Arthritis Rheum 2005;35(1 Suppl 1): 1–10.

29. Amin AR, Dave M, Attur M, et al. COX-2, NO, and cartilage damage and repair. Curr Rheumatol Rep 2000;2:447–53.
30. Moreland LW. Intra-articular hyaluronan (hyaluronic acid) and hylans for the treatment of osteoarthritis: mechanisms of action. Arthritis Res Ther 2003;5:54–67.
31. Altman R, Alarcón G, Appelrouth D, et al. The American College of Rheumatology criteria for the classification and reporting of osteoarthritis of the hip. Arthritis Rheum 1991;34:505–14.
32. Bierma-Zeinstra SM, Oster JD, Bernsen RM, et al. Joint space narrowing and relationship with symptoms and signs in adults consulting for hip pain in primary care. J Rheumatol 2002;29(8):1713–8.
33. Menashe L, Hirko K, Losina E, et al. The diagnostic performance of MRI in osteoarthritis: a systematic review and meta-analysis. Osteoarthritis Cartilage 2012;20(1):13–21.
34. Felson DT, Zhang Y, Anthony JM, et al. Weight loss reduces the risk of symptomatic knee osteoarthritis in women. The Framingham Study. Ann Intern Med 1992;116(7):535–9.
35. Hernández-Molina G, Reichenbach S, Zhang B, et al. Effect of therapeutic exercise for hip osteoarthritis pain: results of a meta-analysis. Arthritis Rheum 2008;59(9):1221–8.
36. Zhang W, Doherty M, Arden N, et al. EULAR evidence based recommendations for the management of hip osteoarthritis: report of a task force of the EULAR Standing Committee for International Clinical Studies Including Therapeutics (ESCISIT). Ann Rheum Dis 2005;64:669–81.
37. Sawitzke AD, Shi H, Finco MF, et al. Clinical efficacy and safety over two years use of glucosamine, chondroitin sulfate, their combination, celecoxib or placebo taken to treat osteoarthritis of the knee: a GAIT report. Ann Rheum Dis 2010;69:1459–64.
38. Wandel S, Jüni P, Tendal B, et al. Effects of glucosamine, chondroitin, or placebo in patients with osteoarthritis of hip or knee: network meta-analysis. BMJ 2010;341:c4675.
39. Towheed TE, Maxwell L, Anastassiades TP, et al. Glucosamine therapy for treating osteoarthritis. Cochrane Database Syst Rev 2005;2:CD002946.
40. Micu MC, Bogdan GD, Fodo D. Steroid injection for hip osteoarthritis: efficacy under ultrasound guidance. Rheumatology 2010;49:1490–4.
41. Lambert RG, Hutchings EJ, Grace MG, et al. Steroid injection for osteoarthritis of the hip: a randomized, double-blind, placebo-controlled trial. Arthritis Rheum 2007;56(7):2278–87.
42. Pozo MA, Balazs EA, Belmonte C. Reduction of sensory responses to passive movements of inflamed knee joints by hylan, a hyaluronan derivative. Exp Brain Res 1997;116:3–9.
43. Migliore A, Massafra U, Bizzi E, et al. Comparative, double-blind, controlled study of intra-articular hyaluronic acid (Hyalubrix) injections versus local anesthetic in osteoarthritis of the hip. Arthritis Res Ther 2009;11(6):R183.
44. Qvistgaard E, Christensen R, Torp-Pedersen S, et al. Intra-articular treatment of hip osteoarthritis: a randomized trial of hyaluronic acid, corticosteroid, and isotonic saline. Osteoarthritis Cartilage 2006;14:163–70.
45. Vissers MM, Bussmann JB, Verhaar JA, et al. Recovery of physical functioning after total hip arthroplasty: systematic review and meta-analysis of the literature. Phys Ther 2011;91(5):615–29.

46. McCarthy JC, Noble PC, Schuck MR, et al. The Otto E. Aufranc Award: the role of labral lesions to development of early degenerative hip disease. Clin Orthop 2001;393:25–37.
47. Narvani AA, Tsiridis E, Kendall S, et al. A preliminary report on prevalence of acetabular labrum tears in sports patients with groin pain. Knee Surg Sports Traumatol Arthrosc 2003;11:403–8.
48. Bharam S. Labral tears, extra-articular injuries, and hip arthroscopy in the athlete. Clin Sports Med 2006;25(2):279–92, ix.
49. Groh MM, Herrera J. A comprehensive review of hip labral tears. Curr Rev Musculoskelet Med 2009;2:105–17.
50. Freehill MT, Safran MR. The labrum of the hip: diagnosis and rationale for surgical correction. Clin Sports Med 2011;30(2):293–315.
51. Lewis CL, Sahrmann SA. Acetabular labral tears. Phys Ther 2006;86:110–21.
52. Smith TO, Hilton G, Toms AP, et al. The diagnostic accuracy of acetabular labral tears using magnetic resonance imaging and magnetic resonance arthrography: a meta-analysis. Eur Radiol 2011;21(4):863–74.
53. Newberg A, Newman J. Imaging the painful hip. Clin Orthop 2003;406:19–28.
54. Huffman GR, Safran M. Arthroscopic treatment of labral tears. Oper Tech Sports Med 2002;10:205–14.
55. Hunt D, Clohisy J, Prather H. Acetabular tears of the hip in women. Phys Med Rehabil Clin N Am 2007;18(3):497–520.
56. Burnett S, Della Rocca G, Prather H, et al. Clinical presentation of patients with tears of the acetabular labrum. J Bone Joint Surg Am 2006;88(7):1448–57.
57. Byrd JW. Clinical Hip arthroscopy in the athlete. N Am J Sports Phys Ther 2007;2(4):217–30.
58. Bharam S, Draovitch P, Fu FH. Return to competition in pro athletes with traumatic labral tears of the hip. Presented at the meeting of the American Orthopaedic Society for Sports Medicine. Orlando, June 23, 2002.
59. Ganz R, Parvizi J, Beck M, et al. Femoroacetabular impingement: a cause for osteoarthritis of the hip. Clin Orthop Relat Res 2003;417:112–20.
60. Lequesne M, Bellaïche L. Anterior femoroacetabular impingement: an update. Joint Bone Spine 2012;79(3):249–55.
61. Gerhardt MB, Romero AA, Silvers HJ, et al. The prevalence of radiographic hip abnormalities in elite soccer players. Am J Sports Med 2012;40(3):584–8.
62. Banerjee P, Mclean C. Femoroacetabular impingement: a review of diagnosis and management. Curr Rev Musculoskelet Med 2011;4:23–32.
63. Ejnisman L, Philippon M, Lertwanich P. Femoroacetabular impingement: the femoral side. Clin Sports Med 2011;30(2):369–77.
64. Leunig M, Casillas MM, Hamlet M, et al. Slipped capital femoral epiphysis: early mechanical damage to the acetabular cartilage by a prominent femoral metaphysis. Acta Orthop Scand 2000;71:370–5.
65. Eijer H, Podeszwa DA, Ganz R, et al. Evaluation and treatment of young adults with femoro-acetabular impingement secondary to Perthes' disease. Hip Int 2006;16:273–80.
66. Ayeni OR, Pruett A, Kelly BT. Arthroscopic management of pincer impingement. In: Kelly BT, Philipon MJ, editors. Arthroscopic techniques in the hip. Theorofare (NJ): SLACK; 2010. p. 69–88.
67. Seldes RM, Tan V, Hunt J, et al. Anatomy, histologic features and vascularity of the adult acetabular labrum. Clin Orthop Relat Res 2001;382:232–40.

68. Philipon MJ, Schenker ML. Arthroscopy for the treatment of femoroacetabular impingement in the athlete. Clin Sports Med 2006;25(2):299–308.
69. Maheshwari A, Malik A, Dorr L. Impingement of the native hip joint. J Bone Joint Surg Am 2007;89(11):2508–18.
70. Kaplan K, Shah M, Youm T. Femoroacetabular impingement: diagnosis and treatment. Bull NYU Hosp Jt Dis 2010;68(2):70–5.
71. Emara K, Samir W, Motasem el H. Conservative treatment for mild femoroacetabular impingement. J Orthop Surg (Hong Kong) 2011;19(1):41–5.
72. Palmer WE. Femoroacetabular impingement: caution is warranted in making imaging-based assumptions and diagnoses. Radiology 2010;257:4–7.
73. Austin AB, Souza RB, Meyer JL, et al. Identification of abnormal hip motion associated with acetabular labral pathology. J Orthop Sports Phys Ther 2008; 38(9):558–65.
74. Larson CM. Arthroscopic management of pincer-type impingement. Sports Med Arthrosc 2010;18(2):100–7.
75. Bathala EA, Bancroft LW, Peterson JJ, et al. Radiologic case study. Femoroacetabular impingement. Orthopedics 2007;30(12):986, 1061–4.
76. Kassarjian A, Brisson M, Palmer WE. Femoroacetabular impingement. Eur J Radiol 2007;63(1):29–35.
77. Notzli HP, Wyss TF, Stoecklin CH, et al. The contour of the femoral head-neck junction as a predictor for the risk of anterior impingement. J Bone Joint Surg Br 2002;84:556–60.
78. Kassarjian A. Hip MR arthrography and femoroacetabular impingement. Semin Musculoskelet Radiol 2006;10:208–19.
79. Byrd JW, Jones KS. Arthroscopic femoroplasty in the management of cam-type femoroacetabular impingement. Clin Orthop Relat Res 2009;467(3):739–46.
80. Matsuda DK, Carlisle JC, Arthurs SC, et al. Comparative systematic review of the open dislocation, mini-open, and arthroscopic surgeries for femoroacetabular impingement. Arthroscopy 2011;27(2):252–69.
81. Randelli F, Pierannunzii L, Banci L, et al. Heterotopic ossifications after arthroscopic management of femoroacetabular impingement: the role of NSAID prophylaxis. J Orthop Traumatol 2010;11(4):245–50.
82. Hawkins RD, Hulse MA, Wilkinson C, et al. The association football medical research programme: an audit of injuries in professional football. Br J Sports Med 2001;35:43–7.
83. Gilmore OJ. Gilmore's groin: ten years experience of groin disruption–a previously unsolved problem in sportsmen. Sports Med Soft Tissue Trauma 1991; 1(3):12–4.
84. Polglase AL, Frydman GM, Farmer KC. Inguinal surgery for debilitating chronic groin pain in athletes. Med J Aust 1991;155:674–7.
85. Litwin DE, Sneider EB, McEnaney PM, et al. Athletic pubalgia (sports hernia). Clin Sports Med 2011;30(2):417–34.
86. Ekberg O, Blomquist P, Olsson S. Positive contrast herniography in adult patients with obscure groin pain. Surgery 1981;89:532–5.
87. Caudill P, Nyland J, Smith C, et al. Sports hernias: a systematic literature review. Br J Sports Med 2008;42:954–64.
88. Zoga AC, Kavanagh EC, Omar IM, et al. Athletic pubalgia and the "sports hernia": MR imaging findings. Radiology 2008;247(3):797–807.
89. Unverzagt CA, Schuemann T, Mathisen J. Differential diagnosis of a sports hernia in a high-school athlete. J Orthop Sports Phys Ther 2008;38:63–70.
90. LeBlanc KE, LeBlanc KA. Groin pain in athletes. Hernia 2003;7:68–71.

91. Biedert RM, Warnke K, Meyer SR. Symphysis syndrome in athletes: surgical treatment for chronic lower abdominal, groin and adductor pain in athletes. Clin J Sport Med 2003;13:278–84.
92. Srinivasan A, Schuricht A. Long-term follow-up of laparoscopic preperitoneal hernia repair in professional athletes. J Laparoendosc Adv Surg Tech A 2002; 12:101–6.
93. Ingoldby CJ. Laparoscopic and conventional repair of groin disruption in sportsmen. Br J Surg 1997;84:213–5.
94. Malycha P, Lovell G. Inguinal surgery in athletes with chronic groin pain: "Sportsman's" hernia. Aust N Z J Surg 1992;62:123–5.
95. Kumar A, Doran J, Batt ME, et al. Results of inguinal canal repair in athletes with sports hernia. J R Coll Surg Edinb 2002;47:561–5.
96. Ahumada LA, Ashruf S, Espinosa-de-los-Monteros A, et al. Athletic pubalgia: definition and surgical treatment. Ann Plast Surg 2005;55:393–6.
97. Canonico S, Benevento R, Della Corte A, et al. Sutureless tension-free hernia repair with human fibrin glue (Tissucol) in soccer players with chronic inguinal pain: initial experience. Int J Sports Med 2007;28(10):873–6.
98. Middleton RG, Carlile RG. The spectrum of osteitis pubis. Compr Ther 1993; 19(3):99–102.
99. Vitanzo PC, McShane JM. Osteitis pubis: solving a perplexing problem. Phys Sportsmed 2001;29:33–48.
100. Beatty T. Osteitis pubis in athletes. Curr Sports Med Rep 2012;11(2):96–8.
101. Verrall GM, Henry L, Fazzalari NL, et al. Bone biopsy of the parasymphyseal pubic bone region in athletes with chronic groin injury demonstrates new woven bone formation consistent with a diagnosis of pubic bone stress injury. Am J Sports Med 2008;36:2425–31.
102. Mandelbaum B, Mora SA. Osteitis pubis. Oper Tech Sports Med 2005;13:62–7.
103. Hiti CJ, Stevens KJ, Jamati MK, et al. Athletic osteitis pubis. Sports Med 2011; 41:361–76.
104. Coventry MB, William MC. Osteitis pubis: observations based on a study of 45 patients. JAMA 1961;178:898–905.
105. O'Connell MJ, Powell T, McCaffrey NM, et al. Symphyseal cleft injection in the diagnosis and treatment of osteitis pubis in athletes. AJR Am J Roentgenol 2002;179:955–9.
106. Harris NH, Murray RO. Lesions of the symphysis in athletes. Br Med J 1974;4: 211–4.
107. Johnson R. Osteitis pubis. Curr Sports Med Rep 2003;2(2):98–102.
108. Verrall GM, Slavotinek JP, Fon GT. Incidence of pubic bone marrow oedema in Australian Rules football players: relation to groin pain. Br J Sports Med 2001; 35:28–33.
109. Jarosz BS. Individualized multi-modal management of osteitis pubis in an Australian Rules footballer. J Chiropr Med 2011;10(2):105–10.
110. Holt MA, Keene JS, Graf BK, et al. Treatment of osteitis pubis in athletes. Results of corticosteroid injections. Am J Sports Med 1995;23(5):601–6.
111. Radic R, Annear P. Use of pubic symphysis curettage for treatment-resistant osteitis pubis in athletes. Am J Sports Med 2008;36(1):122–8.
112. Mulhall KJ, McKenna J, Walsh A, et al. Osteitis pubis in professional soccer players: a report of outcome with symphyseal curettage in cases refractory to conservative management. Clin J Sport Med 2002;12:179–81.
113. Mehin R, Meek R, O'Brien P, et al. Surgery for osteitis pubis. Can J Surg 2006; 49(3):170–6.

114. Grace JN, Sim FH, Shives TC, et al. Wedge resection of the symphysis pubis for the treatment of osteitis pubis. J Bone Joint Surg Am 1989;71:358–64.
115. Williams PR, Thomas DP, Downes EM. Osteitis pubis and instability of the pubic symphysis. When nonoperative measures fail. Am J Sports Med 2000;28:350–5.
116. Tipton JS. Obturator neuropathy. Curr Rev Musculoskelet Med 2008;1:234–7.
117. Morelli V, Weaver V. Groin injuries and groin pain in athletes: part 1. Prim Care 2005;32:163–83.
118. Bradshaw C, McCrory P, Bell S, et al. Obturator neuropathy: a cause of chronic groin pain in athletes. Am J Sports Med 1997;25:402–8.
119. Gutmann L. Pearls and pitfalls in the use of electromyography and nerve conduction studies. Semin Neurol 2003;23(1):77–82.
120. Brukner P, Bradshaw C, McCrory P. Obturator neuropathy. Phys Sportsmed 1999;27(5):1–5.
121. Rigaud J, Labat JJ, Riant T, et al. Obturator nerve entrapment: diagnosis and laparoscopic treatment—technical case report. Neurosurgery 2007;61(l):E175.

Ligamentous Injuries of the Knee

Anterior Cruciate, Medial Collateral, Posterior Cruciate, and Posterolateral Corner Injuries

Vincent Morelli, MD*, Crystal Bright, MD, Ashley Fields, MD, MPH

KEYWORDS

- Athletic injuries of the knee • Anterior cruciate ligament injuries
- Posterior cruciate ligament injuries • Medial collateral ligament injuries
- Posterolateral corner injuries

KEY POINTS

- Best evidence to date validates that conservative management of rupture of the anterior cruciate ligament is a reasonable strategy.
- Current data seem to advocate nonoperative management of posterior cruciate ligament injuries as well.
- All isolated medial collateral ligament injuries, regardless of grade, are usually treated with a brief period of immobilization and symptomatic management.
- Despite surgical literature often advocating surgical treatment of posterolateral corner injuries, there have been no randomized trials substantiating that these injuries are best treated surgically.

ANTERIOR CRUCIATE LIGAMENT

Epidemiology

The annual incidence of anterior cruciate ligament (ACL) injuries in the United States is unknown, but an estimated 100,000 ACL repairs are performed each year.[1] Women are more likely than men to rupture their ACL, with one recent study[2] showing a relative risk of 3.96 in women in comparison with men. There are both extrinsic and intrinsic factors that may contribute to ACL injuries. Examples of extrinsic factors include the type of playing field, the type of shoe and surface,[3,4] weather such as extreme cold[5] or rain,[6] a higher level of competition, and an aggressive playing style. Examples of intrinsic factors include the body size and limb girth,[7] hamstring weakness or quadriceps dominance,[8] leg dominance,[9] Q angle,[10,11] and ligamentous laxity.[12]

Department of Family and Community Medicine, Meharry Medical College, 1005 Dr D. B. Todd Boulevard, Nashville, TN 37208, USA
* Corresponding author.
E-mail address: morellivincent@yahoo.com

Prim Care Clin Office Pract 40 (2013) 335–356
http://dx.doi.org/10.1016/j.pop.2013.02.004 primarycare.theclinics.com
0095-4543/13/$ – see front matter

Mechanism of Injury

ACL injuries can be caused by either contact or noncontact mechanisms, with the majority (70%–84%) being caused by noncontact mechanisms involving deceleration combined with pivoting/changing direction or landing in near extension after a jump. Contact mechanisms of injury usually involve a strong anterior translational force applied to a fixed lower leg.[10,13]

Physical Evaluation

A proper physical examination has been shown to be accurate in assessing ACL ruptures, with sensitivity of 82% and specificity of 94%.[14]

Physical examination tests include the Lachman test, which is most useful in the acute setting (sensitivity 85%–93%, specificity 94%–99%), the anterior drawer test (sensitivity 92%, specificity 91% in chronic injuries but less sensitive in acute injuries), and the pivot shift test (sensitivity of 24%–48%, specificity of 98%).[14,15]

In addition to pain, swelling/hemarthrosis, and the aforementioned physical findings, 17% to 65% of patients with ACL injuries also complain of symptoms of "giving way."[16]

Radiologic Evaluation

Plain films are usually normal in isolated ACL injuries, but a Segond fracture (small avulsion fracture of the lateral tibial eminence) is highly suggestive of ACL rupture and should lead to follow-up magnetic resonance imaging (MRI).

MRI is an accurate method of diagnosing ACL tears, with sensitivity of 86% to 95.9% and specificity of 91% to 95%. However, if the MRI is negative and the clinician still has a high suspicion of an ACL tear, arthroscopy will lead to a definitive diagnosis.[17–19]

Treatment

Operative versus nonoperative treatment

Some controversy exists over whether to treat patients with ruptured ACLs conservatively or operatively. Early studies examining this question were limited by significant methodological shortcomings, and a 2009 Cochrane review[20] found only 2 trials (both of low quality), carried out in the 1980s, that addressed the issue. The Cochrane review concluded that although the conservatively treated knees tended to return to sport sooner, and although surgically treated knees were objectively more stable, there was no significant difference in patient satisfaction or return to previous level of athletic activity. The investigators concluded that as of 2009, there was "insufficient evidence from randomized trials to inform current practice. However, there was some evidence that conservative treatment of acute ACL injuries result[ed] in a satisfactory outcome[s]."

As ACL surgical repair techniques improved and became more standardized in the 1990s, more accurate comparisons between operative and nonoperative treatments became possible.[16] The most recent and well-conducted randomized trial, published in 2010 in the *New England Journal of Medicine*,[21] compared early ACL reconstruction with conservative management (with optional delayed ACL reconstruction) in 121 active adults. The study showed that although 39% of conservatively managed patients eventually chose to have ACL reconstruction, 61% were satisfied with conservative therapy. No differences in symptoms or sports participation were found between groups at 2 years after injury.

In conclusion, the best evidence to date validates that conservative management of ACL ruptures is a reasonable strategy and that up to 61% of patients may be satisfied with such treatment. Because factors such as hamstring strength, quadriceps strength and flexibility, and other individual biomechanical factors[18,22] may influence outcomes, future research should be focused on delineating which subset of patients will do well with conservative management and which subsets will require surgical intervention, thus ensuring that the best intervention is promptly instituted so that the athlete can return to sport as soon as possible.

Issues in Operative Treatment

Choice of autograft used for ACL injuries

The 2 most commonly used tendon autografts (tendons harvested from the patient him/herself) in ACL reconstruction are hamstring and patellar tendon autografts. In 2011, 2 meta-analyses[23,24] examined whether one autograft was better than the other, and demonstrated that patellar tendon autografts showed superior objective stability but were also fraught with more postoperative knee pain. Hamstring autografts, on the other hand, allowed faster recovery and less postoperative pain. Functional outcomes, patient-rated assessment, and rerupture rates did not differ between the 2 autografts.

Autograft versus allograft (cadaver-harvested tendon)

Some surgeons prefer the use of cadaver allografts in ACL repair because of shorter operative times (no time spent harvesting autografts) and less postoperative knee pain (especially when patellar tendon autografts are used). However, allografts have also been shown to incorporate more slowly,[25] possibly requiring as long as 3 years to gain full strength.

The data assessing which grafts provide better clinical results are just beginning to be clarified. The latest (2008), largest (534 patients), and most stringently performed meta-analysis of allograft versus autograft concluded that whereas functional outcomes and return to previous level of athletic activity were similar between groups, patients treated with allograft had a 5 times higher rerupture rate. The investigators did note, however, that no difference in rerupture was observed if only fresh frozen allografts were used (ie, only those allografts sterilized by radiation and treated with acetone drying had an increased risk of rerupture). Subsequent studies[26,27] have demonstrated similarly good functional outcomes but do not report failure or rerupture rates.

Expected rate of ACL rerupture and revision after surgery

The true rate of ACL rerupture after ACL repair is difficult to ascertain because some patients will not seek medical attention for reinjury. However, the most recent and largest study on ACL rerupture and subsequent revision published in 2012[28] followed 12,193 patients with primary ACL repair for 5 years and demonstrated a rerupture with revision rate of 4.1%. The causes of graft failure were new trauma (38%), unknown cause (24%), and poor surgical technique (20%). This study and others[29] have noted that the main risk factor for rerupture was age at the time of primary repair, with patients younger than 20 years being significantly more prone to rerupture.

It should also be noted that early studies have shown double-bundle repairs to have a significantly lower rate of rerupture[30,31] than single-bundle repairs.

Rehabilitation for the operated ACLs

Rehabilitation, including range-of-motion exercises and strengthening, should start preoperatively to ensure the best possible postoperative results. Postoperative rehabilitation should consist of early partial weight bearing, range-of-motion exercises, strengthening the quadriceps, and stretching the hamstrings. In the second rehabilitation phase (~6 weeks postoperatively), goals of therapy should include knee flexion to 120°, further strengthening of the hamstrings and quadriceps, and full weight bearing. Finally (~6–12 weeks postoperatively), patients should achieve full range of motion and strength, and return to jogging and running. At 3 to 6 months postoperatively, patients are usually allowed to begin sport-specific drills and restricted training. At 6 months, with full strength and range of motion and with the surgeon's approval, patients are often allowed to return to sport.

However, it must be remembered that animal studies have demonstrated that at 1 year postoperatively, the load-bearing capacity of autografts reaches only 31% to 47% of normal, and graft stiffness reaches only 35% to 73% of normal.[32–34] The same animal studies demonstrate that histologic remodeling with graft resorption and fibroblast infiltration continues for at least 1 year, and one human case study suggests that remodeling may continue for up to 18 months postoperatively.[35] Together these data attest that the sports medicine physician must keep in mind that although athletes are generally anxious to begin retraining and are usually allowed to return to noncontact sport-specific activities by 6 months, grafts are still undergoing histologic remodeling and have not yet reached optimal tensile strength.

Expected return to high-level competition following operative treatment

A 2011 review of 48 studies and 5770 participants in the *British Journal of Sports Medicine*[36] found that 63% of operated athletes were able to return to their preinjury level of competition. Investigators suggested that psychological factors might have played a role in the relatively low rate of return to high-level competition.

Issues in Nonoperative Treatment

Rehabilitation for the nonoperated ACL injury

Rehabilitation principles for the nonoperated ACL are similar to those already mentioned for operated ACL injuries, and include quadriceps strengthening and hamstring stretching. There are no clear data dictating the optimal length of rehabilitation.[37]

Expected return to high-level competition with nonoperative management

As already noted, best data indicate that 61% of patients may be expected to have satisfactory results after conservative treatment, with 39% returning to previous levels of activity.[21]

The use of bracing in nonoperatively treated patients

The use of knee bracing in ACL-deficient patients remains controversial. At present there is no evidence supporting functional bracing as a means to improve knee stability, prevent reinjury, or prevent posttraumatic osteoarthritis. However, functional knee bracing does provide some athletes with conservatively treated ACL-deficient knees with subjective reassurance.[18,37,38]

Long-Term Follow-Up of the ACL-Deficient Knee

Osteoarthritis

Four long-term studies[39–42] have examined the emergence of osteoarthritis (OA) in ACL-deficient knees. The most recent study (2008)[39] compared surgically treated knees with those treated conservatively and found a 55% prevalence of OA in knees treated surgically, whereas only 39% of those treated conservatively had OA at an 11-year follow-up. In 2004, Lohmander and colleagues[42] again demonstrated a slight increase in OA in patients with operatively treated ACLs at a 12-year follow-up, whereas Fink and colleagues[41] earlier had found no difference in the prevalence of OA between operative and nonoperative treatments. Other long-term studies[43] comparing the incidence of OA in surgically versus conservatively treated patients are of poor quality and offer little additional information.

Neuman and colleagues[40] followed 100 conservatively treated patients (60 with meniscal tears and 40 without meniscal tears) for 15 years, and found that those with meniscal tears had a 46% prevalence of OA whereas those without meniscal tears had no OA.

Meniscal tears

In the aforementioned study, Neuman and colleagues[40] found that of the conservatively treated patients without meniscal injury at presentation, 39% eventually did tear their meniscus, necessitating surgical intervention during the 15-year follow-up.

The latest study by Frobell and colleagues[21] confirms these findings and notes that in their series (with only a 2-year follow-up), 32% of ACL ruptures without meniscal injury at presentation would eventually experience a tear in the meniscus necessitating surgery. Other studies in the nonathletic population have reported a much lower incidence of subsequent meniscal injury/surgery in conservatively treated patients.[44]

In surgically treated ACLs, the incidence of meniscal tears has a lower incidence. Subsequent meniscal tears in repaired ACLs has been noted to range from 3.4%[45] to 8.9%[46] to as high as 26%[28] during long-term (4–10 years) follow-up.

It must be remembered that various individual factors such as severity of injury at presentation, degree of laxity, obesity, participation in high-risk pivoting sports, and concomitant injury must be considered when looking into the best treatment for ACL injuries, as such factors play a role in the development of long-term OA.[41] It also should be kept in mind that the greatest risk factors for developing long-term OA in ACL-deficient knees is the presence of meniscal or chondral damage,[47,48] thus it is now common knowledge among surgeons that preserving as much of the meniscus as possible is of the utmost importance.

In conclusion, the best data to date indicate that surgical treatment of the ACL-deficient knee can be expected to lead to fewer subsequent meniscal tears (3.4%–8.9%) but increased long-term OA (~55%), whereas conservative treatment can be expected to lead to somewhat less OA (~39%) but to increased meniscal tears (32%–39%), noting of course that individual risk factors, concomitant injury, patient preferences, level of activity, and expected outcomes must be taken into consideration when deciding on the best treatment option.

Future Trends

Future trends and areas of research with ACL reconstruction include the use of: (1) extracorporeal shock-wave therapy; (2) platelet-rich plasma (PRP) products; (3) graft alternatives; and (4) stem cells.

Vetrano and colleagues[49] recently demonstrated that extracorporeal shock-wave therapy applied to human tenocytes in vitro promoted cell growth and collagen synthesis. Theoretically, such therapy could hasten healing in patients undergoing ACL repair with autograft, allograft, or scaffolds. However, no such in vivo studies have yet been conducted.

Ongoing research is also examining the use of PRP products to improve graft remodeling and healing in ACL reconstruction. Although an early radiographic trial seemed to show faster healing on MRI,[50] clinical studies have yet to show any significant benefit from the use of PRP.[51,52]

A full discussion of allografts, synthetic grafts or scaffolds is beyond the scope of this article, but although research in early animal studies is promising,[53–55] definitive clinical studies have yet to be performed.

Finally, early animal studies exploring the use of stem cells in ACL reconstruction seem to show positive results[56,57]; however, again clinical usefulness has yet to be established. Though not yet practicable, obviously the use of stem cells in tissue regeneration is an exciting area of future research.

Ongoing research in each of these areas offers an exciting chance to avail patients with new and better treatment options.

POSTERIOR CRUCIATE LIGAMENT

Epidemiology

Because many isolated posterior cruciate ligament (PCL) injuries go unrecognized or unreported, the exact incidence of these injuries is unknown. Studies have reported a wide range of such insults, from fewer than 1% of all injuries in one sports medicine clinic over a 10-year period[58] to 44% of knee injuries presenting with acute knee hemarthrosis in the hospital setting.[59]

The literature reports PCL tears to make up 4% of all knee injuries in college soccer, 2% in college basketball,[60] 3% in professional football,[61] and 4.8% in college wrestling.[62]

Anatomy and Function

The PCL is the main restraint to posterior tibial translation,[63] and secondarily serves to prevent external tibial rotation and hyperextension.[64]

The ligament originates from the intercondylar area of medial femoral condyle and inserts on the posterior aspect of the tibial plateau.[65,66] It has a narrow midsection and is slightly broader at its bony attachments.[67]

Although the precise anatomy of the ligament is not presented consistently in the literature,[68] it is generally considered to be made up of 2 bundles, the anterolateral and posteromedial. The anterolateral bundle is taut during knee flexion while the posteromedial remains lax. During knee extension the reverse is true, with the posteromedial bundle tightening and the anterolateral bundle relaxing.[69] This functional difference has led most surgeons to selectively concentrate on reconstructing the anteromedial bundle when surgery is indicated.

It should also be noted that the PCL lies in close proximity to the structures of the posterolateral corner (PLC) (see the section on PLC injuries), which act collectively as a secondary stabilizer of posterior tibial translation[70] This proximity and similarity in function accounts for the fact that that roughly 60% of significant PCL injuries are associated with PLC disruption.[71,72] Such concomitant injuries must be sought if proper management is to be afforded.

Mechanism of Injury and Classification

PCL injuries are caused by posteriorly directed blows to the proximal tibia, by forced hyperflexion or by hyperextension.[73] Forced hyperflexion is thought to be the most common mechanism for an isolated PCL tear,[74] whereas posteriorly directed blows to the proximal tibia, caused by either athletic or vehicular trauma, commonly result in "PCL combination" injuries (PCL plus concomitant injury).

In the setting of such trauma, up to 90% of PCL tears present as such concomitant injuries, 60% of which are PLC disruptions.[64,75]

Injuries can be classified as grades I, II, or III. Grade I injuries are mild and described as microscopic tears. Grade II injuries are moderate injuries with partial ligament tears, and grade III injuries are complete ligament ruptures. Another classification system grades injuries by the degree of posterior translation, with grade I injuries having a posterior translation from 0 to 5 mm, grade II injuries from 6 to 10 mm posterior translation, and grade III injuries with a posterior translation greater than 10 mm.[76]

Clinical Picture

Signs and symptoms

Patients with acute PCL injuries usually do not feel the typical "pop" felt with ACL tears, and may not even recall the exact mechanism of injury. Patients may complain of posterior knee pain, pain on kneeling, or mild stiffness caused by the moderate hemarthrosis.[63] However, many patients often complain only that the knee "just doesn't feel right."[77] In the chronic setting patients usually will not complain of instability unless other injuries are also present. However, they may complain of "difficulty" walking up or down inclines, pain with deceleration or walking down stairs, or anterior knee pain.[63,75]

Physical examination

In both the acute and chronic setting the physical examination is 96% accurate for diagnosing PCL injuries, with the best single test being the posterior draw test, with sensitivity of 90% and specificity of 99%.[78] To perform this test, the supine patient's knee is flexed 90° and, with the examiner's thumbs on the medial and lateral joint line, a posterior force is applied and the amount of poster translation assessed.[76]

The dial test (tibial external rotation test; see the section on PLC injuries) is performed by applying external rotational forces to the supine patient's flexed leg at both 30° and 90°. If the examiner is able to "dial" the injured leg 10° more than the unaffected side, the possibility of a PCL injury exists.[76] When the examiner is able to "dial" the patient's affected leg at 30° but not at 90°, the patient has an isolated PCL injury. If the increased angular excursion is found at both 30° and 90°, a combined PCL/PLC injury is likely.

Other commonly used tests include the posterior sag test and the quadriceps test.[79]

As already stated, in the setting of acute trauma concomitant injuries, especially PLC disruptions,[64,75] are common, and should be sought and diagnosed if proper management is to be afforded.

Radiographic imaging

MRI is a valuable tool for evaluating PCL injury, and has been shown to have sensitivity of 100% and specificity of 98%.[80] However, chronic grade I and grade II injuries are often missed on MRI and require a high index of suspicion to diagnose.[81] Normally an intact PCL has a broad band of low T1-/T2-weighted signals, whereas the injured PCL will show variations in the signal near the suspected PCL injury.[82]

Treatment

There is no universally agreed treatment for PCL injuries. Instead, care is usually based on the acute/chronic injury periodicity, the degree of the disruption (grade I, II, III), the patient's symptoms and complaints, and/or the patient's activity level or occupation.[83]

Nonoperative treatment

Grade I and grade II isolated PCL injuries are usually treated conservatively, with good results, and most patients are able to return to their previous level of activity.[77]

The same nonoperative approach is usually undertaken with grade III injuries as well, with physical therapy including quadriceps strengthening, stretching, and activity modification begun soon after injury.[83] If patients with grade III injury are unresponsive to therapy or develop significant pain or instability, PCL reconstruction may be considered.[68]

In a 1999 study,[77] 133 patients with ruptured PCLs (grade III tears) were treated conservatively and followed for an average of 5.4 years. At the study's conclusion the investigators noted that 50% of patients returned to their previous level of athletic participation, 32% returned to their sport at a lower level, and 17% had switched to a different sporting activity (it was not noted why the patients switched). Of interest, the degree of objective laxity was not predictive of which knees would fare subjectively better or worse. Nor could the data predict which patients would eventually develop long-term arthritis or which would be unable to return to sport at a high level. The investigators concluded that their research did not support operative intervention for grade III PCL injuries.

The 2 latest studies[84,85] examining conservatively treated PCL injuries were both published in 2007 and substantiated the earlier findings. The first followed 215 PCL patients for 7.8 years, and the second followed 57 PCL patients for 6.8 years. Both studies demonstrated that outcomes and return to sport were independent of objective PCL laxity. No factors could be identified that were able to predict which knees would eventually fare poorly or require surgery.

In addition to the best clinical data seeming to advocate nonoperative management, when discussing treatment options the physician should inform patients that MRI studies have demonstrated spontaneous "healing" of complete PCL ruptures in 66% to 88% of patients after 3 to 12 months,[86–89] with the caveat that those injuries exhibiting greater laxity or concomitant injury are less likely to show MRI healing. This high percentage of PCL "healing" has been demonstrated on MRI but has not, to the best of the authors' knowledge, been confirmed by arthroscopic studies.

Operative treatment

Although there are no clear indications for surgical intervention in PCL injuries, combined injuries involving the PLC, ACL, or avulsion fractures generally require surgical repair.[90,91]

In cases of isolated grade III PCL injury, proponents of operative treatment have argued that more degenerative changes[90,92] and more bothersome symptoms can occur over the long term with conservative treatment.[93,94] However, as stated earlier, the most reliable data to date[93,94] support at least a trial of conservative treatment in all isolated PCL injuries regardless of the laxity or degree of tear.

In conclusion, the preponderance of evidence indicates that all isolated PCL tears should be given an initial trial of conservative management for several months before considering surgical reconstruction. The decision to undergo surgery for isolated PCL injuries should be made only after a trial of conservative treatment, after assessing individual patients' complaints and expectations, and after considering the skill of the involved surgeon.[95] In patients with PCL injuries occurring together with other concomitant injuries, surgical reconstruction is a more reasonable consideration.

MEDIAL COLLATERAL LIGAMENT

The reported incidence of medial collateral ligament (MCL) injuries is 24 per 100,000 athletes per year in the United States.[96] The figure for athletes participating in collegiate (NCAA) athletics is higher, at 2.1 injuries per 1000 athletes per year.[97] However, this incidence is likely a conservative estimate[98] because many mild strains go unreported. Most MCL tears are isolated injuries, occurring mainly in the young athletic population and involving males twice as frequently as females.

Anatomy and Mechanics

Three main anatomic structures constitute the MCL complex: the superficial MCL, extending from the femoral condyle to its 2 distal attachments on the medial tibia; the deep MCL, lying just below the superficial ligament; and the posterior oblique ligament, which arises as a fibrous extension of the distal semimembranosus tendon and courses posteriorly, inserting and reinforcing the posteromedial portion of the joint capsule (**Fig. 1**).

The superficial ligament is the primary restraint to valgus laxity of the knee,[99] and research suggests that when surgical repair of the injured ligament is undertaken, attempts should be made to repair both distal tibial insertions to restore anatomic and functional integrity.[100] The posterior oblique ligament functions to stabilize against rotational and valgus forces, especially in the terminal degrees of extension (especially at 0° of flexion, a fact that aids in testing for compromise of the ligament in the physical examination), and the deep ligament functions as a secondary stabilizer against valgus stress.[101,102]

Physical Examination

Direct palpation of the superficial MCL and the area of the posterior oblique ligament is easily accomplished on physical examination.

In addition, valgus stress applied at both 0° and 30° of flexion will help the clinician detect ligament compromise. A knee that exhibits joint space opening at 30° but not at 0° likely has a torn superficial and deep MCL but an intact posterior oblique ligament. If the knee exhibits opening a both 0° and 30°, all 3 parts of the ligament complex are likely torn.[102] Comparison with the uninjured knee is, of course, necessary. In the American Medical Association classification, an injury is defined by the amount of joint

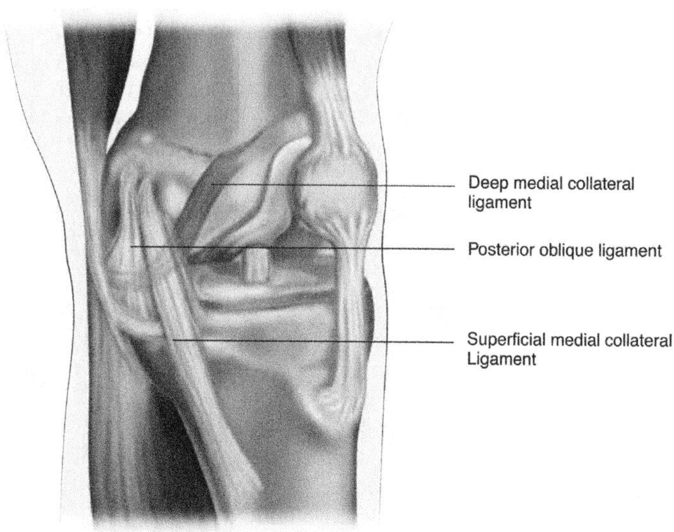

Fig. 1. The 3 main anatomic structures composing the medial collateral ligament complex. The superficial medial collateral ligament extends from the femoral condoyle to its 2 distal attachments on the medial tibia. The deep medial collateral ligament lies just below the superficial ligament. The posterior oblique ligament, which arises as a fibrous extension of the distal semimembranosus tendon and courses posteriorly, inserts and reinforces the posteromedial portion of the joint capsule.

opening with valgus stress: grade I, less than 5 mm of medial joint line opening; grade II, 5 to 10 mm of medial joint line opening; and grade III, greater than 10 mm of medial joint line opening (similar to third-degree injury with no end point).[103]

Fetto and Marshall[104] defined their grade I injuries as those without valgus laxity in both 0° and 30° of flexion, grade II injuries as those with valgus laxity in 30° of flexion but stable in 0° of flexion, and grade III as those with valgus laxity in both 0° and 30° of flexion. Of note, these investigators emphasized the importance of performing the test in 0° of flexion.

The dial test (anteromedial drawer test) is performed with the patient's knee flexed to 90° while the examiner externally rotates the foot, putting external rotatory forces on the medial knee structures. A complete injury to the medial structures (including the posterior oblique ligament) will cause increased external rotation in comparison with the unaffected knee.[105]

Radiographic Studies

Studies have noted MRI to have sensitivity of 56% to 94% and specificity of 82% to 100% in detecting MCL injuries.[106–108] MRI is less useful in addressing the deep MCL or the posterior oblique ligament, and has limited utility in grading the injuries.

Important from a prognostic viewpoint, Miller and colleagues[109] noted a 45% incidence of bone bruising with MCL injuries (half of which occurred with concomitant ACL injuries). Such bruising may delay the usual healing process, requiring up to 4 months to heal.

Treatment

All isolated MCL injuries, regardless of grade, are usually treated with a brief period of immobilization and symptomatic management.

Isolated grade I and grade II MCL injuries

These injuries are universally treated conservatively, with early mobilization and range-of-motion stretching and strengthening, followed by graduated return to sport. Athletes with grade I injuries can usually be allowed to return to play after 10 days and those with grade II injuries by 20 to 30 days.[110,111] In one study, 74% of patients with grade I and grade II injuries returned to preinjury levels of activity by 3 months.[112] Early mobilization and rehabilitation has been well supported both by histologic studies of transected animal MCLs[113,114] and by human clinical trials.[115,116] Ultrasound as adjunctive therapy has also shown to be of benefit in histologic animal studies.[117,118]

Isolated grade III MCL injuries

Despite early controversy regarding the proper treatment of these lesions, several well-designed studies have now confirmed that nonoperative treatment is equally as efficacious as surgical repair.[119,120]

However, surgical intervention is sometimes still undertaken for certain grade III injuries. For example, when the MCL is torn from its tibial insertion with a bony avulsion or if the tibial attachment is torn and becomes displaced outside the pes anserinus tendons, they would be unable to reattach without intervention.[121]

Other surgeons may also occasionally decide on operative repair if the knee exhibits laxity at both 30° and 0° of flexion on initial examination[122] or "if valgus instability remains after an appropriate rehabilitation period."[123] However, this more subjective approach is based on older, small studies and not on high-quality trials.[124]

Rehabilitation of grade III MCL injury, as with grades I and II, consists of pain control, immediate or early mobilization and knee range-of-motion exercises,[125] early weight bearing, and progressive strengthening. Ultrasound has a theoretical benefit based on animal studies. In addition, in grade III injuries the use of a hinged knee brace for 6 weeks to protect against valgus stress is also a consideration. Although data are sparse, athletes with these injuries can be expected to regain 80% of strength by 13 weeks and return to sport within 1 year.

In all MCL injuries, it is important to remember that although clinical healing will occur after some weeks, microscopic remodeling and continued ligament strengthening continues for up to 1 year. This microscopic healing process has been shown to be enhanced by early mobilization.[126]

Combined acute MCL and ACL injuries

Grade I or grade II MCL injuries occurring in conjunction with acute ACL ruptures are treated nonoperatively, often followed by ACL reconstruction once knee stability (MCL healing) has been restored.

Some controversy exists over how best to treat grade III MCL tears that occur alongside ACL ruptures. Early case series[127,128] in which patients had their MCLs surgically repaired at the time of ACL reconstruction reported good results. Other early studies[129] noted that nonoperative treatment of combined ACL/MCL ruptures was successful, with 71% reporting good to excellent results at an average of 3 years, and 70% being able to return to previous levels of athletic activity.

The latest (and only) prospective randomized trial of 47 patients (half of whom were athletes) with these combined injuries found no difference in subjective or objective outcomes, at an average of 27 months, whether the grade III MCL tear was treated conservatively or surgically.[130] To date, the highest-quality data point to a conservative approach in patients with grade III MCL tears in the face of ACL rupture. Whether or not to repair the ACL in these patients is discussed elsewhere in this article.

The rehabilitation of these combined ACL/grade III MCL injuries is initially focused on giving the MCL time to heal and restoring valgus stability. The knee is initially braced in extension to guard against valgus stress for 1 to 2 weeks, after which the brace is adjusted to allow up to 90° of flexion for an additional 4 weeks. Patients are started on immediate range-of-motion and strengthening protocols.[131] This conservative management is then followed by a decision as to whether subsequent ACL reconstruction is warranted.

Chronic MCL injuries

Chronic valgus instability can occur as a result of distal MCL avulsion, entrapment of the MCL into the joint or over the insertion of the pes anserinus, or failed ACL/PCL reconstructions. Resulting instability may affect activities of daily living or limit athletic participation, and require surgical correction. In the chronic condition, MCL edges are often difficult to find or are scarred, necessitating allograft or autograft repair. Short-term outcome studies have shown good results,[132] with a common complication of knee stiffness.

Prophylactic MCL bracing

Many studies have investigated whether prophylactic knee bracing will prevent MCL injuries. Although 2 early epidemiologic studies noted trends of decreased MCL injuries in braced football players,[133,134] more recent reviews have shown no clear benefit.[135] In addition, bracing has been shown to dampen athletic performance by restricting motion and negatively affecting speed and agility.

POSTEROLATERAL CORNER INJURIES

The PLC complex is composed of the arcuate ligament, the lateral collateral ligament (LCL), the popliteus tendon complex, the popliteofibular ligament, the lateral gastrocnemius tendon, and the posterolateral capsule (**Fig. 2**).

The PLC, taken as a whole, functions as a restraint to varus stress, external tibial rotation, and posterior translation of the tibia. The LCL is the primary restraint to varus stress, while the complex together functions as the main stabilizer of external tibial rotation and posterior translation of the tibia.

Isolated injuries to the PLC are uncommon,[136] but have been documented in 63% of those with posterior cruciate ruptures,[137] in 87% of those with multiple ligamentous injuries,[138] and in up to 68% of those with tibial plateau fractures.[139] Unless clinicians maintain a high index of suspicion these injuries are often missed, one study finding that 72% were missed on initial presentation, with a mean delay to diagnosis of 30 months.[140]

The problems of missing a significant PLC injury may be twofold. First, isolated grade III injuries (see later discussion) are said to have a high incidence of late-onset osteoarthritis if left untreated. The second problem concerns those injuries occurring concomitantly with anterior or posterior cruciate injuries. Because the PLC structures are so important in providing dynamic and static stability, when these injuries are unrecognized and untreated they are associated with ACL and PCL graft failure in cases where only the cruciate is repaired.[141,142]

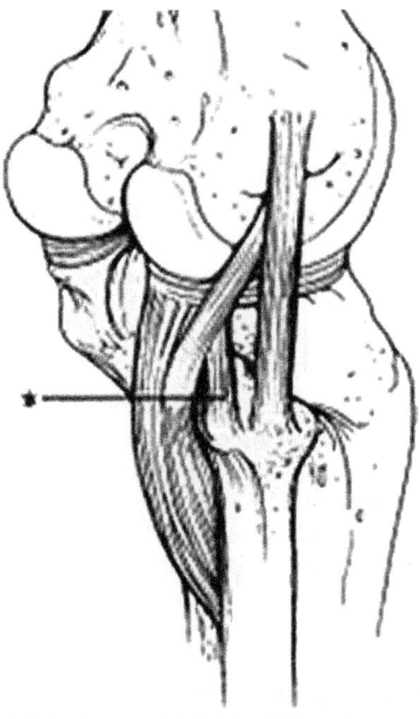

Fig. 2. Arising from the posterior part of the fibula (*asterisk*), the popliteofibular ligament joins the popliteus tendon just superior to the musculotendinous junction. (*From* Veltri DM, Warren RF. Anatomy, biomechanics, and physical findings in posterolateral knee instability. Clin Sports Med 1994;13(3):602; with permission.)

Physical Examination

Clinical evaluation of these injuries includes assessment of both rotational and varus laxity at various degrees of flexion. As described in the section on PCL, the dial test is commonly used to examine rotational laxity. Normal knees (in both males and females) exhibit up to a 5.5° difference in rotational laxity between knees. The dial test is considered positive for posterolateral injury if the affected knee exhibits more than 10° of laxity in comparison with the uninjured knee. A positive test at 30° but not 90° indicates an isolated injury to the PLC. If the test is positive at both 30° and 90°, a combined PLC/PCL injury is likely.[143,144]

Varus laxity is generally tested at 0° and at 30° of flexion. The amount of laxity has been defined by Hughston and colleagues[145] in the following manner: grade I injuries are sprains with little or no varus instability (0–5 mm), grade II injuries exhibit minimal abnormal laxity of 6 to 10 mm (2+), and grade III injuries are complete disruptions with laxity greater than 10 mm (3+).

Imaging

Standard radiographs can suggest PLC injury with findings such as widening of the lateral joint space (especially on stress radiographs), fibular head/tip avulsion fractures, Gerdy tubercle (lateral insertion of the iliotibial band) fractures in iliotibial band injuries, tibial plateau fractures, or Segond fractures (lateral tibial plateau avulsion fracture).

MRI is helpful in identifying concomitant injuries (eg, ACL, PCL, meniscus) and can help identify injured structures in the PLC; however, in some cases it has been noted to have limited sensitivity.[146,147] If performed within the first 12 weeks after injury, MRI has been found to have sensitivity of up to 93%, but if imaging is delayed beyond this, only 26% of injuries may be identified.[140]

Although there are no exact MRI criteria to diagnose clinically relevant posterolateral instability (or grade III injuries for that matter), visualization of complete tears involving 2 or more structures of the PLC on MRI are suggestive of PLC instability, especially in the presence of concomitant tears of the cruciate ligament.

Therefore, despite the usefulness of radiographic findings, surgeons usually rely on physical examination as the ultimate determinant of the need for surgical intervention.[148]

Treatment

Isolated grade I and II injuries

These injuries are generally treated conservatively, with good results.[136,149]

Isolated grade III injuries

Despite the surgical literature often advocating surgical treatment of these injuries,[136,150] there have been no randomized trials substantiating that these injuries are best treated surgically. The most commonly cited study[151] rationalizing surgical treatment of isolated grade III PLC injuries reported a high incidence of osteoarthritis (50% at 8-year follow-up) with conservative management. However, this 1989 study included only 12 patients and included patients who had undergone lateral meniscectomy or had had repeat injuries to the affected knee during the follow-up period, making it impossible to tell whether the arthritis was due to the initial injury, subsequent injury, or surgical meniscectomy. Despite the common claim in the surgical literature that grade III injuries will lead to OA if left untreated, the authors could find no other studies substantiating this claim. Therefore, the authors conclude that the data do not support the idea that conservatively treated isolated grade III injuries will necessarily lead to long-term OA.

The surgical literature[150,152] also commonly states that acute repair of the PLC is generally more successful than if surgery is delayed for more than 3 weeks. Although the literature does report good results with acute repair in case series[152] and case reports,[153] the authors could find no quality data (prospective randomized trials) validating this claim. In other words, it may be that if patients had been treated conservatively in these in "acute" case series they would have fared equally as well as those treated operatively.

Chronic isolated grade III injuries

The literature does, however, support the surgical treatment of knees with chronic instability and symptoms resulting from PLC injury.[154] The one large series of such patients (95 knees with lateral instability and symptoms present for an average of 27 months) was published in 1985 by Hughston and Jacobson,[154] and reported good results in 80% of those managed operatively.

In conclusion, and contrary to what is promulgated in the surgical literature, the data found by the authors do not support operative treatment of isolated grade III injuries to the PLC, but do support delayed surgery as an option if dictated by chronic symptoms and instability.

Grade III injuries with femoral avulsion

A case series (6 patients) reported good results with operative management of patients with grade III injuries and femoral avulsion fractures followed up for as long as 5.1 years.[155]

Grade III injury with concomitant cruciate injury

As noted earlier, the likelihood of PLC injury is high with concomitant cruciate tears, and although no controlled randomized trials exist as guidelines for such combined deficiencies, current practice is to repair both areas because of the possibility of cruciate graft rupture if the PLC structures are not restored.

REFERENCES

1. Miyasaka KC, Daniel DM, Stone ML, et al. The incidence of knee ligament injuries in the general population. Am J Knee Surg 1991;4:3–8.
2. Gwinn DE, Wilckens JH, McDevitt ER, et al. The relative incidence of anterior cruciate ligament injury in men and women at the United States naval academy. Am J Sports Med 2000;28(1):98–102.
3. Bowers KD, Martin RB. Cleat-surface friction on new and old Astroturf. Med Sci Sports 1975;7:123–35.
4. Lambson RB, Barnhill BS, Higgins RW. Football cleat design and its effect on ACL injuries. A three-year prospective study. Am J Sports Med 1996;24:155–9.
5. Orchard JW, Powell JW. Risk of knee and ankle sprains under various weather conditions in American football. Med Sci Sports Exerc 2003;35:1118–23.
6. Orchard J, Seward H, McGivern J, et al. Rainfall, evaporation and the risk of non-contact anterior cruciate ligament injury in the Australian Football League. Med J Aust 1999;170:304–6.
7. Evans KN, Kilcoyne KG, Dickens JF, et al. Predisposing risk factors for non-contact ACL injuries in military subjects. Knee Surg Sports Traumatol Arthrosc 2012;20(8):1554–9.
8. Myer GD, Ford KR, Barber Foss KD, et al. The relationship of hamstrings and quadriceps strength to anterior cruciate ligament injury in female athletes. Clin J Sport Med 2009;19(1):3–8.

9. Ruedl G, Webhofer M, Helle K, et al. Leg dominance is a risk factor for noncontact anterior cruciate ligament injuries in female recreational skiers. Am J Sports Med 2012;40(6):1269–73.
10. Hewett TE, Myer GD, Ford KR. Anterior cruciate ligament injuries in female athletes: part 1, mechanisms and risk factors. Am J Sports Med 2006;34(2):299–311.
11. Alentorn-Geli E, Myer GD, Silvers HJ, et al. Prevention of non-contact anterior cruciate ligament injuries in soccer players. Part 1: mechanisms of injury and underlying risk factors. Knee Surg Sports Traumatol Arthrosc 2009;17(7):705–29.
12. Myer GD, Ford KR, Paterno MV, et al. The effects of generalized joint laxity on risk of anterior cruciate ligament injury in young female athletes. Am J Sports Med 2008;36(6):1073–80.
13. Shimokochi Y, Shultz SJ. Mechanisms of noncontact anterior cruciate ligament injury. J Athl Train 2008;43(4):396–408.
14. Solomon DH, Simel DL, Bates DW, et al. The rational clinical examination. Does this patient have a torn meniscus or ligament of the knee? Value of the physical examination. JAMA 2001;286(13):1610–20.
15. Benjaminse A, Gokeler A, van der Schans CP. Clinical diagnosis of an anterior cruciate ligament rupture: a meta-analysis. J Orthop Sports Phys Ther 2006;36:267.
16. Caborn DN, Johnson BM. The natural history of the anterior cruciate ligament-deficient knee. Clin Sports Med 1993;12(4):625–35.
17. Al-Dadah O, Shepstone L, Marshall TJ, et al. Secondary signs on static stress MRI in anterior cruciate ligament rupture. Knee 2010;18:235–41.
18. Sarraf KM, Sadri A, Thevendran G, et al. Approaching the ruptured anterior cruciate ligament. Emerg Med J 2011;28:644–9.
19. Spindler KP, Wright RW. Clinical practice. Anterior cruciate ligament tear. N Engl J Med 2008;359:2135.
20. Linko E, Harilainen A, Malmivaara A, et al. Surgical versus conservative interventions for anterior cruciate ligament ruptures in adults. Database Syst Rev 2005;(2):CD001356.
21. Frobell RB, Roos EM, Roos HP, et al. A randomized trial of treatment for acute anterior cruciate ligament tears. N Engl J Med 2010;363(4):331–42.
22. Moksnes H, Risberg MA. Performance-based functional evaluation of nonoperative and operative treatment after anterior cruciate ligament injury. Scand J Med Sci Sports 2009;19:345–55.
23. Li S, Su W, Xu Y, et al. A meta-analysis of hamstring autografts versus bone-patellar tendon-bone autografts for reconstruction of the anterior cruciate ligament. Knee 2011;18:287–93.
24. Mohtadi NG, Chan DS, Dainty KN, et al. Patellar tendon versus hamstring tendon autograft for anterior cruciate ligament rupture in adults. Cochrane Bone, Joint and Muscle Trauma Group. Cochrane Database Syst Rev 2011;(9):CD005960.
25. Jackson DW, Corsetti J, Simon TM. Biologic incorporation of allograft anterior cruciate ligament replacements. Clin Orthop Relat Res 1996;324:126–33.
26. Noh JH, Yi SR, Song SJ, et al. Comparison between hamstring autograft and free tendon Achilles allograft: minimum 2-year follow-up after anterior cruciate ligament reconstruction using EndoButton and Intrafix. Knee Surg Sports Traumatol Arthrosc 2011;19(5):816–22.

27. Sun K, Tian SQ, Zhang JH, et al. Anterior cruciate ligament reconstruction with bone-patellar tendon-bone autograft versus allograft. Arthroscopy 2009;25(7): 750–9.
28. Lind M, Menhert F, Pedersen AB. Incidence and outcome after revision anterior cruciate ligament reconstruction: results from the Danish registry for knee ligament reconstructions. Am J Sports Med 2012;40(7):1551–7.
29. Magnussen RA, Lawrence JT, West RL, et al. Graft size and patient age are predictors of early revision after anterior cruciate ligament reconstruction with hamstring autograft. Arthroscopy 2012;28(4):526–31.
30. Suomalainen P, Järvelä T, Paakkala A, et al. Double-bundle versus single-bundle anterior cruciate ligament reconstruction: a prospective randomized study with 5-year results. Am J Sports Med 2012;40(7):1511–8.
31. Suomalainen P, Moisala A, Paakkala A, et al. Double bundle versus single-bundle anterior cruciate ligament reconstruction: randomized clinical and magnetic resonance imaging study with 2-year follow-up. Am J Sports Med 2011;39:1615–22.
32. Ng GY, Oakes BW, Deacon OW, et al. Biomechanics of patellar tendon autograft for reconstruction of the anterior cruciate ligament in the goat: three-year study. J Orthop Res 1995;13:602–8.
33. Weiler A, Peine R, Pashmineh-Azar A, et al. Tendon healing in a bone tunnel, part I: biomechanical results after biodegradable interference fit fixation in a model of anterior cruciate ligament reconstruction in sheep. Arthroscopy 2002;18:113–23.
34. Kondo E, Yasuda K, Katsura T, et al. Biomechanical and histological evaluations of the doubled semitendinosus tendon autograft after anterior cruciate ligament reconstruction in sheep. Am J Sports Med 2012;40(2):315–24.
35. Delay BS, McGrath BE, Mindell ER. Observations on a retrieved patellar tendon autograft used to reconstruct the anterior cruciate ligament: a case report. J Bone Joint Surg Am 2002;84:1433–8.
36. Ardern CL, Webster KE, Taylor NF, et al. Return to sport following anterior cruciate ligament reconstruction surgery: a systematic review and meta-analysis of the state of play. Br J Sports Med 2011;45:596.
37. Williams JS, Bach BR. Operative and nonoperative rehabilitation of the ACL-injured knee. Sports Med Arthrosc Rev 1996;4(1):69–82.
38. Swirtum LR, Jansson A, Renstrom P. The effects of a functional knee brace during early treatment of patients with a non-operated acute anterior cruciate ligament tear: a prospective randomized study. Clin J Sport Med 2005;15: 299–304.
39. Kessler MA, Behrend H, Henz S, et al. Function, osteoarthritis and activity after ACL-rupture: 11 years follow-up results of conservative versus reconstructive treatment. Knee Surg Sports Traumatol Arthrosc 2008;16(5):442–8.
40. Neuman P, Englund M, Kostogiannis I, et al. Prevalence of tibiofemoral osteoarthritis 15 years after nonoperative treatment of anterior cruciate ligament injury: a prospective cohort study. Am J Sports Med 2008;36(9):1717–25.
41. Fink C, Hoser C, Hackl W, et al. Long-term outcome of operative or nonoperative treatment of anterior cruciate ligament rupture: is sports activity a determining variable? Int J Sports Med 2001;22(4):304–9.
42. Lohmander LS, Ostenberg A, Englund M, et al. High prevalence of knee osteoarthritis, pain, and functional limitations in female soccer players twelve years after anterior cruciate ligament injury. Arthritis Rheum 2004;50(10): 3145–52.

43. Mihelic R, Jurdana H, Jotanovic Z, et al. Long-term results of anterior cruciate ligament reconstruction: a comparison with non-operative treatment with a follow-up of 17-20 years. Int Orthop 2011;35:1093–7.
44. Casteleyn PP, Handelberg F. Non-operative management of anterior cruciate ligament injuries in the general population. J Bone Joint Surg Br 1996;78:446–51.
45. Andersson C, Odensten M, Good L, et al. Surgical or non-surgical treatment of acute rupture of the anterior cruciate ligament. A randomized study with long-term follow-up. J Bone Joint Surg Am 1989;71:965–74.
46. Lebel B, Hulet C, Galaud B, et al. Arthroscopic reconstruction of the anterior cruciate ligament using bone-patellar tendon-bone autograft: a minimum 10-year follow-up. Am J Sports Med 2008;36(7):1275–82.
47. Cohen M, Amaro JT, Ejnisman B, et al. Anterior cruciate ligament reconstruction after 10 to 15 years: association between meniscectomy and osteoarthrosis. Arthroscopy 2007;23(6):629–34.
48. Järvelä T, Kannus P, Järvinen M. Anterior cruciate ligament reconstruction in patients with or without accompanying injuries: a re-examination of subjects 5 to 9 years after reconstruction. Arthroscopy 2001;17:818–25.
49. Vetrano M, d'Alessandro F, Torrisi MR, et al. Extracorporeal shock wave therapy promotes cell proliferation and collagen synthesis of primary cultured human tenocytes. Knee Surg Sports Traumatol Arthrosc 2011;19:2159–68.
50. Radice F, Yanez R, Gutierrez V, et al. Comparison of magnetic resonance imaging findings in anterior cruciate ligament grafts with and without autologous platelet-derived growth factors. Arthroscopy 2010;26(1):50–7.
51. Sanchez M, Anitua E, Azofra J, et al. Ligamentization of tendon grafts treated with an endogenous preparation rich in growth factors: gross morphology and histology. Arthroscopy 2010;26(4):470–80.
52. Nin JR, Gasque GM, Azcarate AV, et al. Has platelet-rich plasma any role in anterior cruciate ligament allograft healing? Arthroscopy 2009;25(11):1206–13.
53. Tovar N, Murthy NS, Kohn J, et al. ACL reconstruction using a novel hybrid scaffold composed of polyacrylate fibers and collagen fibers. J Biomed Mater Res A 2012;100(11):2913–20. http://dx.doi.org/10.1002/jbm.a.34229.
54. Walters VI, Kwansa AL, Freeman JW. Design and analysis of braid-twist collagen scaffolds. Connect Tissue Res 2012;53(3):255–66.
55. Laurent CP, Ganghoffer JF, Babin J, et al. Morphological characterization of a novel scaffold for anterior cruciate ligament tissue engineering. J Biomech Eng 2011;133(6):065001.
56. Mifune Y, Matsumoto T, Ota S, et al. Therapeutic potential of anterior cruciate ligament derived stem cells for anterior cruciate ligament reconstruction. Cell Transplant 2012;21(8):1651–65.
57. Matsumoto T, Kubo S, Sasaki K, et al. Acceleration of tendon-bone healing of anterior cruciate ligament graft using autologous ruptured tissue. Am J Sports Med 2012;40(6):1296–302.
58. Majeweski M, Susanne H, Klaus S. Epidemiology of athletic knee injuries: a 10 year study. Knee 2006;13(3):184–8.
59. Fanelli GC. Posterior cruciate ligament injuries in trauma patients. Arthroscopy 1993;9(3):291–4.
60. Arendt E, Dick R. Knee injury patterns among men and women in collegiate basketball and soccer. Am J Sports Med 1995;23(6):694–701.
61. Parolie JM, Bergfeld JA. Long-term results of nonoperative treatment of isolated posterior cruciate ligament injuries in the athlete. Am J Sports Med 1986;14(1):35–8.

62. Jarret GJ, Orwin JF, Dick RW. Injuries in collegiate wrestling. Am J Sports Med 1998;26(5):674–80.
63. Wind W, Bergled J, Parker R. Current concepts: evaluation and treatment of posterior cruciate ligament injuries—revisited. Am J Sports Med 2004;32: 1765–75.
64. Allen CR, Kaplan LD, Fluhme DJ, et al. Posterior cruciate ligament injuries. Curr Opin Rheumatol 2002;14(2):142–9.
65. Hastings DE. Diagnosis and management of acute knee ligament injuries. Can Fam Physician 1990;36:1169–72.
66. Moorman CT 3rd, Murphy Zane MS, Bansai S, et al. Tibial insertion of the posterior cruciate ligament: a sagittal plane analysis using gross, histologic, and radiographic methods. Arthroscopy 2008;24(3):269–75.
67. Bowman K, Sekiya J. Anatomy and biomechanics of the posterior cruciate ligament, medial and lateral sides of the knee. Sports Med Arthrosc Rev 2010;18(4): 222–8.
68. McAllister D, Hussain S. Tibial inlay posterior cruciate ligament reconstruction: surgical technique and results. Sports Med Arthrosc Rev 2010;18:249–53.
69. Takahashi M, Matsubara T, Doi M, et al. Anatomical study of the femoral and tibial insertions of the anterolateral and posteromedial bundles of human posterior cruciate ligament. Knee Surg Sports Traumatol Arthrosc 2006;14: 1055–9.
70. Veltri DM, Warren RF. Anatomy, biomechanics, and physical findings in posterolateral knee instability. Clin Sports Med 1994;13(3):599–614.
71. Miller MD, Cooper DE, Fanelli GC, et al. Posterior cruciate ligament: current concepts. Instr Course Lect 2002;51:347–51.
72. Harner CD, Hoher J. Evaluation and treatment of posterior cruciate ligament injuries. Am J Sports Med 1998;26(3):471–82.
73. Colvin A, Meislin R. Posterior cruciate ligament injuries in the athlete: diagnosis and treatment. Bull NYU Hosp Jt Dis 2009;67(1):45–51.
74. Fowler PJ, Messieh SS. Isolated posterior cruciate ligament injuries in athletes. Am J Sports Med 1987;15(6):553–7.
75. Margheritini F, Rihn J, Musahl V, et al. Posterior cruciate ligament injuries in the athlete. Sports Med 2002;32(6):393–408.
76. Lubowitz J, Bernardini B. Current concept review: comprehensive physical examination for instability of the knee. Am J Sports Med 2008;36(3):577–94.
77. Shelbourne KD, Davis TJ, Patel DV. The natural history of acute, isolated, non operatively treated posterior cruciate ligament injuries. A prospective study. Am J Sports Med 1999;27(3):276–83.
78. Rubinstein RA, Shelbourne KD, McCarroll JD. The accuracy of the clinical examination in the setting of posterior cruciate ligament injuries. Am J Sports Med 1994;22(4):550–7.
79. Voos J, Mauro C, Wente T. Posterior crucial ligament: anatomy, biomechanics, and outcomes. Am J Sports Med 2012;40(1):222–31.
80. Nikolaou VS, Chronopoulos E, Savvidou C. MRI efficacy in diagnosing internal lesions of the knee: a retrospective analysis. J Trauma Manag Outcomes 2008;2(1):4.
81. Servant CT, Ramos JP, Thomas NP. The accuracy of magnetic resonance imaging in diagnosing chronic posterior cruciate ligament injury. Knee 2004; 11:265–70.
82. Roberts C, Towers J, Spangehl M. Advanced MR imaging of the cruciate ligaments. Radiol Clin North Am 2007;45:1003–16.

83. Lopez-Vidriero E, Simon E, Johnson D. Initial evaluation of PCL injuries: history, physical examination, imaging studies, surgical and nonsurgical indication. Sports Med Arthrosc Rev 2010;18(4):230–7.
84. Shelbourne KD, Muthukaruppan Y. Subjective results of nonoperatively treated, acute, isolated posterior cruciate ligament injuries. Arthroscopy 2005;21(4): 457–61.
85. Patel DV, Allen AA. The nonoperative treatment of acute, isolated (partial or complete) posterior cruciate ligament-deficient knees: an intermediate-term follow-up study. HSS J 2007;3(2):137–46.
86. Shelbourne KD, Jennings RW, Vahey TN. Magnetic resonance imaging of posterior cruciate ligament injuries: assessment of healing. Am J Knee Surg 1999;12: 209–13.
87. Tewes DP, Fritts HM, Fields RD, et al. Chronically injured posterior cruciate ligament: magnetic resonance imaging. Clin Orthop Relat Res 1997;335:224–32.
88. Mariani PP, Margheritini F, Camillieri G, et al. Serial magnetic resonance imaging evaluation of the patellar tendon after posterior cruciate ligament reconstruction. Arthroscopy 2002;18:38–45.
89. Jung YB, Jung HJ, Yang JJ. Characterization of spontaneous healing of chronic posterior cruciate ligament injury: analysis of instability and magnetic resonance imaging. J Magn Reson Imaging 2008;27(6):1336–40.
90. Richter M, Kiefer H, Hehl G, et al. Primary repair for posterior cruciate ligament injuries. An eight year followup of fifty-three patients. Am J Sports Med 1996; 24(3):298–305.
91. Torg JS, Barton TM, Pavlov H, et al. Combined PCL with other ligamentous injuries do worse: natural history of the posterior cruciate ligament-deficient knee. Clin Orthop 1989;246:208–16.
92. Clancy WG Jr, Shelbourne KD, Zoellner GB, et al. Treatment of knee joint instability secondary to rupture of the posterior cruciate ligament. Report of a new procedure. J Bone Joint Surg Am 1983;65:310–22.
93. Keller PM, Shelbourne KD, McCarroll JR, et al. Nonoperatively treated isolated posterior cruciate ligament injuries. Am J Sports Med 1993;21:132–6.
94. Boynton MD, Tietjens BR. Long term followup of the untreated isolated posterior cruciate ligament deficient knee. Am J Sports Med 1996;24(3):306–10.
95. Noyes FR, Barber-Westin SD. Posterior cruciate ligament revision reconstruction part 1. Causes of surgical failure in 52 consecutive operations. Am J Sports Med 2005;33(5):646–54.
96. Quarles JD, Hosey RG. Medial and lateral collateral injuries: prognosis and treatment. Prim Care 2004;31(4):957–75.
97. National Collegiate Athletic Association. NCAA Injury Surveillance System for Academic Years 1997–2000. Indianapolis (IN): National Collegiate Athletic Association; 2000.
98. Miyamoto RG, Bosco JA, Sherman OH. Treatment of medial collateral ligament injuries. J Am Acad Orthop Surg 2009;17(3):152–61.
99. Kennedy JC, Fowler PJ. Medial and anterior instability of the knee. An anatomical and clinical study using stress machines. Clin Orthop Relat Res 1995;321:3–9.
100. Griffith CJ, Wijdicks CA, LaPrade RF, et al. Force measurements on the posterior oblique ligament and superficial medial collateral ligament proximal and distal divisions to applied loads. Am J Sports Med 2009;37:140–8.
101. Robinson JR, Bull AM, Thomas RR, et al. The role of the medial collateral ligament and posteromedial capsule in controlling knee laxity. Am J Sports Med 2006;34:1815–23.

102. Griffith CJ, LaPrade RF, Johansen S, et al. Medial knee injury: part 1, static function of the individual components of the main medial knee structures. Am J Sports Med 2009;37:1762–70.
103. American Medical Association. Committee on the Medical Aspects of Sports: standard nomenclature of athletic injuries. Chicago: American Medical Association (AMA); 1966.
104. Fetto JF, Marshall JL. Medial collateral ligament injuries of the knee: a rationale for treatment. Clin Orthop 1978;132:206–18.
105. Grood ES, Stowers SF, Noyes FR. Limits of movement in the human knee. Effect of sectioning the posterior cruciate ligament and posterolateral structures. J Bone Joint Surg Am 1988;70:88–97.
106. Yao L, Dungan D, Seeger LL. MR imaging of tibial collateral ligament injury: comparison with clinical examination. Skeletal Radiol 1994;23:521–4.
107. Lundberg M, Odensten M, Thuomas KA, et al. The diagnostic validity of magnetic resonance imaging in acute knee injuries with hemarthrosis. A single-blinded evaluation in 69 patients using high-field MRI before arthroscopy. Int J Sports Med 1996;17(3):218–22.
108. Schweitzer ME, Tran D, Deely DM, et al. Medial collateral ligament injuries: evaluation of multiple signs, prevalence and location of associated bone bruises, and assessment with MR imaging. Radiology 1995;194(3):825–9.
109. Miller MD, Osborne JR, Gordon WT, et al. The natural history of bone bruises: a prospective study of magnetic resonance imaging detected trabecular microfractures in patients with isolated medial collateral ligament injuries. Am J Sports Med 1998;26:15–9.
110. Derscheid GL, Garrick JG. Medial collateral ligament injuries in football: nonoperative management of grade I and grade II sprains. Am J Sports Med 1981;9:365–8.
111. Holden DL, Eggert AW, Butler JE. The nonoperative treatment of grade I and II medial collateral ligament injuries to the knee. Am J Sports Med 1983;11:340–4.
112. Lundberg M, Messner K. Long-term prognosis of isolated partial medial collateral ligament ruptures: a ten-year clinical and radiographic evaluation of a prospectively observed group of patients. Am J Sports Med 1996;24:160–3.
113. Padgett LR, Dahners LE. Rigid immobilization alters matrix organization in the injured rat medial collateral ligament. J Orthop Res 1992;10:895–900.
114. Woo SL, Gomez MA, Seguchi Y, et al. Measurement of mechanical properties of ligament substance from a bone-ligament-bone preparation. J Orthop Res 1983;1:22–9.
115. Steadman JR. Rehabilitation of first- and second-degree sprains of the medial collateral ligament. Am J Sports Med 1979;7:300–2.
116. Giannotti BF, Rudy T, Graziano J. The non-surgical management of isolated medial collateral ligament injuries of the knee. Sports Med Arthrosc 2006;14(2):74–7.
117. Sparrow KJ, Finucane SD, Owen JR, et al. The effects of low-intensity ultrasound on medial collateral ligament healing in the rabbit model. Am J Sports Med 2005;33:1048–56.
118. Warden SJ, Avin KG, Beck EM, et al. Low intensity pulsed ultrasound accelerates and a nonsteroidal anti-inflammatory drug delays knee ligament healing. Am J Sports Med 2006;34:1094–102.
119. Indelicato PA. Non-operative treatment of complete tears of the medial collateral ligament of the knee. J Bone Joint Surg Am 1983;65:323–9.

120. Reider B, Sathy MR, Talkington J, et al. Treatment of isolated medial collateral ligament injuries in athletes with early functional rehabilitation: a five-year follow-up study. Am J Sports Med 1993;22:470–7.
121. Marchant MH Jr, Tibor LM, Sekiya JK, et al. Management of medial-sided knee injuries, part one medial collateral ligament. Am J Sports Med 2011;39(5): 1102–13.
122. Phisitkul P, James SL, Wolf BR, et al. MCL injuries of the knee: current concepts review. Iowa Orthop J 2006;26:77–90.
123. Grant JA, Tannenbaum E, Miller BS, et al. Treatment of combined complete tears of the anterior cruciate and medial collateral ligaments. Arthroscopy 2012;28(1): 110–22.
124. Kannus P. Long-term results of conservatively treated medial collateral ligament injuries of the knee joint. Clin Orthop 1988;226:103–12.
125. Ballmer PM, Jakob RP. The non operative treatment of isolated complete tears of the medial collateral ligament of the knee. A prospective study. Arch Orthop Trauma Surg 1988;107(5):273–6.
126. Thornton GM, Johnson JC, Maser RV, et al. Strength of medial structures of the knee joint are decreased by the isolated injury to the medial collateral ligament and subsequent joint immobilization. J Orthop Res 2005;23:1191–8.
127. Frölke JP, Oskam J, Vierhout PA. Primary reconstruction of the medial collateral ligament in combined injury of the medial collateral and anterior cruciate ligaments. Short-term results. Knee Surg Sports Traumatol Arthrosc 1998;6(2): 103–6.
128. Andersson C, Gillquist J. Treatment of acute isolated and combined ruptures of the anterior cruciate ligament. A long-term follow-up study. Am J Sports Med 1992;20(1):7–12.
129. Jokl P, Kaplan N, Stovell P. Non-operative treatment of severe injuries to the medial and anterior cruciate ligaments of the knee. J Bone Joint Surg Am 1984;66(5):741–4.
130. Halinen J, Lindahl J, Hirvensalo E, et al. Operative and nonoperative treatments of medial collateral ligament rupture with early anterior cruciate ligament reconstruction. Am J Sports Med 2006;34(7):1134–40.
131. Shelbourne KD, Porter DA. Anterior cruciate ligament-medial collateral ligament injury: nonoperative management of medial collateral ligament tears with anterior cruciate ligament reconstruction: a preliminary report. Am J Sports Med 1992;20:283–6.
132. Yoshiya S, Kuroda R, Mizuno K, et al. Medial collateral ligament reconstruction using autogenous hamstring tendons: technique and results in initial cases. Am J Sports Med 2005;33(9):1380–5.
133. Albright JP, Powell JW, Smith W, et al. Medial collateral ligament knee sprains in college football. Brace wear preferences and injury risk. Am J Sports Med 1994; 22(1):2–11.
134. Albright JP, Powell JW, Smith W, et al. Medial collateral ligament knee sprains in college football. Effectiveness of preventive braces. Am J Sports Med 1994; 22(1):12–8.
135. Najibi S, Albright JP. The use of knee braces, part 1: prophylactic knee braces in contact sports. Am J Sports Med 2005;33(4):602–11.
136. Covey DC. Injuries of the posterolateral corner of the knee. J Bone Joint Surg Am 2001;83:106–18.
137. Fanelli GC, Edson CJ. Posterior cruciate ligament injuries in trauma patients: part II. Arthroscopy 1995;11:526–9.

138. LaPrade RF, Wentorf FA, Fritts H, et al. A prospective magnetic resonance imaging study of the incidence of posterolateral and multiple ligament injuries in acute knee injuries presenting with a hemarthrosis. Arthroscopy 2007; 23(12):1341–7.
139. Gardner MJ, Yacoubian S, Geller D, et al. The incidence of soft tissue injury in operative tibial plateau fractures: a magnetic resonance imaging analysis of 103 patients. J Orthop Trauma 2005;19(2):79–84.
140. Pacheco RJ, Ayre CA, Bollen SR. Posterolateral corner injuries of the knee: a serious injury commonly missed. J Bone Joint Surg Br 2011;93(2):194–7.
141. Harner CD, Vogrin TM, Hoher J, et al. Biomechanical analysis of a posterior cruciate ligament reconstruction: deficiency of the posterolateral structures as a cause of graft failure. Am J Sports Med 2000;28:32–9.
142. LaPrade RF, Resig S, Wentorf F, et al. The effects of grade III posterolateral knee complex injuries on anterior cruciate ligament graft force: a biomechanical analysis. Am J Sports Med 1999;27:469–75.
143. Bleday RM, Fanelli GC, Giannotti BF, et al. Instrumented measurement of the posterolateral corner. Arthroscopy 1998;14(5):489–94.
144. Bae JH, Choi IC, Suh SW, et al. Evaluation of the reliability of the dial test for posterolateral rotatory instability: a cadaveric study using an isotonic rotation machine. Arthroscopy 2008;24:593–8.
145. Hughston JC, Andrews JR, Cross MJ, et al. Classification of knee ligament instabilities: II. The lateral compartment. J Bone Joint Surg Am 1976;58:173–9.
146. Lee J, Papakonstantinou O, Brookenthal KR, et al. Arcuate sign of posterolateral knee injuries: anatomic, radiographic, and MR imaging data related to patterns of injury. Skeletal Radiol 2003;32:619–27.
147. LaPrade RF, Gilbert TJ, Bollom TS, et al. The magnetic resonance imaging appearance of individual structures of the posterolateral knee. A prospective study of normal knees and knees with surgically verified grade III injuries. Am J Sports Med 2000;28(2):191–9.
148. Ranawat A, Baker CL 3rd, Henry S, et al. Posterolateral corner injury of the knee: evaluation and management. J Am Acad Orthop Surg 2008;16(9):506–18.
149. Krukhaug Y, Molster A, Rodt A, et al. Lateral ligament injuries of the knee. Knee Surg Sports Traumatol Arthrosc 1998;6(1):21–5.
150. Ricchetti ET, Sennett BJ, Huffman GR. Acute and chronic management of posterolateral corner injuries of the knee. Orthopedics 2008;31(5):479–88.
151. Kannus P. Nonoperative treatment of grade II and III sprains of the lateral ligament compartment of the knee. Am J Sports Med 1989;17:83–8.
152. DeLee JC, Riley MB, Rockwood CA. Acute posterolateral rotatory instability of the knee. Am J Sports Med 1983;11:199–207.
153. Pavlovich RI, Nafarrate EB. Trivalent reconstruction for posterolateral and lateral knee instability. Arthroscopy 2002;18(1):E1.
154. Hughston JC, Jacobson KE. Chronic posterolateral instability of the knee. J Bone Joint Surg Am 1985;67:351–9.
155. von Heideken J, Mikkelsson C, Boström Windhamre H, et al. Acute injuries to the posterolateral corner of the knee in children: a case series of 6 patients. Am J Sports Med 2011;39(10):2199–205.

Meniscal, Plica, Patellar, and Patellofemoral Injuries of the Knee

Updates, Controversies and Advancements

Vincent Morelli, MD[a,*], Thomas Mark Braxton Jr, MD[b]

KEYWORDS

• Athletic knee injuries • Meniscus tears and cysts • Patellar tendonitis
• Patellofemoral pain syndrome • Plica

KEY POINTS

- Knee injuries common in athletes include meniscus tears and cysts, patellar tendonitis, patellofemoral pain syndrome (PFPS) and plica.
- Peripheral tears and certain vertical and horizontal tears of the meniscus are easy to repair surgically and have good outcomes.
- Radial tears, flap tears, and ragged complex tears are technically more difficult to repair and are less likely to have good outcomes.
- Nonoperative treatment of PFPS, properly focused on the causative factors, can be expected to be successful in most cases.
- The best evidence to date supports the use of physical therapy in the treatment of PFPS with some additional benefit to be expected, at least in the short term, from taping and orthoses.

MENISCUS TEARS AND CYSTS

Epidemiology

The incidence of meniscal tears ranges from 60 to 70 per 100,000 individuals per year.[1,2] They are more common in males (2.5–4:1 males/females)[1] and more than one-third of those in the athletic population are associated with anterior cruciate ligament (ACL) injuries.[3] Lateral meniscal tears are more frequent in cases of acute ACL rupture, whereas chronic ACL deficiency leads more commonly to medial meniscal tears.

[a] Department of Family and Community Medicine, School of Medicine, Meharry Medical College, 1005 Dr D. B. Todd Boulevard, Nashville, TN 37208, USA; [b] Braxton Family and Sports Medicine, Jackson Purchase Medical Center, 1111 Medical Center Circle, Mayfield, KY 42066, USA
* Corresponding author.
E-mail address: morellivincent@yahoo.com

Prim Care Clin Office Pract 40 (2013) 357–382
http://dx.doi.org/10.1016/j.pop.2013.02.014 primarycare.theclinics.com

Meniscal Anatomy and Function

The medial meniscus covers 50% of the tibial plateau in the medial compartment and is firmly attached to the medal collateral ligament. The lateral meniscus covers 70% of the contact area on the lateral side, is more mobile, is not attached to the lateral collateral ligament, and is therefore (except in the case of ACL injury) less likely to be injured than the more fixed medial meniscus.[4] The meniscus functions chiefly as a shock absorber during activity with the lateral meniscus bearing 70% of the load in the lateral compartment, and the medial meniscus bearing 50% of the load in the medial compartment. The meniscus also functions in joint lubrication and plays a significant part (secondary to the ACL) in preventing forward translation of the tibia on the femur. This latter function of the meniscus is especially important in ACL-deficient knees[5] and may explain why ACL-deficient patients have a high incidence of medial meniscus tears. (More stress is borne by the meniscus when the ACL is not present.)[6]

The peripheral meniscus is mainly made up of fibrocartilage (80%); the innermost portion is made up of both hyaline cartilage (60%) and fibrocartilage (40%).[7] The collagen fibers are oriented mainly in a circumferential pattern; however, some radially (perpendicular) oriented fibers do exist, especially along the meniscal surface, and are believed to function in resisting shearing stress and as restraints to longitudinal tearing.

In adults, only the peripheral 25% to 30% of the meniscus is supplied by microvasculature.[8] The remaining inner portion is avascular and thus less likely to heal in repair attempts.

Nerve fibers are also more abundant along the periphery, explaining why peripheral injuries are often more painful than lesions located in the inner portions.[9]

Mechanism of Injury

Tears occur most frequently from noncontact forces (acceleration/deceleration in conjunction with rotation that catches the meniscus between the tibia and femur) but obviously can also occur with contact, especially in conjunction with medial collateral ligament or ACL injuries.[10] In younger patients (<40 years), trauma or twisting injury on a fixed foot is the usual mechanism of injury. Older patients, on the other hand, often get degenerative tears with minimal or no known trauma.[11]

Most acute meniscal tears are longitudinal (vertical), tearing along the natural circumferential lines of the fibrocartilage ring (**Fig. 1**). Radial tears, which tear perpendicular to the natural collagen fiber alignment, generally require a higher impact.[4]

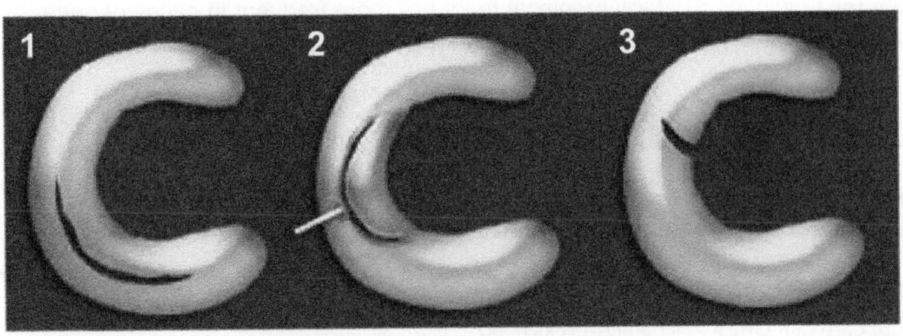

Fig. 1. (1) Vertical/vertical longitudinal; includes bucket handle tears; (2) horizontal tears; (3) radial/transverse/oblique/parrot beak tears.

Clinical Picture

Symptoms

There are no clear data in the literature quantifying the prevalence of individual symptoms of meniscal injury. However, it is known that some patients present with minimal pain and a normal physical examination. Generally, however, patients complain of variable amounts of pain and effusion depending on the size and location of the tear. Larger, more acute, and more peripheral tears tend to cause more symptoms. When swelling develops, it usually does so over the first 24 hours, and patients usually experience joint stiffness from the effusion. Classic mechanical symptoms of popping, catching, locking, or giving way are common but not always present.

Physical examination

The most common physical examination maneuvers for detecting meniscal lesions are presence of an effusion, the Thessaly test, McMurray test, and palpation for joint line tenderness. The Thessaly test, performed by asking the patient to flex the affected knee to 20° while standing, then internally and externally rotate (twist) it, is the most sensitive test with a sensitivity of 60% to 90% and a specificity of 96%. Pain, locking, catching, or inability to twist constitutes a positive test.[12–14] The older McMurray test, the Apley compression test, and joint line palpation are even less sensitive and specific.[15–17]

Despite the variability of symptoms and the shortcomings of physical examination tests, when a good history is combined with a proper examination, it is often more accurate (up to 90%) in diagnosing meniscal tears than magnetic resonance imaging (MRI) or ultrasonography (see later discussion).[18,19] A high clinical suspicion and appropriate patient follow-up of suspected injuries is important.

Radiographic imaging

Xray is not useful in detecting meniscal tears; however, it is helpful in detecting degenerative changes in the joint. The most common imaging modality used to detect meniscal injury is MRI, which has a sensitivity of 47% to 91% and a specificity of 81% to 95% for medial meniscus lesions and a sensitivity of 76% to 100% and specificity of 75% to 95% for lateral meniscal injury.[20–22] This lack of sensitivity on MRI may be because free edge radial tears are often difficult to visualize, as are peripheral tears and detachments of the posterior horns.[11] Further confounding MRI imaging for meniscal injury is that 16% of young asymptomatic patients have evidence of meniscal tears on MRI. This percentage increases to 36% for patients more than 45 years of age. (The natural history/progression of these lesions is unknown.)[23]

Although used less frequently, small studies have found ultrasonography to be 80% sensitive and up to 92% specific for meniscal lesions.[24]

Treatment

General principles

As discussed earlier, not all meniscal tears cause symptoms or problems. Certain tears do not require treatment because they will heal spontaneously or remain asymptomatic; these include short (<10 mm), stable vertical longitudinal tears, stable partial-thickness tears (<50% of the meniscal depth), and small (<3 mm) radial tears.[25]

Chronic degenerative meniscal tears, which occur usually in older patients, are also generally treated conservatively.[26] Studies of patients undergoing arthroscopic meniscectomy for degenerative tears have usually shown no benefit from surgery.[27] In 1 study, only 20% of such patients had good results from meniscectomy at 6-year follow-up.[28]

Factors that influence orthopedists to consider surgical intervention include (1) large complex tears; (2) tears associated with ACL rupture; (3) ongoing symptoms that affect activities of daily living, work, or sports; (4) physical findings of joint effusion, locking, limitation of motion, pain on squatting, or a positive McMurray/Thessaly test; and (5) failure to respond to nonsurgical treatment.

Once surgical intervention is decided on, repair of the meniscus is generally preferable to meniscectomy if the tear is located in an area amenable to repair (the outer vascular portion of the meniscus). Healing rate for the meniscus repair is higher if done in combination with ACL reconstruction. If the meniscus can be restored to its normal or near-normal state, the risk of future osteoarthritis with its debilitating symptoms is diminished. However, although repair is generally favored over meniscectomy, it also requires reoperation in up to 20% of patients, whereas partial meniscectomy requires repeat surgery in only 4% (when followed up for more than 10 years).[29] The recent developments in techniques allowing arthroscopic all-inside meniscal repairs (with no requirement for posterior surgical access for suture anchoring) has minimized the risk of complications.

In cases where meniscectomy is indicated, attempts should be made to preserve as much load-bearing meniscal tissue as possible because meniscectomy increases contact pressures in the knee by as much as 235%,[30] and leads to an increased risk of osteoarthritis by as much as 1400%.[31] The amount of meniscus excised has been shown to be the most important predictor for the development of osteoarthritis.[32] This is especially important in the lateral compartment where the meniscus has a greater load-bearing function.

Treatment based on the shape of tear and presence of meniscal cysts/discoid meniscus

Basic shapes (see **Fig. 1**) include the following:

1. Vertical longitudinal tears are the most common type of tear and can heal with conservative/nonoperative treatment, especially if the tear is along the peripheral one-third. When surgical treatment is indicated (continued symptoms despite trial of conservative treatment) for these vertical peripheral tears, there is increasing evidence supporting meniscal repair (rather than excision) with success rates varying from 63% to 91%.[33–35]
2. Horizontal tears split the meniscus in the horizontal plane and can be associated with meniscal cysts and Baker cysts (see later discussion). They are often treated surgically, especially when associated with mechanical symptoms or meniscal cysts.
3. Radial/transverse/oblique/parrot beak tears are easily excised when small and a rapid resolution of symptoms and return to sport can be expected (see section on rehabilitation). Larger tears, especially in the lateral compartment where load bearing is so critical, may be given a trial of repair, in an attempt to avert long-term arthritis, which occurs so commonly as a complication of lateral meniscectomy.
4. Complex tears (not shown in **Fig. 3**) occur most often as degenerative tears in older patients and occur in multiple planes. Unless locking, giving way, or pain is problematic, conservative treatment is generally recommended.
5. Detachment of the peripheral attachment of the posterior horn of the lateral meniscus (not shown in **Fig. 3**) occurs because the coronary ligaments that secure the posterior lateral meniscus either stretch or tear, leading to instability of the posterior horn. When the knee is flexed, the posterior horn now slides anteriorly into the lateral compartment causing pain, clicking, giving way, and locking. MRI findings in these cases are usually normal; however, arthroscopic diagnosis is easily made

and simple treatment via suturing of the posterior horn to the adjacent capsule is all that is required.

In conclusion, peripheral tears and certain vertical and horizontal tears are easy to repair surgically and have good outcomes. Radial tears, flap tears, and ragged complex tears are technically more difficult to repair, often occur in the avascular region of the meniscus and, thus, are less likely to have good outcomes. These lesions are usually best treated by partial meniscectomy.[7,36]

Treatment of 2 special lesions of the meniscus

Discoid lateral menisci Discoid menisci occur in 1% to 5% of people and are 10 times more common in the lateral meniscus than in the medial meniscus.[37,38] This anatomic anomaly causes excess pressure to be placed on the central portion of the meniscus, increasing the risk of tear. Such tears usually present in children or in teenagers and are usually treated by excision of the tear along with sculpting the remaining meniscus into a normal shape.[11]

Meniscal cysts Meniscal cysts (including Baker cysts) make up 1% to 10% of meniscus lesions and are highly associated with meniscal tears, usually horizontal tears.[39] In a review of 178 parameniscal cysts, those associated with the posterior horn of the lateral meniscus were found to be caused by meniscal tears 100% of the time, whereas cysts associated with the anterior horn of the lateral meniscus were associated with tears only 64% of the time. In contrast, medial meniscal cysts were associated with meniscal tears in 92% of cases regardless of their anterior/posterior location.[40]

Rehabilitation

Rehabilitation for conservatively treated meniscal lesions or after meniscectomy or partial meniscectomy can begin almost immediately. Full weight bearing can begin without delay and strengthening/range of motion (ROM) can start within a week of surgery. Patients treated with meniscectomy can expect a full recovery by around 6 weeks.

On the other hand, rehab following meniscal repair is quite different. Because meniscal healing has been demonstrated by second-look arthroscopy by 4 to 6 weeks,[41] and animal models have shown that repaired meniscus reaches 80% strength only by week 12,[42] rehabilitation after repair is generally much slower. Most surgeons recommend a cautious approach to give the meniscus enough time to heal and strengthen, thus minimizing the risk of repair failure. After surgery, patients are usually on crutches with partial weight bearing for the first 6 weeks with a brace that limits them to 90° of flexion. After 6 weeks, patients can begin a gentle strengthening program and discard the crutches as soon as they are comfortable doing so. Any twisting, running, or impact activity is delayed until at least 3 months and a gradual return to sports can be initiated around this time.

Along with this general conservative approach to rehabilitation after repair, rehabilitation is also individualized as discussed by Cavanaugh and colleagues,[43] and is usually tailored to the patient's weight-bearing status, gait deviations, joint effusion, muscle atrophy, joint alignment, and subjective complaints. Actual protocols also vary depending on the size and severity of the tear and the strength and stability of the repair.

Accelerated rehabilitation is advocated by some investigators[44,45] who have shown that patients (with either isolated meniscus tears or meniscus tears in conjunction with ACL tears) who begin an ROM/strengthening program as soon as their symptoms allow, do equally well in long-term studies as those treated more conservatively (ie, similar clinical success rates and similar rates of reinjury). The early rehabilitation patients in these studies returned to sport significantly sooner that those undergoing a delayed/more conservative approach. Despite these studies, however, and for the reasons stated earlier, most surgeons still follow a conservative rehabilitation protocol.

Recent advances

Recent advances using meniscal scaffolds In attempts to ward off arthritis after partial meniscectomy, artificial scaffolding can be sutured to the remnant meniscal rim to replace the missing meniscus. One of these scaffolds, the Menaflex scaffold (ReGen Biologics, Inc [ReGen], Hackensack, NJ), is made from bovine Achilles tendon that is pressurized and heat-molded into a meniscus shape. It is bioabsorbable and most of the scaffold is resorbed over 18 months. Studies have shown that approximately 50% of the excised meniscal tissue will grow back into the scaffold at 1 year[46] and up to 69% at 6 years.[47] Clinically significant improvements in activity can be expected; however, it is not clear whether pain scores are universally improved at a 6-year follow-up.[48] In the largest randomized trial of 311 patients,[47] no difference in pain scores were noted between patients receiving a Menaflex scaffold and those receiving simple partial meniscectomy. However, despite these less than impressive pain scores, an arresting of articular cartilage damage was noted at 5.8 years follow-up and in other shorter studies.[46] Menaflex scaffolding has yet to receive final US Food and Drug Administration approval for use in the United States.

The Actifit scaffold is a synthetic scaffold that degrades over 5 years. Uncontrolled short-term studies (1 and 2 years) have demonstrated not only native tissue ingrowth[49] but also decreased pain and increased activity levels when implanted in symptomatic patients after previous partial meniscectomy.[50,51] The Actifit studies were done without a partial meniscectomy only control group, several (up to 27%) patients were lost to follow-up, and only short-term results were reported.

With either type of meniscal scaffold, more definitive answers will emerge with longer-term pain and activity monitoring and longer-term follow-up.

Recent advances using meniscal allografts Meniscal allografts (cadaver harvested meniscus) may be used on severely arthritic knees or after meniscectomy in knees lacking a residual meniscal rim. The allografts are appropriately treated so that they can be transplanted without the need for tissue typing/matching or immunosuppressive therapy. The use of allografts began in the late 1980s, and many long-term follow-ups have been encouraging, with more than 70% success rates reported 10 years after intervention.[52–54]

The problem with interpreting these optimistic results, however, is that the procedures have usually been performed on patients who have severe symptoms, multiple contributing pathologic conditions, and have undergone multiple concomitant procedures. For example, allograft transplantation is often done in conjunction with articular cartilage repair/transplantation, ACL reconstruction, or realignment osteotomy. A recent rigorous review[55] found no significant studies of isolated meniscal transplantations in the literature but did note that pain and function seemed improved in the short and intermediate term with the procedure. Despite animal studies demonstrating that meniscal transplantation protects against future arthritis/cartilage damage, to date the literature does not yet demonstrate such prevention/protection in humans.

Future trends in meniscal repair

Future trends to enhance meniscal regrowth and healing include gene therapy, the use of growth factors, platelet-rich plasma (PRP), and the growth factors released from platelet alpha and dense granules, and stem cell therapy.[56–58] Although some early animal studies have been promising,[56] others have been less so.[59] In addition, the complex interactions between the various growth factors and inhibitory cytokines are complex and have yet to be fully elucidated,[60] they are promising and exciting, but not yet ready for clinical use in meniscal injury.

PATELLAR TENDONOPATHY

Patellar tendonopathy or jumper's knee is characterized by activity-related pain at the insertion of patellar tendon near the lower pole of the patella. Because it has been proved histologically that this injury is degenerative and not inflammatory,[61] the term tendinosis is preferred over tendinitis. A career prevalence of up to 22% in high-level athletes has been reported.[62,63] Prevalence is highest in high impact sports such as basketball (55% of players experience symptoms at some point in their career) and volleyball (40%–50%). The average duration of pain and functional impairment is 32 months, but the range is highly variable, ranging from 7 to 57 months.[64] In 1 study of top-level athletes with patellar tendonitis and a 15-year follow-up, 53% of the athletes reported quitting their sports career because of their symptoms.[64] The study also noted that the disease usually causes long-term but mild symptoms that remain even after an athlete's career is over.

Histopathology

The histopathologic changes seen in the injured tendon include tendon microtears, separation of collagen fibers, loss of longitudinal alignment of collagen fibers, mucinoid degeneration between fibers, and fibrocartilaginous change at the inferior patellar pole. In addition, there is cellular proliferation (eg, fibroblasts, endothelial cells) and neovascularization in the area of insult.[65] However, this proliferation ceases abruptly at the site of maximal tendon degeneration, providing evidence of a failed healing response.[66,67]

Diagnosis/Imaging

Patellar tendonopathy remains a clinical diagnosis. However, when confirmatory imaging is considered it is important that the sports physician be aware of the limitations of imaging. Although often used, MRI is limited in its ability to make a definitive diagnosis (limited sensitivity) and ultrasonography may be a better choice. In 1 study of 30 patients diagnosed clinically with patellar tendonitis, MRI was positive only in 57% of patients, whereas ultrasonography diagnosed 87%; specificity was equivalent between the imaging modalities.[68]

Treatment

Conservative treatment

Up to 90% of patients with patellar tendonopathy can be successfully treated conservatively with expectation of good results.[69] The current state of the evidence favors eccentric exercise therapy as the treatment of choice for this injury.[70–74]

One effective method of performing eccentric exercises in patellar tendonopathy, is to do 3 sets of 15 squat repetitions with the affected leg twice daily for 12 weeks. Squatting should progress from straight leg to 60° and should be done on a downhill inclined plane (inclined to 25°). When comparing this incline method of eccentric therapy versus normal noninclined eccentric therapy, evaluations done after 1 year showed a significant decrease in symptoms in the incline group compared with the nonincline group.[75] It may be beneficial for the primary care sports physician to discuss the current best practices with the physical therapists.

Ultrasonography In a recent comprehensive review, ultrasonography was found to be ineffective in the treatment of patellar tendonitis.[76]

Extracorporeal shock wave treatment High-intensity acoustic pulse (as in lithotripsy for kidney stones) applied to the patellar tendon is believed to induce microtrauma in the affected area, which, in turn, promotes increased blood flow and tissue healing. Extracorporeal shockwave therapy (ECST) also induces an inflammatory process in the area, which is believed to aid healing. However, the only good quality randomized placebo-controlled trial with ECST revealed no benefit from ECST over placebo.[77] There is currently no evidence to support ECST in the treatment of patellar tendonopathy.

Minimally invasive therapies

Steroid injection The highest quality trials evaluating steroid injection have demonstrated improvement in the short term (<8 weeks) but this improvement deteriorated in the longer term (follow-up at 12 and 24 weeks).[78,79]

In the most recent review published in the *Lancet*,[80] 41 high-quality studies involving 2672 patients were evaluated. This review was not restricted solely to patellar tendinosis (lateral epicondyle, shoulder and Achilles tendinosis were included) but results from studies on lateral epicondylitis were especially interesting. As in previous studies, these studies revealed the beneficial results of steroid injection in the short term (<8 weeks) but when patients were evaluated at 6 and 12 months, those who received steroid injections actually fared worse than control/placebo groups. It is unknown if physical therapy, in addition to steroid injection, would have ameliorated this late worsening of symptoms. Although this review did not assess isolated patellar tendinopathy (there was an inadequate number of quality studies to evaluate the long-term effects of steroid injections in patellar tendinopathy), these results with lateral epicondylitis should give one pause when considering patellar injection.

In conclusion, current data indicate short-term symptom relief with steroid injection in patellar tendinopathy, but there are no good data to recommend steroid injection in the long-term management of this injury.

Sclerosing injection Sclerosing injection has become increasingly used in cases of chronic tendinosis since 2002,[81] but the theoretic basis for such injections is questionable. Early Doppler studies seemed to show an increased vascularity in the areas of tendinopathy and, thus, provided theoretic justification for sclerosing injections. However, although later histologic studies have shown increased vascularity in the area, a marked decrease in vascularity has been demonstrated in the portion of the tendon exhibiting maximal degeneration.[66]

The most recent study, a 2012 case series of 120 knees, found that injection of sclerosing agent into the affected area of the patellar tendon showed only modest improvement in symptoms after 2 years and only 20% had a clinically significant resolution of symptoms.[82] Most other studies using sclerosing agents are short term or have methodological flaws, thus leaving us with little clinical justification for using sclerosing agents in the treatment of this problematic injury.

Prostaglandin injection Prostaglandin E2, initially believed to contribute to tissue injury in patellar tendinopathy,[83] has been found in experiments on rat tendon to actually improve the structural properties of diseased tendon.[84] Despite this theoretic basis for human trials, none have been conducted so far.

Stem cells In a 2012 pilot study[85] of 8 patients with refractory patellar tendinosis (failed conservative treatment of 6 months), patients were injected with their own bone marrow mononuclear cells and then followed annually for 5 years. Seven of the 8 patients noted significant improvement, were satisfied with the results, and would have the procedure repeated if they sustained a recurrent injury. The investigators noted that "the exact role of implanted stem cells on tendon healing remains uncertain." Stem cells may differentiate into tenocytes or supply growth factors to the healing area. However, because there was no control group in the study and because the natural history of the disease is so variable (see earlier), no conclusive evidence of efficacy can be drawn from this early work. We found no other stem cell trials in the literature.

PRP Platelets are known to contain growth factors and other active metabolites important for tissue repair, thus providing the theoretic basis for injection of PRP in patellar tendinopathy. Early pilot studies without control groups or long-term follow-ups reported encouraging results.[86,87] However, a more recent study[88] was less encouraging. This study followed 15 patients with patellar tendinopathy treated with PRP and 16 controls. At the 6-month follow-up, the investigators noted a significant improvement in the PRP arm. Despite the investigators' conclusions that the results of PRP were encouraging, their work had methodological flaws. In addition, a close look at their data reveals no clinically significant differences between PRP and the control group. At this time, there is no good evidence to promote the use of PRP in patellar tendinopathy.

Surgical treatment

The goal of surgical treatment in patellar tendinopathy is to excise fibrotic and degenerated tissue, disrupt disordered neovascularity in areas surrounding the pathologic tendon, and to stimulate the remaining viable cells to lay down a new healthy matrix and collagen.[65] Animal studies have indeed demonstrated well-ordered proliferation of new blood vessels after surgical intervention, changes postulated to aid healing by increasing delivery of nutrients and repair factors.[89]

Review of studies on surgical treatment Studies on surgical treatment of patellar tendinosis generally report positive results but are usually small and poorly designed.

A comprehensive review of surgical treatment of patellar tendinopathy performed in 2000 revealed a favorable outcome in 46% to 100% of patients. In this review, studies with the poorest methodology reported the best results.[90] No clear difference in outcomes between arthroscopic and open operative procedures was noted.

Since this review, several other studies on surgical treatment have been reported. For example, a recent 2009 study treated 9 patients with refractory patellar tendinosis (refractory to conservative treatment for at least 3 months) with arthroscopic excision of the distill pole of the patella and debridement of the deep patellar tendon. At evaluation 3 months after surgery, 8 of 9 patients had complete resolution of symptoms. However, little clinically useful information can be drawn from this study because the series was so small and no control group existed.[91]

Another, more recent (2012), retrospective analysis studied 23 patients who had failed 6 months of conservative therapy and underwent subsequent surgical debridement of the proximal patellar tendon, the inferior pole of the patella, and the peritenon. Nearly 80% of patients reported that they were able to return to their previous level of activity. However, the study failed to mention the length of time it took patients to return to this level and had no nonoperative control group for comparison.[92]

A final series of 73 knees (2011)[93] treated with arthroscopic debridement of abnormal patellar tendon, debridement of neovascularity in the area adjacent to degenerated tendon, and excision of the lower pole of the patella, found improvement in symptoms at 1-year and 3-year follow-ups in 90% of patients. However, only 19 of the 27 professional athletes were able to return to sport at their previous level of competition. In addition, there was no control group comparing conservative therapy versus operative treatment making definitive conclusions about optimal treatment impossible. In addition, the investigators concluded with a biased and unsubstantiated claim that early return to sport may be achieved.

The only randomized trial comparing surgical treatment versus conservative therapy was published in 2006. Surgical treatment involved debridement of the patellar tendon only (no debridement of the inferior pole of the patella), whereas the conservative treatment group received eccentric exercise therapy.[70] No differences were noted in outcomes between the surgical and conservative treatment groups 1 year after intervention. At the study's conclusion, the investigators stated that conservative treatment should be tried for at least 12 weeks before surgical intervention is considered. The latest study does show, however, that at 1-year after surgery, neither surgery nor conservative treatment worsens symptoms. The 12-week limitation on conservative therapy is entirely arbitrary. The natural history of the disease, as stated earlier, is highly variable and has an average persistence of symptoms of nearly 3 years. Twelve weeks of conservative therapy may be entirely inadequate in some patients. Furthermore, the rush to surgery may have caused both patient and physician to become frustrated with the usual slow progress of the condition and leading to the decision that something must be done.

The best data at this time find no benefit of surgery over conservative treatment of this difficult condition.

Summary

In conclusion, when treating patellar tendinopathy, the primary care physician should educate patients on the natural history of the disease, inform them of the various treatment options, and discuss the expected results of therapy. It is important that treatment decisions are discussed with well-informed patients so that the best plan can be agreed and expectations are realistically set.

PATELLOFEMORAL SYNDROME

Definition

Patellofemoral pain syndrome (PFPS) is defined as anterior knee pain in the absence of any other pathologic condition that is exacerbated by sporting activity, squatting, kneeling, climbing stairs/hills, or prolonged sitting.

Epidemiology

PFPS accounts for 25% to 40% of knee problems presenting to sports medicine clinics[94,95] and up to 25% of the knee problems in the general population.[96] However, the diagnosis is rarely made in general practice[97] suggesting a poor understanding or underreporting of the condition. The syndrome has a female to male ratio of 2:1, and is common in runners; patellofemoral pain is present in 19% to 46% of all knee injuries in this group.[98]

Natural History

A clear picture of the long-term natural history of patients with untreated PFPS is difficult to ascertain; however, 1 study found that 94% of patients with PFPS continued to experience pain 4 years after initial presentation and 25% reported significant symptoms up to 20 years later.[99] Despite this, there is little quality evidence linking PFPS with long-term patellofemoral arthritis.[100]

Pathophysiology

The cause of PFPS is poorly understood and is most likely multifactorial in origin, ultimately resulting in improper patellar tracking, friction, microdamage, inflammation, and pain in the area of the patella and surrounding structures. Imbalance in any of the complex forces acting about the patella may be causative.[101,102] In some cases, a relatively weak vastus medialis is overpowered by lateral forces (tight iliotibial band, tight lateral retinaculum, or overly strong vastus lateralis),[103] causing the patella to be pulled laterally and misaligned. In other cases, a normal static vastus medialis obliquus contracts improperly or in unsynchronized fashion during activity resulting in similar lateral maltracking of the patella.[104,105] Still other cases are brought on by a tight lateral ileotibial band, tight or weak quadriceps,[106] and tight hamstrings, all eventually increasing maltracking and patellofemoral compressive forces.[107] Similarly, excessive pronation from any cause increases the dynamic Q angle and can contribute to lateral maltracking and pain[108] (although static Q angles do not seem to be a causative factor).[109,110]

The lateral retinaculum also may play a role in patients with chronic lateral subluxation of the patella. Lateral subluxation is thought to lead to scarring and shortening of the retinaculum with increased lateral forces and secondary nerve damage.[107]

Decreased strength of hip abduction and decreased strength on femoral external rotation have also been demonstrated in patients with PFPS. These factors contribute to lateral maltracking, again forcing the patella to absorb excessive lateral stresses resulting in painful symptoms (**Fig. 2**).[111,112]

History

Symptoms of peripatellar or retropatellar pain or anterior knee pain usually have an insidious onset. Symptoms may be predominantly felt in the medial (most common), retro or lateral patellar areas and are usually worsened by activities that increase patellofemoral compressive forces (eg, running, jumping, walking uphill, squatting, climbing stairs).[104]

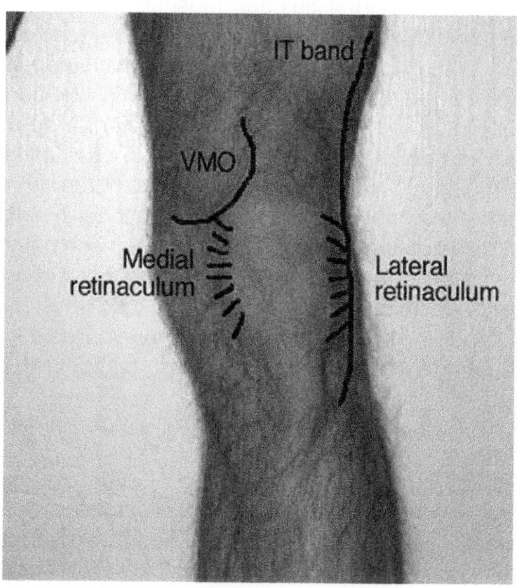

Fig. 2. Result of lateral maltracking. IT, ileotibeal; VMO, vastus medialis obliquus. (*From* LaBella C. Patellofemoral pain syndrome: evaluation and treatment. Prim Care 2004;31(4): 977–1003; with permission.)

Physical Examination

The physical examination should first rule out other causes of anterior knee pain such as patellar tendonitis, bursitis, patellofemoral arthritis, and patellar subluxation.[113]

Once other causes of anterior knee pain have been ruled out, the physician may perform various physical examination maneuvers to try and confirm a diagnosis of PFPS. The most recent and highest quality study assessing physical examination maneuvers in PFPS[114] found that positive findings on 2 of 3 of the following tests were helpful in making the diagnosis: (1) anterior knee pain with quadriceps contraction (patellofemoral grind test); (2) pain during squatting; and (3) pain on palpation of the posteromedial or posterolateral border of the patella.[115] Although the study found no single maneuver helpful in making the diagnosis, 2 commonly performed maneuvers deserve mention. The patellar tilt test is considered positive (supine patient, extended knee) if downward pressure applied to the medial edge of the patella fails to raise the lateral edge to at least a horizontal level, indicating a tight lateral retinaculum. Similarly, the patellar glide test, performed by assessing side-to-side patellar mobility, is positive if the examiner is unable to shift the patella medially more than one-fourth of its width, again indicating excessive tightness of the lateral retinaculum.

Once a diagnosis of PFPS is made, a full static and dynamic biomechanical examination is warranted to search for causative factors. Static alignment may be normal and malalignment may exist only in the dynamic state (ie, abnormal alignment occurring only with activity). Because the syndrome is multifactorial in origin, and because no universal biomechanical/alignment differences between PFP patients and controls have been demonstrated, patient-specific causative factors must be sought.[116,117]

A static biomechanical assessment should assess for factors such as leg length discrepancy, femoral anteversion, abnormal Q angle, genu varum and valgum, patellar tilt, peripatellar tenderness indicating medial or lateral retinacular stress injury, external tibial torsion, and foot and ankle malalignment. A dynamic examination should search for dynamic abnormalities and muscular weakness. Weakness in the hip abductors and external rotators has been shown to lead to excess internal rotation of the femur and tibia and resultant excessive foot pronation during gait, all contributing to excessive lateral patellar forces and PFPS.[118] In addition, a sudden lateral movement of the patella as the knee nears full extension (a positive J-sign) is also considered abnormal and indicates excessive lateral forces acting on the patella as it exits the femoral trochlea.[119] (Alternatively, the patient can flex the knee, causing a sudden medial shift of the patella as it enters the trochlea in early flexion.)

A complete discussion of the assessment for each of these potentially contributory biomechanical factors is beyond the scope of this article, but it is important to emphasize that these patients demand a full static and dynamic physical examination. The clinician is right to keep in mind that the cause of the syndrome is multifactorial and causative and contributing factors must be sought so that proper individualized therapy may be instituted.

Imaging

Radiographs are usually unnecessary in making the diagnosis but may be helpful in ruling out other causes of knee pain (eg, osteochondritis dissecans osteoarthritis, loose bodies), especially if patients fail to improve after a trial of conservative therapy. Radiographs can also occasionally demonstrate contributing factors such as patella alta or baja or a dysplastic/shallow femoral trochlea (trochlear angle >142°), which have been associated with PFPS.[120]

Treatment

Nonoperative treatment, properly focused on causative factors, can be expected to be successful in 75% to 84% of cases.[121,122]

Physical therapy

Improving patellar tracking, decreasing retinacular strain, and decreasing patellofemoral friction are common goals of physical therapy. Combinations of quadriceps and gluteal strengthening, hamstring stretching, iliotibial band stretching, mediolateral patellar mobilization, hip abductor and external rotator strengthening, and deep friction massage have proved effective in achieving these goals and relieving pain in quality trials.[94] Physical therapy has been reported to decrease pain by up to 90% in some trials[123] and has confirmed effectiveness in the only level 1 randomized controlled trial in the literature.[124] This 6-week double-blind study documented a marked benefit of therapy (and taping) over placebo (sham taping and sham ultrasound) in the short-term treatment of PFPS. The study also had a 3-month noncontrolled follow-up period that suggested that the beneficial effects of therapy/home exercise could be maintained over the longer term.

Taping Taping and bracing have been shown to improve abnormal patellar motion in the coronal and transverse planes,[125] beneficially alter patellar tracking,[126,127] decrease patellofemoral compressive forces,[128] improve proprioception,[129] and alter muscle dynamics in a corrective manner.[130]

Kinesio is a taping method that purportedly lifts the skin, increases the space between skin and muscle, reduces patellar pressure, increases peripatellar circulation, and thereby reduces pain.[131,132] It has been shown to be ineffective in a recent (2011) 6-week randomized controlled trial.[133]

McConnell taping, however, a method of taping that pulls the patella medially, has been found to be effective in 66% of patients in the acute setting, with greater improvements in those with a lower body mass index and a large Q angle.[134] Taping is often used in conjunction with physical therapy, the idea being that taping offers temporary realignment until the full effects of physical therapy and muscular realignment can be gained. A recent cohort study confirmed that 2 weeks of taping followed by 3 months of physical therapy was helpful in reducing symptoms,[135] confirming earlier studies.[136,137] However, the latest randomized controlled trial of 31 women with PFPS demonstrated that taping, when added to standardized physical therapy, added no significant additional benefit to therapy alone at 6 weeks (the taping was applied for the full 6-week duration of the study).[133]

Studies also support the use of knee braces in the treatment of PFPS and moderate improvements in pain have been documented with the use of both a patella brace and a neoprene knee sleeve.[138]

Foot orthoses Confirming the effectiveness of off-the-shelf orthoses in cohort studies,[139,140] one randomized controlled in the literature demonstrated a modest benefit of these orthotics in the short-term treatment of PFPS. This study also noted an additional benefit to patients treated with concomitant physical therapy over a 6-week trial period. The study then followed patients for 1 year and found that orthotics alone, physical therapy alone, and orthotics plus physical therapy all provided equal efficacy, each significantly improving more than 80% of patients. The study did not examine whether or not taping could add further benefit in the short or long term.[141] The latest Cochrane review (2011)[142] concluded that orthoses may provide a marginal short-term benefit to patients with PFPS but that patients "treated with orthoses are more likely to complain of mild adverse effects and discomfort."

Surgery Although surgeons have individual approaches to surgery in the treatment of PFPS,[143] the one randomized trial that we could find in the literature[144] compared patients treated with surgery and physical therapy versus patients treated with therapy alone and found no benefit in the surgically treated group.

Summary

The best evidence to date supports the use of physical therapy in the treatment of PFPS with some additional benefit to be expected, at least in the short term, from taping and orthoses. It is possible that proper patient selection and individualized treatment plans may further improve results in patients with PFPS.

PLICA SYNDROME

Introduction

Anterior knee pain is a common and suboptimally treated condition in the athletic population. Studies[99,145] have shown that more than 54% of patients diagnosed with anterior knee pain have continued symptoms at 5.7 years and 25% have continued symptoms at 20 years. These symptoms remain despite proper conservative management and are significant enough to interfere with participation in sports. The lack of success in treating anterior knee pain has led some investigators[146] to speculate that plica syndrome may be an underdiagnosed cause of such symptoms.

The word plica comes from the Latin word meaning fold but the term is misleading as there has been no evidence demonstrating that true folding of the synovial lining actually occurs.

Anatomy

During embryonic development, the knee is divided by synovial membranes into 3 separate compartments. By the third or fourth month of maturation, the membranes are reabsorbed, and the knee becomes a single chamber. If the membranes fail to reabsorb completely embryonic remnants known as synovial plica are left behind. The plica is considered a vestigial structure, in that its presence has no known functional significance.

Four types of plica (see **Fig. 3**) may be present in the knee: the suprapatellar plica, the infrapatellar plica, the medial plica, and the lateral plica. The prevalence of suprapatellar and infrapatellar plica is roughly 86%,[147] the prevalence of medial plica is 72% to 80%[147,148] and the prevalence of lateral plica is 1% to 1.3%.[147,149]

The medial plica (also referred to as the Aoki ledge, Iino band, or medial shelf) lies in the coronal plane on the medial wall of the joint, originating in the suprapatellar area and coursing obliquely down to insert on the infrapatellar fat pad. This plica is the one most likely to cause symptoms in the athletic population.[150]

The suprapatellar plica, partially dividing the suprapatellar pouch from the remainder of the knee, may also cause symptoms on rare occasions. Symptoms include those of nondescript anterior knee pain, suprapatellar bursitis, or even symptoms mimicking internal derangement or chondromalacia patella.[151]

The infrapatellar plica or ligamentum mucosum arises from the femoral intracondylar notch and inserts anteriorly on the infrapatellar fat pad. This plica is commonly encountered by arthroscopists and tends to interfere with visualization of the knee joint during arthroscopy. Although the infrapatellar plica is rarely responsible for symptoms, at least 2 studies have documented the presence of a painful infrapatellar plica syndrome.[146,152]

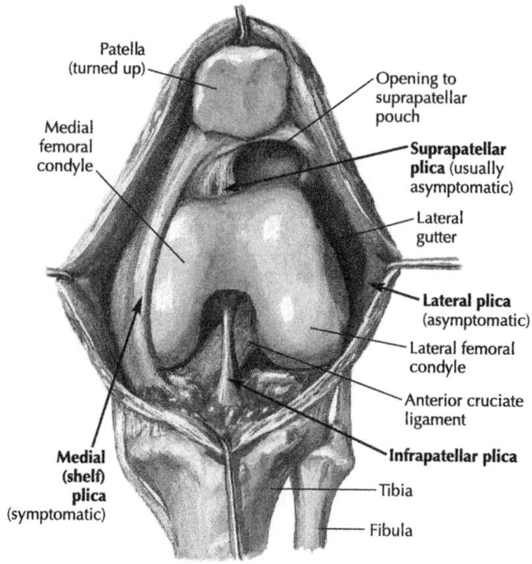

Fig. 3. The 4 types of plica. (Netter illustration from www.netterimages.com. © Elsevier Inc. All rights reserved.)

The lateral synovial plica is the rarest of the plicae (1%–1.3%) and when present, is usually wider and thicker than the medial plica. It arises from the lateral parapatellar synovium and inserts on the lateral patellar facet.

Cause and Histopathology

One cause of plica syndrome is believed to be repetitive stress caused by repetitive friction between an inelastic plica and the femoral condoyle as the patient flexes and extends the knee.[153,154] Direct trauma is another cause, causing the plica to swell and become painful, and eventually may lead to fibrosis.[155] Irritation of the plica may also be caused by loose bodies, altered knee biomechanics as a result of meniscal tears, and infectious/inflammatory conditions. Occasionally, the plica may tear as a result of trauma, which also causes the painful syndrome.[156,157] The most commonly symptomatic plica are the medial plica and the suprapatellar plica.

Normally, plica are soft, wavy, and vascular with synovial-covered edges on arthroscopy. Conversely, examination of plica in symptomatic patients reveals a difference. Histologic samples taken from symptomatic plica initially reveal an edematous hypertrophied synovium. With continued insult, a loss of tissue elasticity, tissue calcification, an ingrowth of hyaline matrix, and fibrosis may occur.[158,159] Continued contact of such a fibrotic plica with the femoral condoyle may lead to erosive chondral lesions of the underlying femoral condoyle or medial pole of the patella.[160]

Clinical Picture

Plica syndrome can occur at any age but is more common during adolescence[161] because of the decreased tissue elasticity that occurs with aging and biomechanical alterations arising from growth spurts.[162]

Making the diagnosis can be difficult because the syndrome can present with symptoms that mimic other common diagnoses, such as patellar tendonosis patellar femoral syndrome, Hoffa syndrome, Sinding-Larsen-Johansson disease, and meniscal tears.

Presenting symptoms include anterior knee pain, locking, catching, clicking, snapping, and giving way. Symptoms are usually aggravated by activity or by prolonged standing, squatting, or sitting.[162]

Physical Examination

Physical examination is crucial in identifying plica syndrome. In most cases, direct palpation over the hypertrophied plica reveals characteristic tenderness. Rovere and colleagues[163] state that a palpably tender plica in the absence of an intra-articular effusion or other pathologic condition conclusively establishes a diagnosis of plica syndrome.

One provocative physical examination test, the mediopatellar plica test (used to detect medial plica syndrome), has reported accuracy and, therefore, deserves mention. This test is conducted with the patient supine and the knee extended. The physician applies pressure to the inferomedial portion of the patellofemoral joint, notes the patient's pain response in this extended position, then flexes the knee to 90°. The test is considered positive when the pain experienced with the knee in extension is eliminated or reduced with flexion. The sensitivity and specificity of this provocative test was reported as 89.5% and 88.7%, respectively, when vetted with arthroscopy.[164]

Occasionally, a positive medial apprehension test of the patella may occur with plica syndrome and, thus, be confused with patellar subluxation. However, with close attention, such tenderness can be properly localized to the plica and patellar instability can be ruled out.

Radiographic Studies

Although most cases of plica syndrome do not require MRI or computed tomography, radiographic examination does play a role in ruling out other causes of knee pain. MRI may show a pathologic plica, if an effusion is present, but more importantly excludes bone bruises, meniscus tears, ligament injuries, cartilage defects, OCD lesions and so forth that may masquerade as plica syndrome. Jee and colleagues,[165] demonstrated that MRI had a 95% sensitivity and 72% specificity; however, plica syndrome was a major research interest at their center and such accuracy has not been reproduced by any other study. The most recent studies[166,167] concur that no useful correlation has been found between MRI findings and confirmation of plica syndrome on arthroscopy.

Dynamic ultrasonography has also initially been reported to be highly effective at detecting abnormalities of medial plica (sensitivity 90%, specificity 83%),[168] but the modality is highly user-dependent and arthroscopy remains the gold standard for definitive diagnosis.[169,170]

Arthroscopic Examination

Some investigators believe that to classify a plica as pathologic, one must not only visualize the plica and impingement but the presence of underlying chondromalacia must also exist in the areas of impingement.

Munzinger and colleagues[171] classified the mediopatellar plica into 4 types based on appearance, as follows:

A - Cordlike
B - Shelflike, does not cover the medial femoral condyle
C - Does cover the medial femoral condyle
D - Double insertion

Jee and colleagues[165] staged medial parapatellar plica according to how far the plica extended into the region of the patellofemoral joint. The following is the system they use:

1+: Does not extend to the medial edge of the patella
2+: Extends to the medial third of medial facet of the patella
3+: Extends over one-third to two-thirds of the medial facet
4+: Extends over more than two-thirds of the medial facet

Treatment

Nonoperative

Conservative treatment involves limiting aggravating activities, correcting any biomechanical abnormalities (eg, tight hamstrings, weak quads), pain relief with nonsteroidal antiinflammatory drugs/cryotherapy, and physical therapy aimed at decreasing compressive forces (increasing quadriceps strength/increasing hamstring flexibility). In 1 study of 136 patients,[172] 60% of patients treated conservatively experienced significant resolution of symptoms after 1 year, whereas the remaining 40% eventually underwent surgery.

Intraplica steroid injection has also been reported to be effective. In 1 small study[173] of 30 patients with established plica syndrome, 73% achieved complete resolution of symptoms and full return to sport after steroid injection. Other investigators, however, question the use of these injections and believe that proper needle placement (and thus delivery of steroids) into the pathologic plica is virtually impossible.[170,174]

However, most investigators would have patients first undergo a trial of conservative therapy for at least 6 to 8 weeks, followed perhaps by a steroid injection, and ultimately, if symptoms persist, surgery. Resected plica will heal back with scar tissue and the procedure has the potential to aggravate symptoms.

Operative treatment

If nonsurgical attempts to reduce symptoms fail, surgery may be indicated. The first goal of the arthroscopic evaluation is to establish that no other intra-articular abnormalities are present. After this, the plica is usually resected back to a point where it no longer impinges on the articular structures. With tough fibrotic plica that drapes over the medial femoral condyle, simple disruption of the tight band may be all that is required to relieve symptoms.

Studies have demonstrated that symptomatic plicae can be successfully treated with arthroscopic resection[175] and excellent results have been documented in up to 70% of patients at follow-ups of up to 8.7 years.[167,176]

One subset of patients seems to do even better in short-term studies. In patients with medial plica syndrome and underlying medial femoral condyle erosive lesions who were treated surgically, excellent results were reported in 94% 6 months after surgery.[177]

Postoperative exercises and rehabilitation can begin shortly after surgery (hours to days) and a full return to sports can usually be expected soon thereafter (within days to 4–6 weeks) Quadriceps strengthening and hamstring flexibility are the mainstay of therapy; correcting any contributing biomechanical abnormalities may also come into play. Therapy advances by gradually including more and more sport-specific exercises until full recovery is achieved.

Interestingly, plica can regrow after resection.

REFERENCES

1. Hede A, Jensen DB, Blyme P, et al. Epidemiology of meniscal lesions in the knee: 1,215 open operations in Copenhagen 1982-84. Acta Orthop Scand 1990;61(5):435–7.

2. Nielsen AB, Yde J. Epidemiology of acute knee injuries: a prospective hospital investigation. J Trauma 1991;31(12):1644–8.
3. Poehling GG, Ruch DS, Chabon SJ. The landscape of meniscal injuries. Clin Sports Med 1990;9(3):539–49.
4. Rath E, John C, Richmond JC. The menisci: basic science and advances in treatment. Br J Sports Med 2000;34:252–7.
5. Seedhom BB, Dowson D. Proceedings: functions of the menisci. A preliminary study. J Bone Joint Surg Br 1974;56:381–2.
6. Duncan JB, Hunter R, Purnell M, et al. Meniscal injuries associated with acute anterior cruciate ligament tears in alpine skiers. Am J Sports Med 1995;23:170–2.
7. Makris EA, Hadidi P, Athanasiou KA. The knee meniscus: structure function, pathophysiology, current repair techniques, and prospects for regeneration. Biomaterials 2011;32(30):7411–31.
8. Arnoczky SP, Warren RF. The microvasculature of the human meniscus. Am J Sports Med 1982;10:90–5.
9. Dye SF, Vaupel GL, Dye CC. Conscious neurosensory mapping of the internal structures of the human knee without intraarticular anesthesia. Am J Sports Med 1998;26:773–7.
10. Levy IM, Torzilli PA, Warren RF. The effect of medial meniscectomy on anterior-posterior motion of the knee. J Bone Joint Surg Am 1982;64(6):883–8.
11. McDermott I. Meniscal tears, repairs and replacement: their relevance to osteoarthritis of the knee. Br J Sports Med 2011;45:292–7.
12. Konan S, Rayan F, Haddad FS. Do physical diagnostic tests accurately detect meniscal tears? Knee Surg Sports Traumatol Arthrosc 2009;17(7):806–11.
13. Karachalios T, Hantes M, Zibis AH, et al. Diagnostic accuracy of a new clinical test (the Thessaly test) for early detection of meniscal tears. J Bone Joint Surg Am 2005;87:955.
14. Harrison BK, Abell BE, Gibson TW. The Thessaly test for detection of meniscal tears: validation of a new physical examination technique for primary care medicine. Clin J Sport Med 2009;19:9.
15. Jackson JL, O'Malley PG, Kroenke K. Evaluation of acute knee pain in primary care. Ann Intern Med 2003;139:575.
16. Solomon DH, Simel DL, Bates DW, et al. The rational clinical examination. Does this patient have a torn meniscus or ligament of the knee? Value of the physical examination. JAMA 2001;286:1610.
17. Ockert B, Haasters F, Polzer H, et al. Value of the clinical examination in suspected meniscal injuries. A meta-analysis. Unfallchirurg 2010;113(4):293–9 [in German].
18. Tarhan NC, Chung CB, Mohana-Borges AV, et al. Meniscal tears: role of axial MRI alone and in combination with other imaging planes. AJR Am J Roentgenol 2004;183:9–15.
19. Terry GC. Reliability of the clinical assessment in predicting the cause of internal derangements of the knee. Arthroscopy 1995;11:568–76.
20. Behairy NH, Dorgham MA, Khaled SA. Accuracy of routine magnetic resonance imaging in meniscal and ligamentous injuries of the knee: comparison with arthroscopy. Int Orthop 2009;33(4):961–7.
21. Fischer SP, Fox JM, Del Pizzo W, et al. Accuracy of diagnoses from magnetic resonance imaging of the knee. A multi-center analysis of one thousand and fourteen patients. J Bone Joint Surg Am 1991;73(1):2–10.
22. Crawford R, Walley G, Bridgman S, et al. Magnetic resonance imaging versus arthroscopy in the diagnosis of knee pathology, concentrating on meniscal lesions and ACL tears: a systematic review. Br Med Bull 2007;84:5–23.

23. Boden SD, Davis DO, Dina TS. A prospective and blinded investigation of magnetic resonance imaging of the knee. Abnormal findings in asymptomatic subjects. Clin Orthop Relat Res 1992;282:177–85.
24. Khan Z, Faruqui Z, Ogyunbiyi O, et al. Ultrasound assessment of internal derangement of the knee. Acta Orthop Belg 2006;72(1):72–6.
25. Greis PE, Bardana DD, Holmstrom MC, et al. Meniscal injury: I. Basic science and evaluation. J Am Acad Orthop Surg 2002;10:168–76.
26. Herrlin S, Hållander M, Wange P, et al. Arthroscopic or conservative treatment of degenerative medial meniscal tears: a prospective randomised trial. Knee Surg Sports Traumatol Arthrosc 2007;15:393–401.
27. Rimington T, Mallik K, Evans D, et al. A prospective study of the nonoperative treatment of degenerative meniscus tears. Orthopedics 2009;32(8). pii.
28. Ménétrey J, Siegrist O, Fritschy D. Medial meniscectomy in patients over the age of fifty: a six year follow-up study. Swiss Surg 2002;8:113–9.
29. Paxton ES, Stock MV, Brophy RH. Meniscal repair versus partial meniscectomy: a systematic review comparing reoperation rates and clinical outcomes. Arthroscopy 2011;27(9):1275–88.
30. Baratz ME. Meniscal tears: the effect of meniscectomy and of repair on intraarticular contact areas and stress in the human knee. A preliminary report. Am J Sports Med 1986;14:270–5.
31. Roos H, Laurén M, Adalberth T, et al. Knee osteoarthritis after meniscectomy: prevalence of radiographic changes after twenty-one years, compared with matched controls. Arthritis Rheum 1998;41:687–93.
32. Papalia R, Del Buono A, Osti L, et al. Meniscectomy as a risk factor for knee osteoarthritis: a systematic review. Br Med Bull 2011;99:89–106.
33. Eggli S, Wegmuller H, Kosina J, et al. Long-term results of arthroscopic meniscal repair. An analysis of isolated tears. Am J Sports Med 1995;23:715–20.
34. Morgan CD, Wojtys EM, Casscells CD, et al. Arthroscopic meniscal repair evaluated by second-look arthroscopy. Am J Sports Med 1991;19:632–7.
35. Scott GA, Jolly BL, Henning CE. Combined posterior incision and arthroscopic intra-articular repair of the meniscus. An examination of factors affecting healing. J Bone Joint Surg Am 1986;68:847–61.
36. Boyd KT, Myers PT. Meniscus preservation; rationale, repair techniques and results. Knee 2003;10(1):1–11.
37. Kramer DE, Micheli LJ. Meniscal tears and discoid meniscus in children: diagnosis and treatment. J Am Acad Orthop Surg 2009;17:698–707.
38. Dickason JM, Del Pizzo W, Blazina ME, et al. A series of ten discoid medial menisci. Clin Orthop Relat Res 1982;168:75–9.
39. Lantz B, Singer KM. Meniscal cysts. Clin Sports Med 1990;9:707–25.
40. De Smet AA, Graf BK, del Rio AM. Association of parameniscal cysts with underlying meniscal tears as identified on MRI and arthroscopy. AJR Am J Roentgenol 2011;196(2):W180–6.
41. McLaughlin J, DeMaio M, Noyes FR. Rehabilitation after meniscus repair. Orthopedics 1994;17:463–71.
42. Kawai Y, Fukubayashi T, Nishino J. Meniscal suture in an experimental study in the dog. Clin Orthop 1989;243:286–93.
43. Cavanaugh JT, Killian SE. Rehabilitation following meniscal repair. Curr Rev Musculoskelet Med 2012;5(1):46–58.
44. Shelbourne KD, Patel DV, Adsit WS. Rehabilitation after meniscus repair. Clin Sports Med 1996;15:595–612.

45. Barber FA. Accelerated rehabilitation for meniscus repairs. Arthroscopy 1994; 10:206–10.
46. Spencer SJ, Saithna A, Carmont MR, et al. Meniscal scaffolds: early experience and review of the literature. Knee 2012;19(6):760–5.
47. Steadman JR, Rodkey WG. Tissue-engineered collagen meniscus implants: 5- to 6-year feasibility study results. Arthroscopy 2005;21(5):515–25.
48. Rodkey WG, DeHaven KE. Comparison of the collagen meniscus implant with partial meniscectomy. A prospective randomized trial. J Bone Joint Surg Am 2008;90:1413–26.
49. Verdonk R, Verdonk P, Huysse W, et al. Tissue ingrowth after implantation of a novel, biodegradable polyurethane scaffold for treatment of partial meniscal lesions. Am J Sports Med 2011;39(4):774–82.
50. Verdonk P. Significant pain reduction functional improvement at 2 years following implantation of a polyurethane meniscus scaffold. Presented at The London Knee Meeting. London, October 14, 2010.
51. Verdonk P, Beaufils P, Bellemans J, et al. Successful treatment of painful irreparable partial meniscal defects with a polyurethane scaffold: two-year safety and clinical outcomes. Am J Sports Med 2012;40(4):844–53.
52. Verdonk PC, Verstraete KL, Almqvist KF, et al. Meniscal allograft transplantation: long-term clinical results with radiological and magnetic resonance imaging correlations. Knee Surg Sports Traumatol Arthrosc 2006;14:694–706.
53. van der Wal RJ, Thomassen BJ, van Arkel ER. Long-term clinical outcome of open meniscal allograft transplantation. Am J Sports Med 2009;37:2134–9.
54. Stone KR, Adelson WS, Pelsis JR, et al. Long-term survival of concurrent meniscus allograft transplantation and repair of the articular cartilage: a prospective two- to 12-year follow-up report. J Bone Joint Surg Br 2010;92:941–8.
55. Crook TB, Ardolino A, Williams LA, et al. Meniscal allograft transplantation: a review of the current literature. Ann R Coll Surg Engl 2009;91(5):361–5.
56. Zellner J, Mueller M, Berner A, et al. Role of mesenchymal stem cells in tissue engineering of meniscus. J Biomed Mater Res A 2010;94(4):1150–61.
57. Pereira H, Frias AM, Oliveira JM, et al. Tissue engineering and regenerative medicine strategies in meniscus lesions. Arthroscopy 2011;27(12):1706–19.
58. Delos D, Rodeo SA. Enhancing meniscal repair through biology: platelet-rich plasma as an alternative strategy. Instr Course Lect 2011;60:453–60.
59. Kopf S, Birkenfeld F, Becker R, et al. Local treatment of meniscal lesions with vascular endothelial growth factor. J Bone Joint Surg Am 2010;92(16):2682–91.
60. McNulty AL, Guilak F. Integrative repair of the meniscus: lessons from in vitro studies. Biorheology 2008;45(3–4):487–500.
61. Khan KM, Cook JL, Bonar F, et al. Histopathology of common tendinopathies. Update and implications for clinical management. Sports Med 1999;27(6): 393–408.
62. Ferretti A, Puddu G, Mariani PP, et al. The natural history of jumper's knee: patellar or quadriceps tendonitis. Int Orthop 1985;8(4):239–42.
63. Lian OB, Engebretsen L, Bahr R. Prevalence of jumper's knee among elite athletes from different sports: a cross-sectional study. Am J Sports Med 2005;33(4): 561–7.
64. Kettunen JA, Kvist M, Alanen E, et al. Long term prognosis for jumper's knee in male athletes. A prospective follow-up study. Am J Sports Med 2002;30(5): 689–92.
65. Rees JD, Maffulli N, Cook J. Management of tendinopathy. Am J Sports Med 2009;37(9):1855–67.

66. Khan KM, Bonar F, Desmond PM, et al. Patellar tendinosis (jumper's knee): findings at histopathologic examination, US, and MR imaging, Victorian Institute of Sport Tendon Study Group. Radiology 1996;200(3):821–7.
67. Riley GP, Goddard MJ, Hazleman BL. Histopathological assessment and pathological significance of matrix degeneration in supraspinatus tendons. Rheumatology (Oxford) 2001;40(2):229–30.
68. Warden SJ, Kiss ZS, Malara FA, et al. Comparative accuracy of magnetic resonance imaging and ultrasonography in confirming clinically diagnosed patellar tendinopathy. Am J Sports Med 2007;35(3):427–36.
69. Eifert-Mangine M, Brewster C, Wong M, et al. Patellar tendinitis in the recreational athlete. Orthopedics 1992;15(11):1359–67.
70. Bahr R, Fossan B, Loken S, et al. Surgical treatment compared with eccentric training for patellar tendinopathy (jumper's knee). A randomized, controlled trial. J Bone Joint Surg Am 2006;88(8):1689–98.
71. Mafi N, Lorentzon R, Alfredson H. Superior short-term results with eccentric calf muscle training compared to concentric training in a randomized prospective multicenter study on patients with chronic Achilles tendinosis. Knee Surg Sports Traumatol Arthrosc 2001;9:42–7.
72. Cannell LJ, Taunton JE, Clement DB, et al. A randomised clinical trial of the efficacy of drop squats or leg – extension/leg curl exercises to treat clinically diagnosed jumper's knee in athletes: pilot study. Br J Sports Med 2001;35(1):60–4.
73. Frohm A, Saartok T, Halvorsen K, et al. Eccentric treatment for patellar tendinopathy: a prospective randomised short-term pilot study of two rehabilitation protocols. Br J Sports Med 2007;41(7):e7.
74. Jonsson P, Alfredson H. Superior results with eccentric compared to concentric quadriceps training in patients with jumper's knee: a prospective randomised study. Br J Sports Med 2005;39(11):847–50.
75. Young MA, Cook JL, Purdam CR, et al. Eccentric decline squat protocol offers superior results at 12 months compared with traditional eccentric protocol forpatellar tendinopathy in volleyball players. Br J Sports Med 2005;39(2):102–5.
76. Larsson ME, Käll I, Nilsson-Helander K. Treatment of patellar tendinopathy–a systematic review of randomized controlled trials. Knee Surg Sports Traumatol Arthrosc 2012;20(8):1632–46.
77. Zwerver J, Hartgens F, Verhagen E, et al. No effect of extracorporeal shockwave therapy on patellar tendinopathy in jumping athletes during the competitive season: a randomized clinical trial. Am J Sports Med 2011;39(6):1191–9.
78. Kongsgaard M, Kovanen V, Aagaard P, et al. Corticosteroid injections, eccentric decline squat training and heavy slow resistance training in patellar tendinopathy. Scand J Med Sci Sports 2009;19:790–802.
79. Capasso G, Testa V, Maffulli N, et al. Aprotinin, corticosteroids and normosaline in the management of patellar tendinopathy in athletes: a prospective randomized study. Sports Exerc Inj 1997;3:111–5.
80. Coombes BK, Bisset L, Vicenzino B. Efficacy and safety of corticosteroid injections and other injections for management of tendinopathy: a systematic review of randomised controlled trials. Lancet 2010;376(9754):1751–67.
81. Ohberg L, Alfredson H. Ultrasound guided sclerosis of neovessels in painful chronic Achilles tendinosis: pilot study of a new treatment. Br J Sports Med 2002;36:173–7.
82. Hoksrud A, Torgalsen T, Harstad H, et al. Ultrasound-guided sclerosis of neovessels in patellar tendinopathy: a prospective study of 101 patients. Am J Sports Med 2012;40(3):542–7.

83. Wang JH, Iosifidis MI, Fu FH. Biomechanical basis for tendinopathy. Clin Orthop Relat Res 2006;443:320–32.
84. Ferry ST, Afshari HM, Lee JA, et al. Effect of prostaglandin E2 injection on the structural properties of the rat patellar tendon. Sports Med Arthrosc Rehabil Ther Technol 2012;4(1):2.
85. Pascual-Garrido C, Rolón A, Makino A. Treatment of chronic patellar tendinopathy with autologous bone marrow stem cells: a 5-year-followup. Stem Cells Int 2012;2012:953510.
86. Kon E, Filardo G, Delcogliano M, et al. Platelet-rich plasma: new clinical application: a pilot study for treatment of jumper's knee. Injury 2009;40(6):598–603.
87. Volpi P, Marinoni L, Bait C, et al. Treatment of chronic patellar tendinosis with buffered platelet rich plasma: a preliminary study. Med Sport 2007;60:595–603.
88. Filardo G, Kon E, Della Villa S, et al. Use of platelet-rich plasma for the treatment of refractory jumper's knee. Int Orthop 2010;34(6):909–15.
89. Friedrich T, Schmidt W, Jungmichel D, et al. Histopathology in rabbit Achilles tendon after operative tenolysis (longitudinal fiber incisions). Scand J Med Sci Sports 2001;11:4–8.
90. Coleman BD, Khan KM, Kiss ZS, et al. Open and arthroscopic patellar tenotomy for chronic patellar tendinopathy: a retrospective outcome study. Victorian Institute of Sport Tendon Study Group. Am J Sports Med 2000;28:183–90.
91. Kelly JD 4th. Arthroscopic excision of distal pole of patella for refractory patellar tendinitis. Orthopedics 2009;32(7):504.
92. Santander J, Zarba E, Iraporda H, et al. Can arthroscopically assisted treatment of chronic patellar tendinopathy reduce pain and restore function? Clin Orthop Relat Res 2012;470(4):993–7.
93. Pascarella A, Alam M, Pascarella F, et al. Arthroscopic management of chronic patellar tendinopathy. Am J Sports Med 2011;39(9):1975–83.
94. Bizzini M, Childs JD, Piva SR, et al. Systematic review of the quality of randomized controlled trials for patellofemoral pain syndrome. J Orthop Sports Phys Ther 2003;33:4–20.
95. Chesworth BM, Culham EG, Tata GE, et al. Validation of outcome measures in patients with patellofemoral pain syndrome. J Orthop Sports Phys Ther 1989;10:302–8.
96. McConnell J. The management of chondromalacia patellae: a long term solution. Aust J Physiother 1986;32:215–23.
97. Wood L, Muller S, Peat G. The epidemiology of patellofemoral disorders in adulthood: a review of routine general practice morbidity recording. Prim Health Care Res Dev 2011;12(2):157–64.
98. Taunton JE, Ryan MB, Clement DB, et al. A retrospective case-control analysis of 2002 running injuries. Br J Sports Med 2002;36:95–101.
99. Nimon G, Murray D, Sandow M, et al. Natural history of anterior knee pain: a 14- to 20-year follow-up of nonoperative management. J Pediatr Orthop 1998;18:118–22.
100. Thomas MJ, Wood L, Selfe J, et al. Anterior knee pain in younger adults as a precursor to subsequent patellofemoral osteoarthritis: a systematic review. BMC Musculoskelet Disord 2010;11:201.
101. Earl JE, Vetter CS. Patellofemoral pain. Phys Med Rehabil Clin N Am 2007;18:439–58.
102. Witvrouw E, Lysens R, Bellemans J, et al. Intrinsic risk factors for the development of anterior knee pain in an athletic population. A two-year prospective study. Am J Sports Med 2000;28:480–9.

103. Fredericson M, Powers CM. Practical management of patellofemoral pain. Clin J Sport Med 2002;12:36–8.
104. Powers CM. Rehabilitation of patellofemoral joint disorders: a critical review. J Orthop Sports Phys Ther 1998;28(5):345–54.
105. Van Tiggelen D, Cowan S, Coorevits P, et al. Delayed vastus medialis obliquus to vastus lateralis onset timing contributes to the development of patellofemoral pain in previously healthy men: a prospective study. Am J Sports Med 2009; 37(6):1099–105.
106. Lankhorst NE, Bierma-Zeinstra SM, van Middelkoop M. Risk factors for PFS. J Orthop Sports Phys Ther 2012;42(2):81–94.
107. Sanchis-Alfonso V, Rosello-Sastre E, Martinez-Sanjuan V. Pathogenesis of anterior knee pain syndrome and functional patellofemoral instability in the active young. Am J Knee Surg 1999;12:29–40.
108. James SL, Jones DC. Biomechanical aspects of distance running injuries. In: Cavanagh PR, editor. Biomechanics of distance running. Champaign (IL): Human Kinetics Books; 1990. p. 249–69.
109. Herrington L, Nester C. Q-angle undervalued? The relationship between Q-angle and medio-lateral position of the patella. Clin Biomech 2004;19:1070–3.
110. Boling MC, Padua DA, Marshall SW, et al. A prospective investigation of biomechanical risk factors for patellofemoral pain syndrome: the Joint Undertaking to Monitor and Prevent ACL Injury (JUMP-ACL) cohort. Am J Sports Med 2009; 37(11):2108–16.
111. Powers CM. The influence of abnormal hip mechanics on knee injury: a biomechanical perspective. J Orthop Sports Phys Ther 2010;40(2):42–51.
112. Powers CM. The influence of altered lower-extremity kinematics on patellofemoral joint dysfunction: a theoretical perspective. J Orthop Sports Phys Ther 2003;33(11):639–46.
113. LaBella C. Patellofemoral pain syndrome: evaluation and treatment. Prim Care 2004;31(4):977–1003.
114. Cook C, Hegedus E, Hawkins R, et al. Diagnostic accuracy and association to disability of clinical test findings associated with patellofemoral pain syndrome. Physiother Can 2010;62:17–24.
115. Nijs J, van Geel C, van der Auwera C, et al. Diagnostic value of five clinical tests in patellofemoral pain syndrome. Man Ther 2006;11:69–77.
116. Thomee R, Renstrom P, Karlsson J, et al. Patellofemoral pain syndrome in young women. I. A clinical analysis of alignment, pain, parameters, common symptoms and functional activity level. Scand J Med Sci Sports 1995;5(4):237–44.
117. Kannus P, Nittymaki S. Which factors predict outcome in the nonoperative treatment of patellofemoral pain syndrome? A prospective follow-up study. Med Sci Sports Exerc 1994;26(3):289–96.
118. Host J, Craig R, Lehman R. Patellofemoral dysfunction in tennis players: a dynamic problem. Clin Sports Med 1995;14:177–203.
119. Fulkerson JP, Kalenak A, Rosenberg TD, et al. Patellofemoral pain. Instructional course outlines. Rosemount (IL): American Academy of Orthopaedic Surgeons; 1994. 57–71.
120. Fulkerson J. Disorders of the patellofemoral joint. 3rd edition. Baltimore (MD): Williams & Wilkins; 1997. p. 153–4.
121. Douchette SA, Goble EM. The effect of exercise on patellar tracking in lateral patellar compression syndrome. Am J Sports Med 1992;20:434–40.
122. DeHaven KE, Dolan WA, Mayer PJ. Chondromalacia patellae in athletes. Clinical presentation and conservative management. Am J Sports Med 1979;7:5–11.

123. Dursun N, Dursun E, Kilic Z. Electromyographic biofeedback- Controlled exercise versus conservative care for patellofemoral pain syndrome. Arch Phys Med Rehabil 2001;82:1692–5.
124. Crossley KM, Bennell KL, Green S, et al. Physical therapy for patellofemoral pain. A randomized, double-blinded, placebo-controlled trial. Am J Sports Med 2002; 30(6):857–65.
125. Selfe J, Thewlis D, Hill S, et al. A clinical study of the biomechanics of step descent using different treatment modalities for patellofemoral pain. Gait Posture 2011; 34(1):92–6.
126. Derasari A, Brindle TJ, Alter KE, et al. McConnell taping shifts the patella inferiorly in patients with patellofemoral pain: a dynamic magnetic resonance imaging study. Phys Ther 2010;90(3):411–9.
127. Herrington L. The effect of corrective taping of the patella on patella position as defined by MRI. Res Sports Med 2006;14(3):215–23.
128. Mostamand J, Bader DL, Hudson Z. The effect of patellar taping on joint reaction forces during squatting in subjects with patellofemoral pain syndrome (PFPS). J Bodyw Mov Ther 2010;14(4):375–81.
129. Callaghan MJ, Selfe J, McHenry A, et al. Effects of patellar taping on knee joint proprioception in patients with patellofemoral pain syndrome. Man Ther 2008; 13(3):192–9.
130. Mostamand J, Bader DL, Hudson Z. The effect of patellar taping on EMG activity of vasti muscles during squatting in individuals with patellofemoral pain syndrome. J Sports Sci 2011;29(2):197–205.
131. Chen PL, Hong WH, Lin CH, et al. Biomechanics effects of kinesio taping for persons with patellofemoral pain syndrome during stair climbing. In: Abu Osman NA, Ibrahim F, Wan Abas WA, et al, editors. Biomed 2008, Proceedings 21. Berlin: Springer; 2008. p. 395–7.
132. Chen WC, Hong WH, Huang TF, et al. Effects of kinesio taping on the timing and ratio of vastus medialis obliquus and vastus lateralis muscle for person with patellofemoral pain. J Biomech 2007;40:318, XXI ISB Congress, 1–5 July 2007, Taiwan, Podium Sessions.
133. Akbaş E, Atay AO, Yüksel I. The effects of additional kinesio taping over exercise in the treatment of patellofemoral pain syndrome. Acta Orthop Traumatol Turc 2011;45(5):335–41.
134. Lan TY, Lin WP, Jiang CC, et al. Immediate effect and predictors of effectiveness of taping for patellofemoral pain syndrome: a prospective cohort study. Am J Sports Med 2010;38(8):1626–30.
135. Paoloni M, Fratocchi G, Mangone M, et al. Long-term efficacy of a short period of taping followed by an exercise program in a cohort of patients with patellofemoral pain syndrome. Clin Rheumatol 2012;31(3):535–9.
136. Clark DI, Downing N, Mitchell J, et al. Physiotherapy for anterior knee pain: a randomised controlled trial. Ann Rheum Dis 2000;59:700–4.
137. Whittingham M, Palmer S, Macmillan F. Effects of taping on pain and function in patellofemoral pain syndrome: a randomized controlled trial. J Orthop Sports Phys Ther 2004;34(9):504–10.
138. Lun VM, Wiley JP, Meeuwisse WH, et al. Effectiveness of patellar bracing for treatment of patellofemoral pain syndrome. Clin J Sport Med 2005;15(4): 235–40.
139. Barton CJ, Menz HB, Crossley KM. Effects of prefabricated foot orthoses on pain and function in individuals with patellofemoral pain syndrome: a cohort study. Phys Ther Sport 2011;12(2):70–5.

140. Barton CJ, Menz HB, Crossley KM. The immediate effects of foot orthoses on functional performance in individuals with patellofemoral pain syndrome. Br J Sports Med 2011;45(3):193–7.
141. Collins N, Crossley K, Beller E, et al. Foot orthoses and physiotherapy in the treatment of patellofemoral pain syndrome: randomised clinical trial. Br J Sports Med 2009;43(3):169–71.
142. Hossain M, Alexander P, Burls A, et al. Foot orthoses for patellofemoral pain in adults. Cochrane Database Syst Rev 2011;(1):CD008402.
143. Teitge RA. Patellofemoral syndrome a paradigm for current surgical strategies. Orthop Clin North Am 2008;39(3):287–311, v.
144. Kettunen JA, Harilainen A, Sandelin J, et al. Knee arthroscopy and exercise versus exercise only for chronic patellofemoral pain syndrome: a randomized controlled trial. BMC Med 2007;13(5):38.
145. Blønd L, Hansen L. Patellofemoral pain syndrome in athletes: a 5.7-year retrospective follow-up study of 250 athletes. Acta Orthop Belg 1998;64(4):393–400.
146. Boyd CR, Eakin C, Matheson GO. Infrapatellar plica as a cause of anterior knee pain. Clin J Sport Med 2005;15:98–103.
147. Kim SJ, Choe WS. Arthroscopic findings of the synovial plicae of the knee. Arthroscopy 1997;13:33–41.
148. Nakayama A, Sugita T, Aizawa T, et al. Incidence of medial plica in 3,889 knee joints in the Japanese population. Arthroscopy 2011;27(11):1523–7.
149. Dupont JY. Synovial plicae of the knee. Controversies and review. Clin Sports Med 1997;16(1):87–122.
150. Sznajderman T, Smorgick Y, Lindner D, et al. Medial plica syndrome. Isr Med Assoc J 2009;11(1):54–7.
151. Pipkin G. Knee injuries: the role of the suprapatellar plica and suprapatellar bursa in simulating internal derangements. Clin Orthop 1971;74:161–76.
152. Demirag B, Ozturk C, Karakayali M. Symptomatic infrapatellar plica. Knee Surg Sports Traumatol Arthrosc 2006;14(2):156–60.
153. Lyu SR. Relationship of medial plica and medial femoral condyle during flexion. Clin Biomech (Bristol, Avon) 2007;22:1013–6.
154. Hardaker WT, Whipple TL, Bassett FH 3rd. Diagnosis and treatment of the plica syndrome of the knee. J Bone Joint Surg Am 1980;62(2):221–5.
155. Kim SJ, Kim JY, Lee JW. Pathologic infrapatellar plica. Arthroscopy 2002;18:E25.
156. Kerimoglu S, Citlak A, Cavusoglu S, et al. Bucket-handle tear of medial plica. Knee 2005;12:239–41.
157. Hansen H, Boe S. The pathological plica in the knee. Results after arthroscopic resection. Arch Orthop Trauma Surg 1989;108:282–4.
158. Lyu SR, Tzeng JE, Kuo CY, et al. Mechanical strength of mediopatellar plica—the influence of its fiber content. Clin Biomech 2006;21:860–3.
159. Farkas C, Hargitai Z, Gaspar L, et al. Histological changes in the symptomatic mediopatellar plica. Knee 2004;11:103–8.
160. Christoforakis J, Sanchez-Ballester N, Hunt R, et al. Synovial shelves of the knee: association with chondral lesions. Knee Surg Sports Traumatol Arthrosc 2006;14:1292–8.
161. Irha E, Vrdoljak J. Medial synovial plica syndrome of the knee: a diagnostic pitfall in adolescent athletes. J Pediatr Orthop B 2003;12(1):44–8.
162. Duri ZA, Patel DV, Aichroth PM. The immature athlete. Clin Sports Med 2002;21(3):461–82, ix.
163. Rovere GD, Nichols AW. Frequency, associated factors, and treatment of breaststroker's knee in competitive swimmers. Am J Sports Med 1985;13(2):99–104.

164. Kim SJ, Lee DH, Kim TE. The relationship between the MPP test and arthoscopically found medial patellar plica pathology. Arthroscopy 2007;23:1303–8.
165. Jee WH, Choe BY, Kim JM, et al. The plica syndrome: diagnostic value of MRI with arthroscopic correlation. J Comput Assist Tomogr 1998;22:814–8.
166. Boles CA, Butler J, Lee JA, et al. Magnetic resonance characteristics of medial plica of the knee: correlation with arthroscopic resection. J Comput Assist Tomogr 2004;28:397–401.
167. Weckström M, Niva MH, Lamminen A, et al. Arthroscopic resection of medial plica of the knee in young adults. Knee 2010;17(2):103–7.
168. Paczesny L, Kruczynski J. Medial plica syndrome of the knee: diagnosis with dynamic sonography. Radiology 2009;251:439–46.
169. Shetty VD, Vowler SL, Krishnamurthy S, et al. Clinical diagnosis of medial plica syndrome of the knee: a prospective study. J Knee Surg 2007;20(4):277–80.
170. Johnson DP, Eastwood DM, Witherow PJ. Symptomatic synovial plicae of the knee. J Bone Joint Surg Am 1993;75:1485–96.
171. Munzinger U, Ruckstuhl J, Scherrer H, et al. Internal derangement of the knee joint due to pathologic synovial folds: the mediopatellar plica syndrome. Clin Orthop 1981;155:59–64.
172. Amatuzzi MM, Fazzi A, Varella MH. Pathologic synovial plica of the knee. Results of conservative treatment. Am J Sports Med 1990;18:466–9.
173. Rovere GD, Adair DM. Medial synovial shelf plica syndrome. Treatment by intraplical steroid injection. Am J Sports Med 1985;13:382–6.
174. Griffith CJ, LaPrade RF. Medial plica irritation: diagnosis and treatment. Curr Rev Musculoskelet Med 2008;1(1):53–60.
175. Dorchak JD, Barrack RL, Kneisl JS. Arthroscopic treatment of symptomatic synovial plica of the knee. Long-term followup. Am J Sports Med 1991;19:503–7.
176. Flanagan JP, Trakru S, Meyer M, et al. Arthroscopic excision of symptomatic medial plica. A study of 118 knees with 1–4 year follow-up. Acta Orthop Scand 1994;65:408–11.
177. Guney A, Bilal O, Oner M, et al. Short- and mid-term results of plica excision in patients with mediopatellar plica and associated cartilage degeneration. Knee Surg Sports Traumatol Arthrosc 2010;18(11):1526–31.

Foot and Ankle Update

Ahmed Saleh, MD[a], Ramin Sadeghpour, MD[b],
John Munyak, MD[c,d,*]

KEYWORDS

• Achilles • Tendon rupture • Thompson test • Ankle sprain • High ankle sprain
• Jones fracture • Fifth metatarsal • Lisfranc

KEY POINTS

- In patients with acute ruptures of the Achilles tendon, surgical management decreases rerupture rates, but is associated with an increased rate of complications, primarily in higher-risk populations.
- All acute ankle sprains should be treated conservatively regardless of grade; however, patients with multiple recurrent sprains or functional instability should be considered for surgical intervention.
- In patients with suspected syndesmotic injuries, full length tibia/fibula radiographs in addition to 3 views of the ankle should be considered to rule out a proximal fibula fracture.
- In patients with proximal fifth metatarsal fractures, the exact location of the fracture line will dictate the treatment.
- Lisfranc injuries are perhaps the most commonly missed orthopedic injury of the foot. Accurate diagnosis is crucial, as missed injuries may lead to long-term disability.
- Most stress fractures of the foot and ankle are generally uncomplicated, and can be managed by brief periods of immobilization and non–weight bearing.
- A few high-risk stress fractures (medial malleolus, tarsal navicular, sesamoid, and base of the fifth metatarsal) must be distinguished from their low-risk counterparts, as they have a higher likelihood of progressing to nonunion and/or delayed union.

RUPTURES OF THE ACHILLES TENDON

Introduction

The Achilles tendon is the largest tendon in the body. It is a confluence of the gastrocnemius and soleus muscles, and inserts on the most posterior aspect of the calcaneus. The tendon works as the primary plantar flexor of the foot. The tendon rotates

The authors of this text have no financial relationships to disclose.
[a] PGY-3, Department of Orthopaedic Surgery, Maimonides Medical Center, 927 49th Street, Brooklyn, NY 11219, USA; [b] Department of Orthopaedic Surgery, Maimonides Medical Center, 927 49th Street, Brooklyn, NY 11219, USA; [c] Sports Medicine, Department of Orthopaedic Surgery, Maimonides Medical Center, 927 49th Street, Brooklyn, NY 11219, USA; [d] Brooklyn Nets Basketball, 927 49th Street, Brooklyn, NY 11219, USA
* Corresponding author. Sports Medicine, Department of Orthopaedic Surgery, Maimonides Medical Center, 927 49th Street, Brooklyn, NY 11219.
E-mail address: jmunyak@maimonidesmed.org

Prim Care Clin Office Pract 40 (2013) 383–406
http://dx.doi.org/10.1016/j.pop.2013.02.015 primarycare.theclinics.com
0095-4543/13/$ – see front matter

as it inserts onto the calcaneus. There is a relatively avascular section of the tendon approximately 2 to 6 cm from its insertion site.[1] This area of the tendon is the most likely to rupture.

Nature of the Problem

Achilles tendinopathy is usually secondary to overuse injuries. It is commonly seen in runners. Adults in their third to fifth decades of life are most susceptible to ruptures of the Achilles tendon. These injuries occur more commonly in men.[2] In patients with suspected ruptures, a thorough history should be taken, including:

- History of inflammatory disorders
- Recent fluoroquinolone usage
- Local steroid injections[3]

Symptom Criteria

Patients with acute ruptures of the Achilles tendon often complain of a sensation of being struck in the back of the leg during the time of rupture. Often they experience preceding pain at the site of the tendon. Mechanisms of injury include maximal dorsiflexion of the foot, or forced dorsiflexion of a plantarflexed foot.[1] Some patients may experience retrocalcaneal pain before a rupture, secondary to chronic tendonitis/tendinosis.[4]

Clinical Findings

Inspection:

- Significant swelling and ecchymosis may be present on the back of the leg.
- A palpable gap may also be present at the site of the rupture.

Physical Examination:

- Decreased strength in plantarflexion.
- *Thompson test:* Place the patient in the prone position and have them flex the knee up. Next squeeze the calf; a positive test reveals no plantarflexion of the foot, indicating a ruptured tendon.[5]

Imaging

To aid in the diagnosis of ruptures of the Achilles tendon, several imaging modalities may be considered.

- *Radiography*. Although the tendon cannot be directly visualized on a plain film, a radiograph does help to rule out any other causes of heel pain, including fractures.
- *Ultrasonography* will directly visualize the tendon and aid in the diagnosis of a tendon rupture. It is also helpful in dynamically evaluating the tear during a full range of motion for nonsurgical and surgical intervention.
- *Magnetic resonance imaging (MRI)* can also directly visualize the tendon. MRI may be helpful before surgical intervention to help identify the length of the gap between both ends of the tendon. In chronic tears, it may also reveal the length of tendinosis of the tendon, which may once again help guide surgical treatment.[4]

Treatment

There are significant controversies as to how acute ruptures of the Achilles tendon should be treated. A thorough discussion with the patients regarding their goals and preferences is important to help guide their treatment.

- *Nonsurgical treatment*. Ruptures of the Achilles tendon may be treated nonoperatively with the use of a cast or by keeping the foot in a plantarflexed position (**Table 1**). Nonoperative treatment is associated with higher rerupture rates is surgery. For athletes, return to sports should be no sooner than 3 months, but may take as long as 6 months for complete activity. Some patients may require physical therapy to help regain full range of motion and strength after treatment.[1]
- *Surgical treatment*. The gold standard of surgical treatment is an open end-to-end repair of the tendon. Limited open and percutaneous procedures are also described; however, there are no definite recommendations favoring the use of one technique over another.[5] Patients treated surgically have a lower rerupture rate than patients treated nonoperatively; however, they have increased rates of complications from surgery such as skin sloughing, sural nerve damage, and wound infections.[6,7] High-risk groups for developing complications from surgery are smokers, diabetics, and elderly patients.[5]
    - Patients with chronic tears with gaps between the two ends of the tendons may require more extensive surgical procedures, such as a V-Y advancement of the gastrocnemius or a flexor hallucis longus (FHL) autograft transfer. In some cases an allograft may also be used.[4]

Current Controversies

- There is no consensus as to whether casting is more superior to a boot with heel lift. However, there are some preliminary studies suggesting that patients treated with functional bracing with early range of motion therapy have rerupture rates approaching those of surgical treatment.[3]
- Although most providers protect the weight bearing of the patient after casting or bracing, there is no consensus regarding how long a patient's weight-bearing status should be protected.
- At present, there is no evidence suggesting superiority of open Achilles tendon repair when compared with percutaneous techniques. Rerupture rates appear to be similar, with decreased wound complications with percutaneous techniques.[3,6]

ANKLE SPRAINS

Introduction

Ankle sprains are one of the most commonly encountered musculoskeletal injuries. It is estimated that 1 out of every 10 people in the United States experiences an ankle sprain at some time. Most of these injuries occur during athletic activity, but many also occur with other activities such as walking on uneven ground. Men between the ages of 15 and 24 years are more likely than their female counterparts to experience an ankle sprain. However, women older than 30 years are more likely than men to sprain their ankles.[8] Ankle sprains occur secondary to an inversion and/or twisting

Table 1
Treatment of Achilles tendon rupture and guidelines for return to play

	Treatment and Return-to-Play Guidelines
Nonoperative treatment	1. Non–weight bearing in a cast in plantarflexion for 6 wk 2. Walking boot with heel lift for 6 wk (may begin therapy for range of motion at this time) 3. At 12 wk, patient may begin to walk unprotected 4. At 4–6 mo, patient may begin running 5. After 6 mo, patient may return to sports

injury of the ankle. The most common mechanism of injury is inversion of a plantar-flexed foot, which puts a strain primarily on the lateral ligaments of the ankle.[9]

Nature of the Problem

The ankle is a very complex joint comprising several bony articulations, which are stabilized by multiple different ligaments.[9–11] There are 3 primary ligamentous complexes that help stabilize the ankle (**Table 2**).

The lateral ligaments are 10 times more likely than the medial ligaments to be injured during an ankle sprain. Because of the inversion nature of the injuries around the ankle, the anterior talofibular ligament (ATFL) is the most commonly injured ligament, but severe injuries may also cause tears of the calcaneofibular ligament (CFL) or even fractures of the distal fibula. Lateral ankle sprains may be graded according to the severity of the injury to the ATFL (**Table 3**).[9]

Symptom Criteria

As for all musculoskeletal injuries, a thorough history should be taken to understand the nature of the injury. The mechanism of the injury and the position of the foot at the time of the injury are important facts to elicit from the patient, as it can provide clues as to which ligament was injured. Inversion of the foot leads to lateral ligament injuries, whereas eversion injuries lead to syndesmotic or deltoid ligament injuries, and fractures may result from both mechanisms.[9]

Symptoms can differ greatly according to the severity of the sprain. For grade 1 sprains, patients usually present with mild to moderate pain at the anterolateral aspect of ankle. Patients with more severe sprains may present with difficulty ambulating or even bearing weight on that extremity. Swelling and ecchymosis is commonly seen.

For patients with recurrent or chronic ankle sprains one should attempt to elicit a history of functional instability, defined as a subjective feeling of ankle instability or a feeling of the ankle giving way with normal daily activities.[12]

Differential Diagnosis

Because of the complex anatomy of the foot, other injuries around the foot and ankle may be mistaken for an ankle sprain. Other common injuries that may be mistaken for ankle sprains are[3]:

- Ankle fractures
- Syndesmotic injuries
- Lateral process of the talus fractures (snowboarder's fracture)
- Anterior process of the calcaneus fractures

Table 2
The 3 ligamentous complexes of the ankle

Lateral ligamentous complex (lateral ankle sprain)	Anterior talofibular ligament (ATFL) Calcaneofibular ligament (CFL) Posterior talofibular ligament (PTFL)
Medial ligamentous complex (medial ankle sprain)	Superficial and deep deltoid ligaments
Syndesmotic ligaments (high ankle sprain)	Anterior inferior tibiofibular ligament (AITFL) Posterior inferior tibiofibular ligament (PITFL) Interosseous membrane Inferior transverse ligament

Table 3
Lateral ankle sprain grading

Grade 1	Stretching of the fibers of the ATFL
Grade 2	Partial tear of the fibers of the ATFL
Grade 3	Complete rupture of the ATFL

- Jones fractures: fifth metatarsal fracture at the metaphyseal-diaphyseal junction
- Pseudo-Jones fractures: fifth metatarsal tuberosity avulsion fracture
- Osteochondral defects of the talus
- Achilles tendon tears
- Peroneal tendon tears or strains

Clinical Findings

Inspection. On visual inspection of the injured foot, significant swelling and ecchymosis may be noted.

Physical examination. As with all musculoskeletal injuries, a thorough neurovascular examination should be performed. Next, all bony prominences should be palpated to help aid in ruling out a fracture. The lateral malleolus, lateral process of the talus, medial malleolus, base of the fifth metatarsal, and the fibula from proximal to distal should be palpated. The strength of the Achilles tendon and peroneal tendons should be tested as well.

- Anterior drawer test: This physical-examination maneuver tests the competency of the ATFL to prevent anterior translation of the foot. The test is performed by plantarflexing the foot about 20° and pulling forward on the heel, noting how much anterior translation of the foot occurs. A positive anterior drawer test is when there is more translation on the injured side than there is on the noninjured side, or about a 3- to 5-mm difference.[9] It may be difficult to perform this test in an acute setting secondary to pain and swelling.
- Talar tilt/inversion/varus test: This physical-examination maneuver is used in the evaluation of an ankle sprain involving both the ATFL and the CFL to test their competency in preventing inversion of the talus. Testing the ankle in neutral or slight dorsiflexion primarily assesses the CFL, whereas positioning the ankle in plantarflexion primarily assesses the ATFL. When performing this test it is important to grasp the leg just proximal to the malleoli with one hand and apply the inversion force while grasping the hindfoot/lateral aspect of the talus, to ensure that the talus is tilting. A combined injury to the ATFL and CFL results in increased talar tilt on the injured side in comparison with the noninjured side, with minimal increases in talar tilt when only the ATFL is injured. An angulation greater than 23° or a difference of more than 10° when compared with the uninjured ankle indicates injuries to the ATFL and CFL.[9]

Imaging

- *Radiography*. Because ankle sprains are so common and radiographic findings are lacking in most patients, the Ottawa Ankle Rules are often used to determine whether a radiograph is indicated for a patient. If the patient has pain around one of the malleoli and any 1 of these other 3 criteria, an ankle radiograph is indicated[13]:
  - Bony tenderness along the most distal 6 cm of the posterior aspect of the lateral or medial malleoli

- Age over 55 years
- Inability to bear weight on the injured extremity for 4 steps

Radiographs should be thoroughly examined to help identify other commonly missed injuries such as the ones described above.

- *MRI*. MRI may be useful in patients with persistent ankle pain with no significant radiographic findings. MRI may help reveal occult fractures, tendon tears, or talar dome osteochondral defects, and can even help delineate the extent of ligament tears. In patients with chronic or recurrent ankle sprains, there may also be a case for obtaining an MRI.[14]

Treatment of Acute Ankle Sprains

- *Nonsurgical treatment*. The treatment of ankle sprains can vary widely according to the severity of the injury. The mainstay of most ankle sprains is Rest, Ice, Compression, and Elevation (RICE).[9,14] However, for more severe injuries, casting, taping, bracing, or CAM-boot immobilization may be used in the treatment of ankle sprains. Treatment is usually continued until the patient is asymptomatic; however cast immobilization should not be continued for more than 2 to 3 weeks, owing to residual ankle stiffness. Some studies reveal that patients treated with functional bracing and therapy have an earlier return to sports than patients treated with cast immobilization. There was also no significant difference in the recurrence of ankle sprains between these 2 groups.[15]

After an initial period of immobilization, patients should undergo therapy on the ankle with a focus on range of motion, strengthening, and proprioceptive exercises. These exercises have been shown to decrease recurrent ankle sprains in athletes (**Table 4**).[15]

- *Surgical treatment*. Surgical management of an acute ankle sprain is rarely indicated.

Treatment of Recurrent/Chronic Ankle Sprains

Patients who experience recurrent ankle sprains with minimal trauma and are having symptoms of ankle instability have likely developed incompetence of the ATFL.[9,14] The ligament may be so severely attenuated that even if it has healed, it provides little to no functional benefit. Patients who are experiencing these symptoms may require surgical treatment to help repair or reconstruct this ligamentous complex. In such patients, it is important to elicit a history of recurrent sprains, even with minimal trauma to the ankle.

Table 4
Treatment of ankle sprain and guidelines for return to play

	Treatment and Return-to-Play Guidelines
Ankle sprain	1. RICE protocol 2. Protected weight bearing if necessary 3. Rarely, severe sprains may benefit from brief cast or air CAM boot immobilization 4. Physical therapy (including range of motion, strength, and proprioception) 5. Return to play when pain and swelling have completely resolved

- *Nonsurgical treatment*. For patients with recurrent ankle sprains, a trial of nonoperative management can be attempted before the exploration of surgical options. Patients can be treated in a short leg cast for 4 to 6 weeks, followed by a walking boot, and proprioceptive physical therapy exercises.
- *Surgical treatment*. Surgical management of ankle sprains is reserved only for patients who have failed conservative management. These patients often complain of multiple ankle sprains, even with minimal activity, as well as functional instability.
  - Broström procedure: Direct repair of a torn or attenuated ATFL ligament. In some patients, the ligament must be cut and shortened to restore anatomic alignment.[14]
  - Evans, Watson-Jones, Chrismann-Snook procedures: Reconstructive procedures whereby the tendon of the peroneus brevis is brought through the fibula to help stabilize the lateral column of the ankle.[14]

A recent study revealed that patients treated with surgery had rates of return to activity similar to those who were treated with functional therapy. However, there was a significant increase in the reinjury rate of patients treated with functional therapy when compared with patients treated with surgery.[15,16]

Current Controversies

- There is good evidence to support the use of ankle orthoses for both primary and secondary prevention of ankle sprains. However, there is currently no consensus in the orthopedic literature regarding the most superior ankle orthotic to use after an ankle sprain. Studies are currently being conducted comparing patients treated with taping of the ankle, ankle bracing, and no ankle support at all.[17]

SYNDESMOTIC INJURY (HIGH ANKLE SPRAINS)

Introduction

Whereas ankle sprains are one of the most commonly encountered musculoskeletal injuries, the syndesmotic injuries, otherwise known as high ankle sprains, account for only about 1% of all ankle sprains. The diagnosis of these injuries can easily be missed, and proper treatment can be delayed. Syndesmotic injuries usually occur in athletes. Unlike the common ankle sprain, which is usually secondary to an inversion injury of the foot, most syndesmotic injuries occur as a result of an eversion and external rotation injury of the foot.[11] These injuries occur in sports when the foot is planted and the tibia internally rotates in relation to the foot.

Nature of the Problem

The ankle is a very complex joint comprising several bony articulations, which are stabilized by multiple different ligaments.[9–11] As previously mentioned, there are 3 primary ligamentous complexes that help stabilize the ankle: the lateral, medial, and syndesmotic ligaments.

The syndesmotic ligaments play a crucial role in stabilizing the ankle joint. The function of these ligaments is to stabilize the fibula to the tibia. The anterior-inferior tibiofibular ligament (AITFL) attaches from the distal anterior tibia to the distal anterior fibula. The posterior-inferior tibiofibular ligament (PITFL) attaches from the distal posterior tibia to the distal posterior fibula. The interosseous membrane runs between the fibula and tibia along nearly the entire length of the two bones. Incompetence of the syndesmosis will cause instability between the tibia and fibula, primarily in the anterior to posterior direction.[10,11,18]

Syndesmotic injures are usually purely ligamentous injuries, but the ligaments can also be compromised in conjunction with fractures around the ankle. Fractures of the medial malleolus or ruptures of the deltoid ligament may be associated with syndesmotic injuries.[11] Although ruptures of the syndesmotic ligaments are more common, avulsion fractures from their insertion sites may also occur. An avulsion of the AITFL from the tibial side creates a Chaput fragment, whereas an avulsion from the fibular side is known as a Wagstaffe fragment. An avulsion of the PITFL is known as a Volkmann fragment.[10]

Symptom Criteria

Syndesmotic injuries may be difficult to diagnose. As with all musculoskeletal disorders, a thorough history detailing the mechanism of injury is important in aiding a diagnosis. It is important to determine the position of the foot during the time of injury, and whether it was an inversion or eversion injury. As with all ankle sprains, the extent of a patient's symptoms may differ greatly according the extent of the injury. Patients may experience pain, swelling, and ecchymosis of the ankle. The patient may not be able to bear weight on the injured extremity, or may have a sensation of ankle instability.

Clinical Findings

Physical examination. As with all musculoskeletal injuries, a thorough neuromuscular examination should be performed. All bony prominences should be palpated, special attention being paid to the medial malleolus and the entire length of the fibula. The location of the AITFL and PITFL can also be palpated. Pain directly over this area can point to a syndesmotic injury. Some physical-examination maneuvers that can help with the diagnosis are:

- Squeeze test: This test is performed by squeezing the proximal tibia and fibula together at the level of the calf. This maneuver places stress on the distal syndesmotic ligaments, therefore in a positive test the patient's pain is reproduced over the distal syndesmotic ligaments.[11,19]
- External rotation stress test: This test is performed by flexing the knee and placing the foot in a neutral position. The foot is then externally rotated as the knee is stabilized. A positive test causes the patient to feel pain over the distal syndesmotic ligaments.[11]

Imaging

- *Radiography*. In patients with suspected syndesmotic injuries, radiographs are an integral part of obtaining a diagnosis. As previously mentioned, syndesmotic injuries can often accompany fractures. Providers should obtain 3 views of the ankle, including anteroposterior (AP), lateral, and mortise views. Radiographs should be examined carefully to rule out any fractures, most commonly of the medial malleolus and distal fibula. Even if no fractures are present, several radiographic parameters suggest syndesmotic ligament injury.
  - Medial clear space: The medial clear space is observed on the mortise radiograph. The clear space between the talus and the medial malleolus should be equivalent to the space between the talus and the tibial plafond, or less than 4 mm. Evidence of widening of the medial clear space signifies a rupture of the deltoid ligament.[10,19]
  - Tibiofibular clear space (**Fig. 1**): This radiographic parameter is observed on an AP radiograph of the ankle and is measured 1 cm above the joint line. There should be a gap of no more than 6 mm between the medial border of the fibula

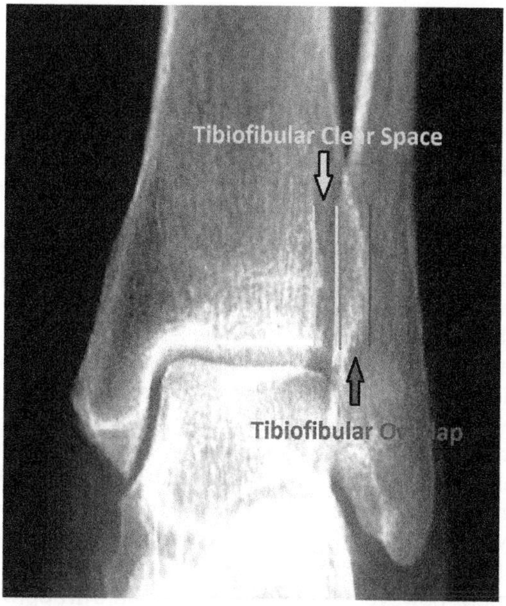

Fig. 1. Tibiofibular clear space and tibiofibular overlap on a normal ankle radiograph.

and the posterior edge of the tibia. A gap greater than 6 mm suggests a widening of the syndesmosis. A gap greater than 10 mm is a syndesmotic injury.[10,19]

- Tibiofibular overlap (see **Fig. 1**): This radiographic parameter is observed on an AP radiograph of the ankle. There should be a minimum of 6 mm of overlap between the fibula and tibia. An overlap of less than 6 mm suggests a syndesmotic injury.[10,19]

- Another extremely important radiograph to obtain for ankle fractures is a full-length tibia/fibula radiograph. Because of its mechanism, it is possible that the energy of the injury travels up the interosseous membrane and exits at the proximal fibula, causing a proximal fibula fracture. When this fracture occurs in conjunction with a deltoid ligament rupture causing widening of the medial clear space, this fracture is classically termed a Maisonneuve fracture.
- *MRI*. MRI may have some utility in the diagnosis of syndesmotic injuries. Patients with persistent ankle pain with no radiographic findings may benefit from an MRI. MRIs can reveal the fine anatomy of the syndesmotic ligaments as well as that of the interosseous membrane, and can also aid in the diagnosis of occult fractures.[10,19]

Treatment

The treatment of syndesmotic injuries can vary greatly from nonsurgical to surgical, according to the severity of the injury.

- *Nonsurgical management*. Patients with symptoms of a syndesmotic injury or high ankle sprain, with no evidence of radiographic widening, can be treated nonoperatively. These injuries are notorious for taking a longer time to heal than normal ankle sprains. Patients with these injuries can be treated in a cast or air walking boot. For minor sprains, some providers will keep the patient non–weight bearing for approximately 3 to 4 weeks, then begin protected weight bearing and therapy on that extremity.[11,19]

- For patients with more severe sprains, or even patients with minimal evidence of syndesmotic widening on radiographs, treatment usually consists of a short leg cast for 6 weeks, provided that the syndesmosis remains reduced on the postcasting radiographs.[10]

- *Surgical management*. There are several indications for surgery in patients with syndesmotic injuries. Patients with gross widening of the syndesmosis should have the syndesmosis surgically reduced and stabilized. Patients with a medial malleolus fracture should also have the fracture surgically stabilized. Associated distal fibula fractures are also surgically stabilized.[10–17]
  - Several techniques and implants can be used in stabilization of the syndesmosis; however, no single technique or implant has been shown to be more superior in vivo. In general, fixation of the syndesmosis is obtained by fixing the distal fibula to the distal tibia with the use of screws, plates, or suture "tightrope" constructs. Fixation is placed 2 to 4 cm proximal to the joint. After surgery, patients are kept non–weight bearing for approximately 10 to 12 weeks.[19]
  - With the onset of weight bearing, these screws can and usually do break. Studies have shown that there is no difference in outcome for patients with broken implants, because by that time the syndesmosis should be fully healed. Some providers, however, will remove the hardware at approximately 12 weeks to avoid this issue.[19]

Current Controversies

There are many controversies regarding the treatment of syndesmotic injuries. Although studies looking at each of these issues are ongoing, to date there is no consensus in the literature regarding these issues.

- To avoid removal of the syndesmotic screw, some providers have started to use bioabsorbable screws, which begin to degrade after the 3-month period for which they are needed to help the syndesmosis heal. These screws have been shown to be equivalent to metal screws in syndesmotic fixation.[10]
- Some providers advocate suture or "tightrope" fixation techniques for syndesmotic fixation. The idea is that the distal tibiofibular articulation is a joint that even under nonpathologic conditions allows for some movement. The suture technique holds the syndesmosis together long enough to allow the syndesmosis to heal, but still allows a small amount of physiologic movement.[19] There is also no need for removal of hardware when patients undergo suture fixation.
- There is also significant controversy regarding the number of screws, the size of the screws, whether or not a plate should be used, and how many cortices the screw should penetrate. Biomechanical studies have shown stronger fixation with larger screws, more screws, and more cortices, but to date these have not been shown to affect patient outcomes.[10]

FIFTH METATARSAL FRACTURES

Introduction

Fractures of the proximal fifth metatarsal are a commonly encountered cause of foot pain in the clinical setting. For such a small location, there are several different fracture patterns that are imperative for the clinician to be able to differentiate. Each fracture pattern is treated differently. A thorough understanding of the anatomy and pathology is necessary to help correctly guide treatment of these fractures.

Nature of the Problem

The proximal fifth metatarsal has two articulations, one with the cuboid and the other with the fourth metatarsal. There are several soft-tissue attachments to this small area as well. The peroneus brevis and lateral band of the plantar fascia attach proximally on the fifth metatarsal, and the peroneus tertius attaches a little more distally at the metaphyseal-diaphyseal junction of the fifth metatarsal.[20] These articulations help to separate the 3 most common fractures of the proximal fifth metatarsal.

The Torg classification is often used to describe fractures of the fifth metatarsal (**Fig. 2**). Zone 1, or proximal tuberosity fractures, is the most common fracture pattern. This fracture is often referred to as a pseudo-Jones fracture.[20,21] These fractures are usually caused by an avulsion of either the peroneus brevis or lateral band of the plantar fascia.[20] Depending on the size of the fragment, the fracture may or may not extend into the fifth metatarsocuboid joint. In Zone 2 or Jones fractures, the fracture line is slightly more distal and extends into the fourth/fifth metatarsal joint. Fractures distal to the fourth/fifth metatarsal joint are Zone 3 fractures, and are usually diaphyseal stress fractures (**Table 5**).[20,21]

The vascularity of the proximal fifth metatarsal is supplied proximally by a metaphyseal arcade and more distally by a diaphyseal nutrient artery. This process causes a watershed zone of decreased vascularity at the location of the metaphyseal-diaphyseal junction at the level where Jones fractures commonly occur.[22] This configuration explains the high rate of nonunion of Jones fractures, and why 2 fractures in such close proximity are treated very differently. More distal fractures disrupt the vascularity because of rupture of the nutrient artery.[22]

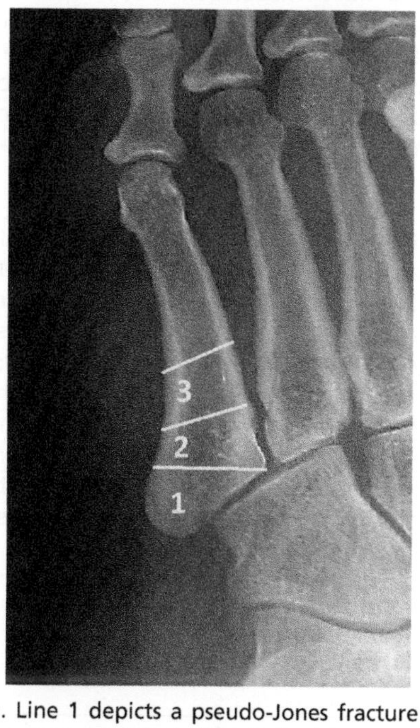

Fig. 2. Torg classification. Line 1 depicts a pseudo-Jones fracture or zone 1 injury. Line 2 depicts a Jones fracture or zone 2 injury. Line 3 depicts a metatarsal shaft fracture or zone 3 injury.

Table 5
Torg classification for fractures of base of the fifth metatarsal

Fracture	Torg Classification	Fracture Line
Tuberosity fracture (pseudo-Jones fracture)	Zone 1	Distal avulsion fracture, may propagate into the fifth metatarsocuboid joint
Jones fracture	Zone 2	Fracture line extends into the fourth/fifth metatarsal joint
Diaphyseal stress fracture	Zone 3	Fracture line is distal to the fourth/fifth metatarsal joint

Symptom Criteria

A thorough history is an important part of the diagnosis of these fractures. Patients who have repetitive cyclical loading of their foot are at a higher risk for developing these fractures. These types of fracture are common in athletes and runners, but can often occur secondary to a twisting injury of the foot.[22,23] Patients present with pain at the lateral aspect of their foot. It is important to determine the chronicity of the pain. Tuberosity and Jones fractures are usually secondary to an acute injury, whereas diaphyseal stress fractures are usually preceded by prodromal pain.[22,23]

Clinical Findings

Although the physical signs may be subtle, swelling and ecchymosis may be present. In patients with stress fractures, there may be no significant physical examination findings other than tenderness along the fifth metatarsal.

Physical examination. As with all musculoskeletal complaints, a thorough neurovascular examination should be performed. Muscle strength should be assessed to rule out any tendon abnormality. All bony prominences should be palpated to determine the point of maximal tenderness. These fractures can often be missed, or mistaken for ankle sprains. Palpation of the lateral and medial malleoli is important to help rule out an ankle fracture.

Imaging

- *Radiography*. In patients with a suspected fifth metatarsal fracture, 3 views of the foot are indicated, as previously mentioned. It is important to determine the exact location of the fracture line, as this will help dictate the treatment of the fracture. In some patients with stress fractures there may be no significant radiographic appearance initially. In patients with a high index of suspicion of a stress fracture with no radiographic abnormalities, close follow-up with repeat radiographs is recommended.[24] Radiography follow-up is also important in patients with Jones fractures to assess adequate healing and callus formation. If this is not apparent after treatment, the provider must consider the possibility of a nonunion. A computed tomography (CT) scan can sometimes be useful to help determine the extent of bony healing that has occurred.
- *MRI*. MRI can be very useful in patients with a suspected stress fracture with no radiographic abnormalities. An exact fracture line can often be observed with a high-quality MRI.[24]

Treatment

- Tuberosity fractures (pseudo-Jones fractures): Because of the location of these fractures, and the ample blood supply from the metaphyseal vessels, they tend to heal at a high rate. These fractures are usually treated symptomatically. Patients can be treated with a hard-sole shoe or walking boot as well as rest and activity modification until symptoms resolve. If the patient has a significant amount of pain, weight bearing may be protected for a short period of time.[20–23]

- Jones fractures: These fractures occur through the watershed zone of the fifth metatarsal, and therefore are treated very differently to tuberosity fractures.
  - Nonoperative management: Patients should be placed in a short leg cast, and kept non–weight bearing for 6 to 8 weeks. If radiographic healing is evident, the patient can be transitioned into a fracture brace or walking boot.[25]
  - Surgical management: Because of the high rates of nonunion, high-demand athletes should be treated with surgery. Surgical fixation is achieved with intramedullary screw fixation. Also, patients with little to no evidence of healing after 6 to 8 weeks of casting and non–weight bearing should be considered for surgical intervention.[20–25]
- Diaphyseal stress fractures: These fractures are also very common in athletes, and can also be very difficult to treat. It is important to determine the chronicity of the fracture. Many of these fractures have to be treated surgically to achieve full healing.
  - Nonoperative treatment: Patients should be placed in a short leg cast and kept non–weight bearing for 6 to 8 weeks. If radiographic healing is evident, the patient can be transitioned into a fracture brace or walking boot.[22,23]
  - Operative treatment is indicated in these fractures in athletes, owing to a high nonunion rate. Patients with a lengthy prodromal course before diagnosis will also likely require surgical management. As with the treatment of Jones fractures, fixation is usually achieved with intramedullary screw fixation. However, open reduction and bone-grafting techniques have also been described.[22,23]

Current Controversies

There are many controversies regarding the treatment of fractures of the fifth metatarsal.

- Some providers advocate fixation of tuberosity fractures that are intra-articular and have significant step-off of the fifth metatarsal cuboid joint, whereas others advocate a removal of the bony fragment with preservation of the peroneus brevis insertion.[20]
- There has also been some recent evidence suggesting that shock-wave therapy can be as efficacious as surgery in the treatment of Jones fractures.[26]
- Because fracture healing can take as long as 20 weeks in some patients, there are no definite guidelines as to how long a patient should stay immobilized and non–weight bearing. Cast immobilization for 6 to 8 weeks is generally recommended; however, the risks of joint stiffness and prolonged immobilization must be considered.

LISFRANC INJURIES

Introduction

The Lisfranc joint complex includes the medial, middle, and lateral cuneiforms, along with the cuboid, and the articulations with the 5 metatarsal bases. The unique anatomy of the Lisfranc joint makes it a vital structure in both the transverse and longitudinal arches of the foot. The trapezoidal shape of the middle 3 metatarsal bases and their associated cuneiforms produce a stable arch referred to as the transverse arch or Roman arch (**Fig. 3**). The keystone to this arch is the second tarsometatarsal joint,

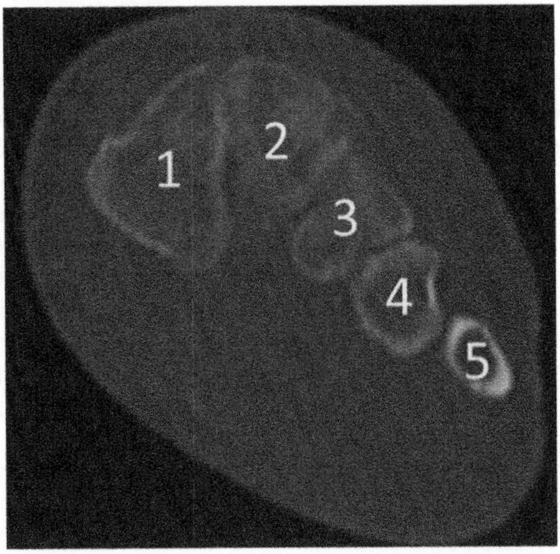

Fig. 3. Roman arch configuration of the metatarsals. Corresponding metatarsals are labeled 1 to 5, with great toe labeled as 1.

which has inherent longitudinal stability owing to its position within the recessed middle cuneiform. The Lisfranc ligament, which is the strongest ligament of the tarsometatarsal joint complex, runs from the medial cuneiform to the base of the second metatarsal. Injuries to the Lisfranc joint can be very easy to miss, given their rarity and subtle findings on examination. Also, the lack of obvious radiographic findings in up to 33% of cases and the lack of familiarity with these injuries by treating physicians adds to the difficulty with regard to proper diagnosis.[27,28] Although these injuries are uncommon, the importance of accurate diagnosis is crucial because missed injuries may lead to long-term disability. To properly diagnose these injuries, the treating physician must have a high index of suspicion for this type of injury, and know the clinical examination findings and appropriate imaging studies to order.

Nature of the Problem

Injuries to the tarsometatarsal joint occur in 1 out of every 55,000 people in the United States, accounting for 0.2% of all fractures.[29] Nearly 20% of these injuries are missed or misdiagnosed on initial radiographic assessment.[30] Physicians must be suspicious for a Lisfranc injury in certain clinical scenarios so that they may avoid the devastating complications of misdiagnosis such as posttraumatic arthritis and flatfoot deformity. Injuries to the Lisfranc joint may be grouped as direct and indirect injuries. With direct injuries, such as a crush injury to the foot, the clinician's index of suspicion is already very high, and these injuries are often easier to pick up. These high-energy direct injuries are often associated with significant soft-tissue trauma, vascular compromise, and compartment syndrome.[31] Indirect injuries are often the result of low-energy mechanisms and require a higher index of suspicion. Indirect injuries are most commonly the result of a longitudinal force on the forefoot, which then undergoes rotation and compression.[32] Any mechanism of injury that involves excessive abduction and plantarflexion should also raise suspicion for possible indirect Lisfranc disruption. Excessive plantarflexion can be seen in the patient who misses a step or unexpectedly catches his or her heel on a curb as they are stepping down. Another classic scenario to be aware of is the football player who, while lying prone, has another player land on his heel. This impact leads to an excessive external rotation force on the fixed prone forefoot that can lead to severe ligamentous injury.[33] Other examples of indirect injuries with excessive abduction forces occur in such sports that require foot straps or stirrups. Horseback riding and windsurfing are 2 sports commonly associated with Lisfranc injuries. In these injuries, the forefoot is abducted around a fixed hindfoot that can lead to dislocation of the second tarsometatarsal joint, as well as the so-called nutcracker fracture of the cuboid as it is compressed during extreme abduction. Treating physicians must be aware that these low-energy mechanisms of injury often have a presentation similar to that of other soft-tissue sprains, and have a high index of suspicion for Lisfranc injury. Investigators have reported Lisfranc injuries to be the injury most commonly missed in the emergency department.[34]

Symptom Criteria

Patients will often complain of difficulty with ambulation and pain in the midfoot/forefoot region. Some patients may recall feeling a pop when the injury occurred. A clinician must be wary of pain out of proportion to examination, as compartment syndrome may occur with these injuries.

Clinical Findings

Inspection:

- Significant swelling of the midfoot or entire foot may be present.
- Plantar ecchymosis is considered to be pathognomonic for a Lisfranc injury.
- Dorsal ecchymosis may be present as well.

Physical examination:

- Test for inability to bear weight on the foot.
- Passively pronate and abduct the foot to see if any pain is elicited. Make sure to keep the hindfoot fixed during this test.
- Piano key test: The physician grasps the first and second metatarsals and dorsiflexes/plantarflexes/adducts/abducts them to test for any instability or pain.
- Compartment syndrome should be considered in these patients.
- Always assess for the dorsalis pedis pulse, as it may be injured with dislocations.

Imaging

To properly diagnose Lisfranc injuries, an understanding of normal radiographic foot anatomy is needed. Of vital importance is determining whether the injury is stable or unstable. If not obvious from standard radiographs, standing (stress) views of the foot should be taken to assess for stability. Most investigators set a threshold of displacement of more than 2 mm compared with the contralateral side.[19]

- *Radiography*. AP, lateral, and 30° oblique views of the injured foot taken parallel to the midfoot joint should be obtained. If concern for a subtle injury is suspected, weight-bearing radiographs of bilateral feet should be obtained for comparison, thus providing a stress view of the foot. On the AP view, diastasis of greater than 2.7 mm between the first and second metatarsal is considered abnormal.[35] Also on the AP, the medial aspect of the second metatarsal should line up with the medial aspect of the middle cuneiform (**Fig. 4**A). On the oblique view, the medial aspect of the fourth metatarsal should line up with the medial aspect of the cuboid (see **Fig. 4**B). Also, one should always look for the fleck sign (**Fig. 5**), pathognomonic for Lisfranc injury, on the AP and oblique views, as this represents an avulsion of the Lisfranc ligament from either the medial cuneiform or

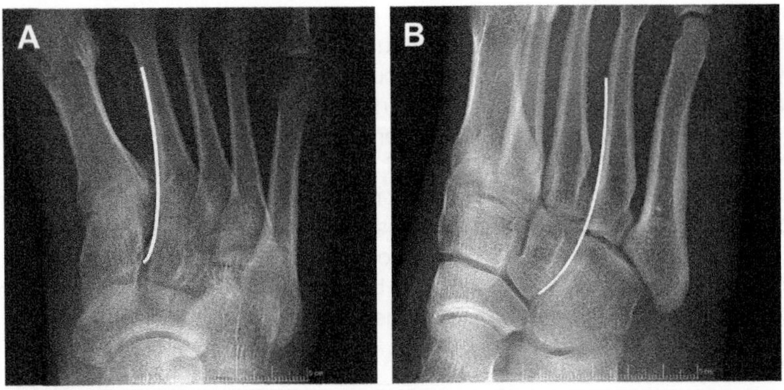

Fig. 4. (*A*) Proper anatomic relationship of the medial aspect of the second metatarsal lining up with the medial aspect of the middle cuneiform. (*B*) Normal anatomic relationship of the medial aspect of the fourth metatarsal lining up with the medial aspect of the cuboid.

second metatarsal base. On the lateral view there should be no step-off, dorsal or plantar, between the metatarsal shafts and their respective tarsal bones (**Fig. 6**B).

- *CT scan*. CT may be used in any instance when further fracture delineation is needed. These scans often help assess for comminution and intra-articular extension that may help plan for surgery. An important aspect to note is that CT scans are non–weight bearing and therefore are not helpful on assessing stability of the midfoot after injury.
- *MRI*. When physical examination and plain radiographs are equivocal, MRI can be used to evaluate the soft tissues. Also, in the high-level athlete MRI findings

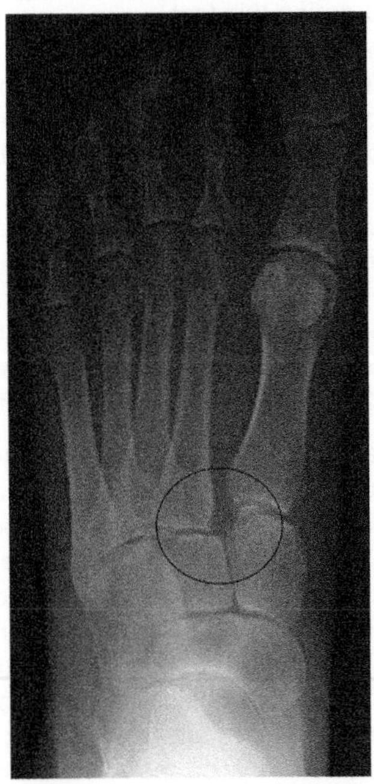

Fig. 5. The fleck sign (*circled*) that is pathognomonic for a Lisfranc injury.

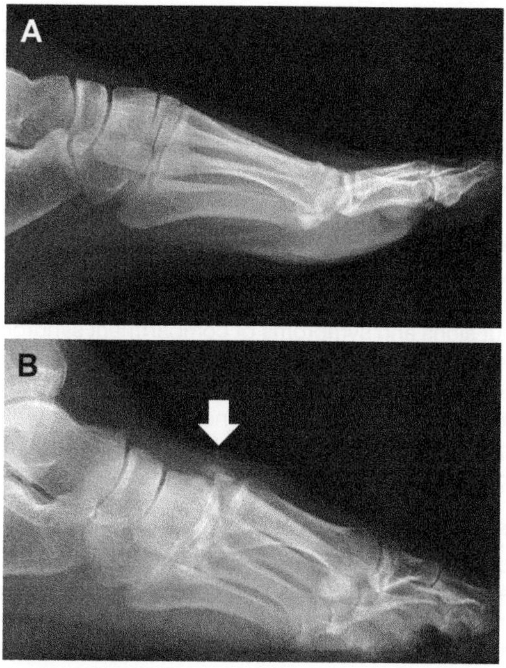

Fig. 6. (*A*) Normal anatomic relationships without step-off between the metatarsal and tarsal bones. (*B*) Obvious step-off (*arrow*) noted at the tarsometatarsal joint secondary to a Lisfranc injury.

may be helpful in determining return-to-play status.[33] Lisfranc ligament injuries can be classified as grade I (pain at the joint, with minimal swelling and no instability) or grade II (increased pain and swelling at the joint, with mild laxity but no instability). The more severe grade III sprain represents complete ligamentous disruption and may represent fracture-dislocation.[36] In a recent study, Raikin and colleagues[37] found that rupture or grade II sprains of the Lisfranc ligament found on MRI are highly predictive of midfoot instability, and that these patients should undergo surgery (**Table 6**).

- *Ultrasonography*. The current role of ultrasonography in diagnosing Lisfranc injuries is under investigation. A recent case series has demonstrated that sonographic features might prove successful in predicting unstable joints requiring intervention.[34]

Table 6
Grading and treatment guidelines for sprain of Lisfranc ligament complex

Grade I Lisfranc sprain	Pain at the joint, minimal swelling, no instability	No weight bearing in cast for minimum 3–6 wk followed by progressive weight bearing
Grade II Lisfranc sprain	Pain and swelling at joint, mild laxity, but no instability	No weight bearing for 6 wk followed by progressive weight bearing
Grade III Lisfranc sprain	Complete ligamentous disruption and/or fracture-dislocation	Surgical intervention required

Treatment

Once a Lisfranc injury is diagnosed, the decision of surgical versus nonsurgical stabilization must be made. In either case the goal of treatment is to obtain a stable, painless, plantigrade foot.[27]

- *Nonsurgical treatment*. Nonoperative treatment is reserved for nondisplaced and stable injuries only. It is imperative to demonstrate weight-bearing stability if nonoperative treatment is to be undertaken.[38] A well-padded short leg cast or boot is applied, and the patient is made non–weight bearing for 4 to 6 weeks. Progressive weight bearing is as tolerated, and follow-up weight-bearing radiographs are taken approximately 2 to 3 weeks after injury. Patients should be educated about signs and symptoms of compartment syndrome, and instructed to come immediately to the emergency room should they occur.
- *Surgical treatment*. With any degree of displacement, anatomic reduction becomes essential.[38] All unstable injuries, including subtle ones, should be treated surgically, and referral to an orthopedic surgeon should be within 7 days. Surgical treatment involves either open reduction and internal fixation or fusion.

Current Controversies

- Most of the controversy surrounding Lisfranc injuries concerns surgical treatment and the decision to perform open reduction and internal fixation rather than fusion for primary Lisfranc injury. However, there is no controversy regarding treatment of these injuries by operative versus nonoperative treatment. Any unstable and/or displaced injury needs surgical intervention.

Summary

- Lisfranc injury is a rare orthopedic injury that is often missed on initial presentation.
- If missed or misdiagnosed, it may lead to devastating posttraumatic arthritis and flatfoot deformities.
- The treating clinician must have a high index of suspicion for this type of injury and should know the mechanism of injury, clinical examination findings, and appropriate imaging studies to order.
- It is imperative to demonstrate weight-bearing stability if nonoperative treatment is to be undertaken.
- If any instability exists or there is significant displacement (>2 mm), referral to an orthopedic surgeon is indicated.

STRESS FRACTURES

Introduction

Stress fractures are relatively common injuries in the athletic and military population. The reported incidence in the sports population has been recorded at 1%, although in runners it is as high as 20%.[39] Common areas of stress fractures in the foot and ankle include the medial malleolus, tarsal bones, metatarsals, and sesamoids. Most of these stress fractures are uncomplicated and can be managed by brief periods of immobilization and non–weight bearing. However, there does exist a subset of high-risk fractures that must be distinguished from their low-risk counterparts, as they have a higher likelihood of progressing to nonunion and or delayed union. These high-risk fractures include fractures of the medial malleolus, tarsal navicular, sesamoid, and proximal fifth metatarsal fractures. Proximal fifth metatarsal fractures are discussed in the section on fifth metatarsal fractures.

Nature of the Problem

Stress fractures result from repetitive, excessive, submaximal loads on bones that cause an imbalance between bone resorption and formation.[39] Both intrinsic and extrinsic factors can contribute to the development of stress fractures. The clinician should be very thorough with history taking and inquire about:

- Recent increase in physical activity, footwear, and playing surfaces
- Medical history (diabetes, endocrinopathies, autoimmune disorders)
- Menstrual cycle, always being aware of the female athlete triad, which includes amenorrhea, anorexia, and osteoporosis[24]
- Dietary history including calcium, vitamin D, protein, and alcohol consumption

Symptom Criteria

Patients with stress fractures often complain of a 2- to 3-week history of insidious pain, generally correlated with a recent increase in activity, training habits, and shoe wear.[40] There is typically a history of acute and or repetitive trauma to the foot.[41] The symptoms are generally exacerbated with activity and alleviated by rest. Mechanisms of injury vary, depending on the site of stress fracture. More important to the treating clinician is to be aware of certain patient populations such as runners, military recruits, and ballet dancers, who are especially at risk for stress fractures.

Clinical Findings

Inspection:

- Superficial stress fractures may exhibit local swelling and palpable periosteal thickening.
- Ecchymosis and severe swelling may be present with displaced fractures.

Physical examination:

- Bone tenderness by direct palpation is the most consistent physical examination finding.[42–44]
- Percussion of the bone away from the site of injury may cause pain at the fracture site.
- A single leg-hop test can also elicit pain.

Imaging

Although a stress fracture may be diagnosed based on a thorough history and physical examination, specific imaging studies may be helpful in confirming the diagnosis.

- *Radiography*. Plain radiography is the most useful imaging modality for initial radiographic assessment of stress fractures of the lower extremity.[24] Early radiographic findings may include a subtle linear radiolucency or poor definition of the cortex. Radiographic findings typically lag several weeks behind clinical symptoms, and may not appear at all if activity has been modified.[45] If initial radiographs are negative and a stress fracture is suspected, repeat radiographs should be obtained in 2 weeks, as they may reveal a fracture or periosteal reaction. If a more urgent diagnosis is needed, a bone scan or MRI may be ordered.[46]
- *Bone scan*. This highly sensitive test can detect fractures days to weeks earlier than radiographs. One of the shortcomings of the bone scan is that it is not very specific and can pick up any process that remodels bone such as tumor, infection, or stress reaction. The additional use of a single-photon emission CT scan can improve specificity.

- *MRI*. Highly sensitive and specific, MRI allows evaluation of soft tissues and provides greater anatomic detail than plain radiography. MRI is highly sensitive for endosteal marrow edema and periosteal edema, which are typically the first features of stress fractures.[47] It is considered to be as sensitive as and more specific than a bone scan in detecting stress fractures.[48]
- *CT scan*. CT is rarely used in initial diagnosis of stress fractures, secondary to high radiation doses in comparison with conventional radiography and lower sensitivity compared with MRI. CT is usually reserved for cases where detailed osseous anatomy is needed and in evaluation of nonunion.

Treatment

The first step of treatment is to determine any predisposing factors for injury and to correct them. A full medical evaluation may be needed for patients with hormonal or nutritional abnormalities. For most cases of stress fractures, treatment consists of rest and immobilization. It is important to classify the fracture as low-risk or high-risk to help with appropriate nonoperative or operative treatment.[24]

- *Low-risk fractures* (**Table 7**). These fractures are usually diagnosed through history, examination, and plain radiographs. Appropriate initial treatment is with activity restriction and rest for 1 to 6 weeks, with progressive weight bearing begun thereafter. Once the patient can tolerate low-impact activities, gradual transition to higher-impact activities is begun.
- *High-risk fractures* (**Table 8**). High-risk stress fractures have a predilection for progressing to complete fracture, delayed union, or nonunion; therefore, they present treatment challenges and require a more aggressive treatment approach.[39] These fractures include medial malleolus fractures, tarsal navicular, fifth metatarsal, and great toe sesamoid fractures. Suspected high-risk stress fractures with negative radiographs and a positive bone scan should be given an initial trial of aggressive nonoperative treatment with cast immobilization of the extremity. The exception to this rule is the high-performance athlete who wants to return to play. In this case, surgical intervention may be warranted. Any displaced stress fractures, fractures that have failed nonoperative treatment, and fractures with chronic radiographic findings such as cystic changes or sclerosis also require operative intervention.[19]
- *Preventive measures*. Ideally the best management of these injuries is prevention. It is important to counsel patients on excessive training, and appropriate shoe wear and training surfaces. Athletes, military recruits, and coaches should also

Table 7
Low-risk stress fractures of the foot and ankle: guidelines for treatment and return to play

Low-Risk Fracture	Nonoperative	Surgical	Return to Play
Distal 2–4 metatarsal	Weight bearing as tolerated in walking boot	Only needed if fractures displace or go on to nonunion	4–6 wk
Proximal 2–4 metatarsal (higher risk compared with distal fracture)	4–6 wk non–weight bearing in short leg cast	Displaced fractures, nonunion and delayed union	4–6 wk
Calcaneus	Weight bearing as tolerated in boot	Displaced fractures, malunion, delayed union	4–6 wk

Table 8
High-risk stress fractures of the foot and ankle: guidelines for treatment and return to play

High-Risk Fracture	Nonoperative Treatment (Nondisplaced Fractures)	Surgical Treatment	Return to Play
Medial malleolus	Cast immobilization and avoidance of impact activities for 4–6 wk	Indicated for failed nonoperative treatment, nonunion or high-level athlete. Internal fixation with malleolar screws	*Nonsurgical:* May take 2–5 mo to fully heal *Surgical:* 6–8 wk
Proximal fifth metatarsal	Cast immobilization and strict non–weight bearing for minimum 6–8 wk, followed by fracture brace or walking boot for 6–8 wk	Failed nonoperative treatment and high-level athlete/dancer. Intramedullary screw fixation	*Nonsurgical:* 3–6 mo *Surgical:* 3–6 mo (decreased rate of nonunion compared with nonsurgical)
Navicular	Cast immobilization and strict non–weight bearing for 6 wk, transfer to walking boot for 6 wk, rehab 6 wk	Displaced, nonunion, and delayed unions. Internal fixation with compression screws. Non–weight bearing for 4 wk postoperatively followed by progressive weight bearing	*Nonsurgical:* 5–6 mo *Surgical:* 8–12 wk postsurgery. Radiograph before athletic return encouraged
Great toe sesamoids	Cast immobilization and strict non–weight bearing for 6 wk (ensure to cast distal to toes to prevent dorsiflexion). Progressive weight bearing in postoperative shoe for 2 wk	Displaced, nonunions, and delayed unions. Surgical options include sesamoidectomy and bone grafting. Postoperative cast 2 wk	*Nonsurgical:* 6 wk *Surgical:* 2–6 wk

be educated about the importance of rest days and (with female athletes) the importance of eating habits.

Current Controversies

- Recent interest has been shown in the development of pharmacologic agents to assist in fracture healing. Several studies involving the administration of bisphosphonates to aid in the healing of stress fractures have been published. Unfortunately, to date there are no well-designed clinical trials to support their use.
- Studies involving pulsed ultrasound as well as extracorporeal shock-wave therapy as adjuncts to aid in stress-fracture healing have also been the topic of recent interest. Again, there is insufficient evidence at this time to support the use of either modality as an adjunct to treating stress fractures of the foot and ankle.

SUMMARY

- Stress fractures commonly occur in the foot and ankle, and may result in significantly delayed healing if not treated appropriately.
- Both intrinsic and extrinsic factors should be sought after as causes of stress fractures; therefore, a thorough history is imperative.

- Distinguishing between low-risk and high-risk stress fractures is crucial to providing appropriate treatment.
- Excellent results have been obtained with conservative treatment of low-risk fractures, and even high-risk fractures, with activity restrictions and limited weight bearing.
- Surgical intervention may be required in high-risk athletes who desire to return to work soon and in those whose conservative treatment has failed.

REFERENCES

1. Saltzman CL, Tearse DS. Achilles tendon injuries. J Am Acad Orthop Surg 1998; 6:316–25.
2. Jones MP, Khan RJ, Carey Smith RL. Surgical interventions for treating Achilles tendon rupture: key findings from a recent Cochrane review. J Bone Joint Surg Am 2012;94(1–6):e88.
3. Pinzur MS. Orthopaedic knowledge update: foot and ankle 4. Rosemont (IL): American Academy of Orthopaedic Surgeons; 2008.
4. Reddy SS, Pedowitz DI, Parekh SG, et al. Surgical treatment for chronic disease and disorders of the Achilles tendon. J Am Acad Orthop Surg 2009;17:3–14.
5. Chiodo CP, Glazebrook M. AAOS clinical practice guideline summary: diagnosis and treatment of acute Achilles tendon ruptures. J Am Acad Orthop Surg 2010; 18:503–10.
6. Zhou HM, Yu GR, Yang YF, et al. Outcomes and complications of operative versus nonoperative treatment of acute Achilles tendon ruptures: a meta-analysis. Chin Med J 2011;124(23):4050–5.
7. Soroceanu A, Sidhwa F, Aarabi S, et al. Surgical versus nonsurgical treatment of acute Achilles tendon rupture: a meta-analysis of randomized trials. J Bone Joint Surg Am 2012;94:2136–43.
8. Waterman BR, Owens BD. The epidemiology of ankle sprains in the United States. J Bone Joint Surg Am 2010;92:2279–84.
9. Colville M. Surgical treatment of the unstable ankle. J Am Acad Orthop Surg 1998;6:368–77.
10. Zalavras C, Thordarson D. Ankle syndesmotic injury. J Am Acad Orthop Surg 2007;15:330–9.
11. Wuest TK. Injuries to the distal lower extremity syndesmosis. J Am Acad Orthop Surg 1997;5:172–81.
12. Renström PA. Persistently painful sprained ankle. J Am Acad Orthop Surg 1994; 2:270–80.
13. Stiell IG, Greenberg GH. Decision rules for the use of radiography in acute ankle injuries: refinement and prospective validation. JAMA 1993;269:1127–32.
14. Maffulli N, Ferran NA. Management of acute and chronic ankle instability. J Am Acad Orthop Surg 2008;16:608–15.
15. Pihlajamaki H, Hietaniemi K. Surgical versus functional treatment for acute ruptures of the lateral ligament complex of the ankle in young men: a randomized controlled trial. J Bone Joint Surg Am 2010;92:2367–74.
16. Zheng TH, Yu XM, et al. Comparison of surgical intervention with functional treatment of ruptures of lateral ankle ligament: a meta-analysis. Asian Pac J Trop Med 2012;5(5):396–401.
17. Witjes S, Gresnigt F, van den Bekerom MP, et al. The ANKLE trial (Ankle Treatment after injuries of the Ankle Ligaments): what is the benefit of external support

devices in the functional treatment of acute ankle sprains?: a randomized controlled trial. BMC Musculoskelet Disord 2012;13(21):1–7.
18. Xenos JS, Hopkinson WJ, Hopkinson WJ, et al. The tibiofibular syndesmosis: evaluation of the ligamentous structures, method of fixation, and radiographic assessment. J Bone Joint Surg Am 1995;77(6):847–56.
19. Anderson RB, Hunt KJ, McCormick JJ. Management of common sports-related injuries about the foot and ankle. J Am Acad Orthop Surg 2010;18(9):546–56.
20. Rosenberg GA, Sferra JJ. Treatment strategies for acute fractures and nonunions of the proximal fifth metatarsal. J Am Acad Orthop Surg 2000;8:332–8.
21. Hartog BD. Fracture of the proximal fifth metatarsal. J Am Acad Orthop Surg 2009;17:458–64.
22. Dameron TB. Fractures of the proximal fifth metatarsal: selecting the best treatment option. J Am Acad Orthop Surg 1995;3:110–4.
23. Dameron TB. Fractures and anatomical variations of the proximal portion of the fifth metatarsal. J Bone Joint Surg Am 1975;57(6):788–92.
24. Shindle MK, Endo Y, Warren RF, et al. Stress fractures about the tibia, foot, and ankle. J Am Acad Orthop Surg 2012;20:167–76.
25. Torg JS, Balduini FC, Zelko RR, et al. Fractures of the base of the fifth metatarsal distal to the tuberosity. J Bone Joint Surg Am 1984;66(4):209–14.
26. Furia JP, Juliano PJ, Wade AM, et al. Shock wave therapy compared with intramedullary screw fixation for nonunion of proximal fifth metatarsal metaphyseal-diaphyseal fractures. J Bone Joint Surg Am 2010;92:846–54.
27. Benirschke SK, Meinberg E, Anderson SA, et al. Fractures and dislocations of the midfoot: Chopart and Lisfranc injuries. J Bone Joint Surg Am 2012;94(14):1326–37.
28. Myerson MS, Cerrato RA. Current management of tarsometatarsal injuries in the athlete. J Bone Joint Surg Am 2008;90(11):2522–33.
29. Mantas JP, Burks RT. Lisfranc injuries in the athlete. Clin Sports Med 1994;13(4):719–30.
30. Trevino SG, Kodros S. Controversies in tarsometatarsal injuries. Orthop Clin North Am 1995;26(2):229–38.
31. Myerson MS. The diagnosis and treatment of injury to the tarsometatarsal joint complex. J Bone Joint Surg Br 1999;81(5):756–63, 1998;19(7):438–46.
32. Hatem SF, Davis A, Sundaram M. Your diagnosis? midfoot sprain: Lisfranc ligament disruption. Orthopedics 2005;28(1):2, 75–7.
33. Watson TS, Shurnas PS, Denker J. Treatment of Lisfranc joint injury: current concepts. J Am Acad Orthop Surg 2010;18:718–28.
34. Mayich DJ, Mayich MS, Daniels TR. Effective detection and management of low-velocity Lisfranc injuries in the emergency setting. Can Fam Physician 2012;58(11):1199–204.
35. Faciszewski T, Burks RT, Manaster BJ. Subtle injuries of the Lisfranc joint. J Bone Joint Surg Am 1990;72(10):1519–22.
36. Kraeger DR. Foot injuries. In: Lillegard WA, Rucker KS, editors. Handbook of sports medicine: a symptom- oriented approach. Boston: Andover Medical; 1993. p. 159–71.
37. Raikin SM, Elias I, Dheer S, et al. Prediction of midfoot instability in the subtle Lisfranc injury: comparison of magnetic resonance imaging with intraoperative findings. J Bone Joint Surg Am 2009;91(4):892–9.
38. Schenck RC, Heckman JD. Fractures and dislocations of the forefoot: operative versus non-operative treatment. J Am Acad Orthop Surg 1995;3:70–8.

39. Boden BP, Osbahr DC. High risk stress fractures: evaluation and treatment. J Am Acad Orthop Surg 2000;8:344–53.
40. Fetzer GB, Wright RW. Metatarsal shaft fractures and fractures of the proximal fifth metatarsal. Clin Sports Med 2006;25:139–50.
41. Early JS. Fractures and dislocations of the midfoot and forefoot. In: Buckholz RW, Heck-man JD, editors. Fractures in adults. 5th edition. Philadelphia: Lippincott Williams and Wilkins; 2001. p. 2215–28.
42. Bishop AJ, Palanca AA, Bellino MJ, et al. Assessment of compromised fracture healing. J Am Acad Orthop Surg 2012;20:273–82.
43. Micheli LJ, Sohn RS. Stress fracture of the second metatarsal involving Lisfranc's joint in ballet dancers. J Bone Joint Surg Am 1985;67:1372–5.
44. Eisele SA, Sammarco GJ. Fatigue fractures of the foot and ankle in an athlete. J Bone Joint Surg Am 1993;75:290–8.
45. Sofka CM. Imaging of stress fractures. Clin Sports Med 2006;25(1):53–62, viii.
46. O'Malley MJ, Hamilton WG, Munyak J. Stress fractures at the base of the second metatarsal in ballet dancers. Foot Ankle Int 1996;17(2):89–94.
47. Kiuru MJ, Niva M, Reponen A, et al. Bone stress injuries in asymptomatic elite recruits: a clinical and magnetic resonance imaging study. Am J Sports Med 2005;33(2):272–6.
48. Gaeta M, Minutoli F, Scribano E, et al. CT and MR imaging findings in athletes with early tibial stress injuries: comparison with bone scintigraphy findings and emphasis on cortical abnormalities. Radiology 2005;235(2):553–61.

The Evaluation and Treatment of Elbow Injuries

Mark E. Lavallee, MD, CSCS[a,*], Kari Sears, MD[b], Amy Corrigan, DO[b]

KEYWORDS

• Olecranon • Epicondyle • Physis • Ulnar • Median nerve • Radius

KEY POINTS

- Location and mechanism of injury should be considered when approaching an elbow injury.
- Due to the numerous growth plates (physis) around the elbow, the skeletally-immature individual needs to be assessed very carefully.
- Chronic and acute injuries around the elbow often follow very different treatment protocols.

ANTERIOR ELBOW INJURIES

Distal Biceps Rupture

Mechanism of injury

A distal biceps rupture can occur proximally off of the superior glenoid but more commonly occurs at the insertion of the biceps tendon on the radial tuberosity. It occurs when an eccentric load is applied to the forearm, resulting in forced extension, resisted at the elbow. The tendon is most at risk when the elbow is flexed and the forearm supinated. Biceps tendon rupture occurs most commonly in middle-aged men and tends to be an acute injury with sudden onset of symptoms. A noticeable pop is often felt or heard. Although much less common than Achilles tendon rupture, biceps tendon rupture has been associated with fluoroquinolone use, especially in conjunction with chronic corticosteroid use, and with anabolic steroid use.[1,2]

Physical examination

The patient may complain of sudden-onset sharp pain in the anterior elbow, and may describe a tearing or popping sensation. Examination will reveal swelling and ecchymosis over the antecubital fossa. The examiner may be able to observe a "Popeye"

[a] South Bend-Notre Dame Sports Medicine Fellowship, 111 West Jefferson Boulevard, Suite 100, South Bend, IN 46601, USA; [b] Memorial Family Medicine Residency, 714 North Michigan Avenue, South Bend, IN 46601, USA

* Corresponding author.

E-mail address: mlavallee@memorialsb.org

Prim Care Clin Office Pract 40 (2013) 407–429
http://dx.doi.org/10.1016/j.pop.2013.02.010 **primarycare.theclinics.com**
0095-4543/13/$ – see front matter

deformity with both proximal or distal tendon rupture caused by the retraction of the biceps muscle proximally and may be able to palpate a defect distal to the retracted muscle. However, in the acute setting this is often obscured by significant edema. Because the bicep is the primary forearm supinator and secondary elbow flexor, strength testing may reveal weakness of both. Active and passive range of motion (ROM) are usually full, unless limited by pain. Specific tests that are both sensitive and specific to biceps tendon rupture include the biceps squeeze test and hook test. The squeeze test is done by compressing the biceps at the musculotendinous junction, which results in pronation of the forearm if the biceps tendon is intact or partially torn but no movement of the forearm if it is completely ruptured. The hook test is performed on the patient by holding his or her arm in about 45° of flexion. The examiner should be able to hook his or her index finger under the biceps tendon in the antecubital fossa if it is intact. If ruptured, the tendon will be noticeably absent.

Imaging

Frequently, diagnosis of a biceps tendon rupture will be apparent with only clinical history and examination. However, confirmation of the diagnosis can be made with both ultrasound and MRI. The biceps tendon can be visualized longitudinally on MRI or ultrasound with specific positioning of the arm. If there is suspicion of a biceps tendon rupture, MRI should be done with the elbow slightly flexed, shoulder abducted, and forearm supinated (FABS). Ultrasound will show either the absence of biceps tendon, in complete rupture, or disruption of the fibers with surrounding edema, in a partial tear.

Differential diagnosis

Differential diagnosis should include cubital bursitis, biceps tendonitis, entrapment of lateral antebrachial cutaneous nerve, and posterior interosseous nerve (PIN) syndrome.

Treatment

Acute partial tears, as well as old partial or complete tears, may be treated conservatively with rest, ice, nonsteroidal anti-inflammatory drugs (NSAIDs), and a gradual strengthening and ROM program with physical therapy (PT). Conservative management may also be the best treatment approach for all injuries in elderly patients or those who are not good surgical candidates. However, most patients with a significant injury to the distal biceps tendon warrant surgery. Nonsurgical treatment of a complete biceps tendon rupture can result in a 40% loss of supination strength and 30% loss of flexion strength, and an even more significant loss in muscle endurance.[3–5]

Referral

Referral is indicated in patients with complete tendon rupture who can tolerate surgery, especially competitive, younger athletes or those physically demanding jobs. Patients with greater than 50% partial tears who wish to return to activity faster, without strength compromise, may also consider surgery.

Prognosis and return to play

If repaired within 2 weeks following injury, patients generally return to normal sporting activity within 6 months. Injuries that are treated conservatively may have more protracted recoveries and patients may have permanent loss of strength but should retain full ROM.

Pronator Syndrome (Median Nerve Entrapment)

Mechanism of injury

Compression of the median nerve courses across the elbow can occur at several sites. The three most common sites are

1. Between the two heads of the pronator teres
2. Under the proximal superficial edge of the pronator teres
3. Under the proximal edge of the flexor digitorum superficialis.

Chronic repetitive pronation can result in hypertrophy of these muscles or repetitive trauma to the median nerve resulting in chronic compression.

Physical examination

Patients with pronator syndrome generally complain of insidious onset of aching pain in the anterior proximal forearm. They may have paresthesias in the hand consistent with a median nerve distribution of the hand, including the thumb, index, and third fingers, and half of the fourth finger (**Table 1**). Patients will have pain with resisted pronation of the forearm, especially if the elbow is extended. Pain with resisted flexion of the third finger suggests entrapment at the flexor digitorum superficialis. Pronator syndrome can sometimes be difficult to distinguish from carpal tunnel syndrome because of the similarities of hand symptoms. Distinguishing features for the diagnosis of pronator syndrome include loss of sensation over the palmar cutaneous nerve distribution (thenar eminence), forearm pain, no nighttime symptoms, and a negative Tinel sign.

Imaging

Nerve conduction studies are the most useful diagnostic tool if symptoms have been present for 3 to 4 weeks and can help determine the location of impingement. Rarely, these symptoms can be caused by nerve compression due to anatomic variant or mass, in which case MRI may be useful.

Differential diagnosis

Differential diagnosis should include carpal tunnel syndrome and proximal median nerve injury.

Treatment

Conservative treatment is the mainstay of treatment for pronator syndrome. Rest and limitation of the precipitating activity will result in resolution of symptoms in most patients. NSAIDs can also be useful in initial therapy. Ultrasound evaluation and hydro-dissection, which is a process preformed in the office under ultrasound guidance in which the entrapped nerve is visualized and a needle is directed in close proximity

Table 1
Pronator syndrome symptoms

	Pronator Syndrome	Carpel Tunnel Syndrome
Sensory deficit in fingers	+	+
Sensory deficit thenar eminence	+	–
Tinel sign	–	+
Night symptoms	–	+
Forearm pain	+	–

of the nerve and the area of entrapment using the fluid's (ie, normal saline, D5W, or lidocaine) hydrostatic pressure to stretch out the tissue entrapping the nerve, can be performed and often precludes need for surgery.[6–10]

Referral

Surgical decompression or exploration is only indicated in refractory cases that have failed conservative therapy after 3 to 6 months, or if physical examination or imaging is concerning for mass.

Prognosis and return to play

Most patients have complete resolution of their symptoms with conservative treatment. Because symptoms are primarily sensory, and not motor, permanent disability is rare.

Distal Biceps Tendinopathy

Mechanism of injury

The mechanism of injury for distal biceps tendinopathy is repetitive flexion or supination.

History

Patients frequently complain of pain and weakness with flexion or supination motions. The pain of biceps tendonitis usually has a gradual onset compared with the sudden onset of pain after a specific injury with biceps rupture.

Physical examination

Patients will exhibit tenderness over the distal biceps tendon and pain with resisted flexion and supination. The hook test at the proximal biceps should be negative.

Imaging

Ultrasound can be useful in diagnosing biceps tendinopathy, mostly to distinguish it from a partial or complete tendon tear. Dynamically, ultrasound very helpful in assessing the increased cross-sectional area seen in tendinosis (shoulder). Because the biceps tendon has no synovial sheath, it can be difficult to distinguish anatomic structures and may be hard to tell tendonitis from cubital bursitis.

Differential diagnosis

Differential diagnosis should include partial biceps tendon rupture, cubital bursitis, and brachioradialis tendonitis.

Treatment

Treatment consists of discontinuation of provoking activity, ice, NSAIDs, and PT (ie, ROM, strengthening, modalities, eccentrics exercises). Because of the extensive neurovascular structures at the insertion of the biceps tendon, as well as lack of synovial sheath to contain medication, steroid injections are not recommended.

Referral

Referral is rarely indicated.

Prognosis and return to play

Distal biceps tendinopathy is rarely a serious injury, although it can cause significant pain. Return to play is limited by the athlete's tolerance of sport-specific activity and return to play should be dictated by the effectiveness and safety of an athlete's participation in a game-like situation.

POSTERIOR ELBOW PAIN

Distal Triceps Rupture or Olecranon Avulsion

Mechanism of injury

The triceps tendon can rupture at its insertion on the olecranon process of the ulna or there can be an avulsion of the olecranon process from the ulna with the triceps tendon still attached. Overall, the injury is rare; however, it occurs more frequently in men and can happen at any age. This injury typically occurs after a fall onto an outstretched hand in which the triceps muscle is contracting and flexion is forced, causing it to avulse off of the olecranon.[11,12] Direct trauma can also cause a rupture. If the rupture is spontaneous, consider anabolic steroid use, corticosteroid injections, fluoroquinolone use, metabolic bone disorders, renal dysfunction, lupus, or hyperparathyroidism as possible causes.[13]

Physical examination

Patients may complain of acute weakness in arm extension, pain, or swelling and bruising at the posterior elbow. On examination, ecchymosis, edema, and a palpable defect of the triceps tendon or a step off at the olecranon may be noted. The elbow will be tender to palpate over the posterior olecranon and distal triceps tendon. The patient will have normal ROM but overall weakness with extension and will be unable to hold his or her elbow in extension against gravity. In complete tears, there will be no active extension of the elbow. A modified Thompson squeeze test does not cause elbow extension.

Imaging

In 80% of cases, plain radiographs may show a "flake sign" which is a small bony avulsion fragment from the olecranon or a large olecranon fragment. Radiographs are also useful in ruling out radial head or distal humerus fractures. MRI or ultrasound can aid diagnosis by localizing and determining the degree of tear.[13]

Differential diagnosis

Differential diagnosis should include triceps tendonitis, olecranon bursitis, olecranon stress fracture, posterior elbow impingement, and brachial plexopathy involving nerve root.

Treatment

Nonoperative treatment by immobilizing the elbow in 30° of flexion for 4 weeks with a splint is recommended for elderly patients with complete tears or for younger patients with partial tears.[11] Some studies have shown that partial tears involving up to 75% of the tendon have the capacity to heal.[13] Operative treatment is recommended within 2 weeks of injury if there is complete tear; however, partial tears can be repaired in a delayed manner if symptoms persist.[13] Postoperatively, the patient's arm will need to be immobilized in 30° to 45° of flexion for 3 to 4 weeks. Then the patient should gradually begin PT to work on passive ROM. The patient may begin active ROM exercises 6 weeks after surgery but should avoid lifting weights for at least 4 to 6 months.[11]

Prognosis and return to play

This type of injury is likely a season-ending injury that requires 6 months of recovery. Bracing that has the ability to lockout certain ROMs should also be considered for protection once an athlete returns to play.[13]

Olecranon Impingement Syndrome

Mechanism of injury

Also referred to as valgus extension overload, olecranon fossitis, or "boxer's elbow," olecranon impingement syndrome is caused from overuse and repetitive valgus extension from throwing or boxing, causing the medial aspect of the olecranon process to be pushed against the medial wall of the olecranon fossa. This mechanism of injury results in inflammation, thickening, insufficiency of the ulnar collateral ligament (UCL), and microtrauma.[14] The injury is seen in stable elbows or in athletes, such as overhead throwers, who have insufficient UCLs .

Physical examination

Patients will complain of insidious onset of posterior medial elbow pain while extending the elbow and may notice the elbow catching or locking in extension. Throwers will complain of loss of pitching velocity or control. The examiner will notice tenderness and swelling at the posterior medial elbow. The patient my be unable to fully extend the elbow and will experience pain with forced valgus extension that may also produce crepitus. Loose bodies may be palpated and there may be laxity of UCL with valgus stress.

Imaging

Plain films, including anteroposterior (AP), lateral, and axial views, will show hypertrophy of the olecranon, spurring of the medial olecranon tip, and/or loose bodies. MRI can be useful to assess and visualize thickening, tearing, or degeneration of the UCL, olecranon osteophytes, chondromalacia of olecranon fossa, loose bodies, or osteochondritis dissecans of the RC joint. Ultrasound may also be valuable to assess function of UCL with valgus stress.[14]

Differential diagnosis

Differential diagnosis should include olecranon bursitis, olecranon stress fracture, triceps tendonitis, and osteochondral fragment.

Treatment

Conservative treatment is recommended and includes rest, NSAIDs, ice, and PT aimed to increase flexibility and strength of the wrist flexors and extensors, as well as the scapular stabilizers and core. It is also important to correct poor throwing mechanics to prevent future injuries. Surgical removal of the olecranon tip, osteophytes, and loose bodies via arthroscopy or posterior arthrotomy may be an option in patients who fail conservative treatment.

Prognosis and return to play

Patients who have stable elbows do well following arthroscopic debridement and can expect full return to play. Patients who have instability do well in the short term with surgery; however, up to 25% of high-level throwers will need revision with UCL reconstruction.

Olecranon Stress Fracture

Mechanism of injury

A microfracture of the proximal ulna is a result of overuse and repetitive tension of the proximal ulna from throwing or weightbearing in gymnastics.

Physical examination

Patients will complain of gradual onset of pain in the posterior or lateral elbow that occurs during the acceleration phase of throwing. It is more common in adolescents and older children. Patients will have a normal neurologic examination and full ROM. There will be focal point tenderness to palpation over the olecranon without tenderness over the triceps tendon moving proximally and no crepitus on examination. Pain with resisted extension may also be present.

Imaging

Typically, plain films are negative. If an occult fracture is suspected, a CT scan may be ordered. When no fracture line is seen, an MRI is often needed to see bone marrow edema. A bone scan could also be considered as an alternative option. In skeletally immature athletes, comparison radiographs may be useful to look for widening of the olecranon apophysis.

Differential diagnosis

Differential diagnosis should include olecranon apophysitis, triceps tendonitis, olecranon bursitis, and posterior impingement syndrome.

Treatment

Athletes must immediately stop throwing and not bear weight in the affected arm regardless of treatment choice. Conservative treatment or percutaneous screw fixation are the two options. If choosing conservative treatment, the patient needs to not bear weight and stay out of play until tenderness stops and, then, may gradually start rehabilitating the injury. If symptoms return during rehabilitation, operative treatment should be considered. After surgery, once radiographs show evidence of healing, the patient can start working on ROM and strengthening.

Prognosis and return to play

With appropriate treatment, patients can generally return to play after 3 to 4 months.

Triceps Tendinopathy

Mechanism of injury

The mechanism of injury for triceps tendinopathy is inflammation of the triceps tendon at its insertion on the olecranon process due to overuse from repetitive extension and hyperextension of the elbow.

Physical examination

Triceps tendinopathy is often seen in baseball players and weightlifters. Normally, no acute trauma is reported. Patients complain of pain at the insertion of the triceps tendon. Focal pain is noted at the triceps insertion on the olecranon and pain occurs with resisted elbow extension. Normal ROM is preserved and no defects can be palpated on examination.

Imaging

Plain radiographs typically are normal but traction osteophytes or calcific deposits can be seen on lateral views. MRI or ultrasound can be useful to help distinguish between tendon degeneration and partial triceps tendon tear.

Differential diagnosis

Differential diagnosis should include olecranon bursitis, olecranon stress fracture, fracture of an olecranon osteophyte, and partial tendon tear.

Treatment

Conservative treatment includes rest, ice, NSAIDs, and rehabilitation that includes gradual stretching and strengthening, as well as core and scapular stabilization. Consider corticosteroid injections in refractory cases but use caution because of increased risk of triceps tendon rupture. Surgical debridement can be sought to remove degenerative tissue and help stimulate healing in cases where symptoms persist following conservative treatment for greater than 1 year.

Prognosis and return to play

Patients can continue to participate in activities but should rest and undergo focused rehabilitation during off season.

Olecranon Bursitis

Mechanism of injury

Olecranon bursitis, also known as miner's or student's elbow is due do inflammation of the bursa over the olecranon. Bursitis can be acute or chronic and septic or aseptic. Bursitis is a result of either direct trauma to the posterior elbow from a single blow (fall onto the elbow) or repetitive trauma (leaning on the elbow) that damages the superficial tissues leading to inflammation. If there is contamination of the bursa from a closely approximated skin wound or dermatitis, the patient may develop a septic bursa.

Physical examination

The patient may complain of either acute or gradual onset of swelling. Pain is associated with acute or septic bursitis, whereas chronic bursitis is often painless. This is an injury often seen in football or hockey players. The examiner will notice posterior elbow swelling and can palpate a mobile, fluctuant mass that changes size. There will be a normal neurovascular examination and full ROM. With septic bursitis, erythema, heat, and drainage may be present.

Imaging

Plain radiographs may show calcifications at the bursa or an olecranon spur; otherwise they are negative. Aspirating the bursa in acute and chronic cases and sending fluid for cell count, differential diagnosis, Gram stain and culture, and crystal analysis can be helpful. *Staphylococcus aureus* is the most common bacterial cause of septic bursitis. Aseptic fluid will have a low white blood cell count with a high percentage of monocytes (>80%). Gouty crystals may also be seen in fluid on analysis. Ultrasound can also be helpful in diagnosis.

Differential diagnosis

Differential diagnosis should include gouty tophus, calcium pyrophosphate deposition, septic elbow arthritis, and cellulitis.

Treatment

In the acute setting, treat olecranon bursitis with rest, short-term immobilization of 3 to 5 days, compressive dressing, ice, and NSAIDs. In chronic cases, aspirate and inject with corticosteroids, then apply compressive dressing for 2 to 3 weeks. Interventional ultrasound can be helpful in treatment by guiding injections. If there is high suspicion of a septic bursitis drain, excise and administer intravenous antibiotics for 1 to 3 weeks and follow with 2 weeks of oral antibiotics. Bursa sacs can also be excised in cases of chronic aseptic cases; however, skin healing is difficult over the olecranon.

Prognosis and return to play

If surgically excised, expect a 6 week absence from sport. Aseptic bursitis should not affect play; however, the patient should wear a protective elbow pad and may be at risk for recurrence or septic conversion.

Elbow Dislocations

Mechanism of injury

The mechanism of injury for elbow dislocation is discontinuity of the ulnohumeral articulation with associated radiocapitellar joint disruption with or without proximal radioulnar disruption. There are simple and complex elbow dislocations. Complex elbow dislocations involve either open or closed fractures. Posterior elbow dislocations are the most common; however, they can also be displaced anteriorly, laterally, medially, or in some combination. Typically, the lateral ligaments tear first, followed by the anterior and posterior capsules. The medial collateral ligament is the last to be injured and typically remains intact but with posterolateral rotatory instability.[15,16]

Physical examination

The examiner will notice a visible deformity on inspection. The median and ulnar nerves should be evaluated because they can be compromised. When there is a proximal radial fracture present, there may also be a radial nerve injury. Despite arterial injury, the patient may have ulnar or radial pulses because of collateral circulation.

Imaging

Plain radiographs with AP and lateral views help determine the nature and scope of the dislocation. Oblique views can help with a tomographic view of the radial head. If complex, consider CT imaging or MRI to help identify ligamentous or cartilaginous injuries.

Differential diagnosis

Differential diagnosis should include elbow fracture, elbow subluxation, and tendon rupture.

Treatment

In simple dislocations, depending on the time between dislocation or relocation, age and willingness of the patient, and skill of the physician, one can consider local anesthetic, conscious sedation, or complete sedation in the operating room to perform a closed reduction. The authors have noted that rapid reduction within 15 minutes of dislocation can often occur with anesthesia. Conversely, however, patients who are young, scared, or noncompliant often need some form of anesthesia. After reducing the elbow, assess ROM and stability. Then, repeat radiographs because fractures can be missed on initial films. If there is limitation or crepitus with motion, this could be due to an impinging fracture fragment or an osteochondral lesion. Fluoroscopy and, sometimes, musculoskeletal ultrasound can be helpful in determining joint stability. Once the elbow is stable, apply a broad arm sling and encourage mobilization. NSAIDs may be useful to control pain. Open reduction is often not needed in simple posterior dislocations. Complex elbow dislocations involve fractures and may need closed reduction, open reduction internal fixation, repair of ligaments, and/or dynamic external fixation to obtain stability.

In simple dislocations in which the elbow is stable, a broad arm sling is used for comfort and the patient is encouraged to mobilize the joint as comfort allows. In cases where there is instability after reduction, the patient may need a block splint, which limits extension, keeps forearm in full pronation, and allows active flexion. Extension is gradually increased over 3 to 4 weeks. The patient should be re-examined and have repeat radiographs 5 to 7 days after reduction.[15]

Prognosis and return to play
Fixed flexion contractures can occur if the elbow is immobilized for a prolonged period of greater than 3 weeks. Patients could be at risk for developing arthrosis. Loss of extension is a common complication and the authors recommend using a skilled physical therapist or occupational therapist to help guide patient rehabilitation.

Fractures

Mechanism of injury
A fracture of the proximal radius, ulna, or distal humerus can occur with or without dislocation or subluxation of the elbow. A Monteggia fracture is a fracture of the proximal third of the ulna with dislocation of the head of the radius. A Galeazzi fracture is a fracture of the radius with dislocation of the distal radioulnar joint. It classically involves an isolated fracture of the junction of the distal third and middle third of the radius with associated subluxation or dislocation of the distal radioulnar joint. The injury disrupts the forearm axis joint. The most common mechanism of injury is trauma from falling on an outstretched hand.

Physical examination
The patient will have a history of an acute trauma, complain of severe pain that is exacerbated by movements, and may notice instability and crepitus. They often hold the injured arm tight to chest in flexed position. There may be a deformity, tenderness, swelling, ecchymosis, crepitus, limited ROM, and severe pain. The patient may or may not have a normal neurovascular examination and varus or valgus instability.

Imaging
Plain radiograph (AP and lateral) films may show a fracture of the radial head or neck, olecranon, coronoid, or distal humerus. The fat pads are very helpful in the case of subtle fractures. An elevated anterior fat pad or any visible posterior fat pad indicates a hemarthrosis and, therefore, a fracture. Radiographs can also show dislocations with or without fractures. Some associated dislocations with fractures of the proximal ulna fracture with radial head dislocations are referred to as a Monteggia fractures. The authors suggest considering CT or MRI to asses bone and ligament damage if radiographs are inconclusive.

Differential diagnosis
Differential diagnosis should include ligament injury, elbow subluxation, and elbow dislocation.

Treatment
It is important to document the neurovascular examination. Attempt a reduction immediately if neurovascular compromise is present; then immobilize with a splint. After reduction, immediately repeat radiographs. Treatment may require either no reduction, closed reduction, or open reduction, as well as internal fixation.

Prognosis and return to play
Typically, a fracture is a season-ending injury and will require an extensive course of treatment and rehabilitation. With simple dislocations without fractures, it is important to begin early ROM exercises. In cases in which there is a complex fracture and dislocation, it is unlikely that the player will return to her or his previous level of play.

MEDIAL ELBOW INJURIES

Medial Epicondylitis (aka Golfer's Elbow)

Mechanism of injury

The mechanism of injury for medial epicondylitis is degenerative changes of the wrist flexor tendons at their origin on the medial epicondyle, which is a result of repetitive overloading and stress with repetition of wrist flexion and forearm pronation. This is caused by failure of a normal tendon to repair itself along with angiofibroblastic degeneration.[17,18] Less commonly, it can be a result of direct trauma or sudden eccentric contraction.[15] This injury is seen in pitchers, golfers, bowlers, weightlifters, javelin throwers, and football players, as well as in carpenters, plumbers, or any labor involving repetitive forearm, wrist, and hand motions.

Physical examination

Medial epicondylitis is less common than lateral epicondylitis. Pain is at the medial epicondyle. Occasionally patients can have associated ulnar neuropathy, triceps tendonitis, loose body formations, or UCL injuries, along with their medial epicondylitis. Pain will be noted at the medial epicondyle and over the flexor tendon origin. There is weakness and pain with resisted wrist flexion and forearm pronation when performed in full extension. A positive Tinel sign with percussion of flexor pronator is consistent with a cubital tunnel syndrome. There may also be localized swelling or warmth.

Imaging

Radiographs will be normal. Calcifications in the flexor-pronator tendon often present in long-standing chronic cases. Electromyography is recommended in patients with neurologic deficits but are normal in the case epicondylitis. MRI arthrogram or ultrasound can be useful to evaluate the UCL or determine traumatic tears to flexor pronator origin at the epicondyle.[15]

Differential diagnosis

Differential diagnosis should include UCL sprain, flexor-pronator tear, and ulnar neuritis.

Treatment

Conservative treatment consists of rest, ice for 15 to 20 minutes three times a day, activity modification, counterforce elbow bracing, wrist bracing (wrist in flexion), pain control with NSAIDs, and PT aimed at stretching and strengthening the flexor pronator, especially with eccentric exercises. Complete immobilization should be avoided to prevent atrophy.[15] Corticosteroid injections can be considered in refractory cases; however, caution must be taken to avoid the ulnar nerve and limit injections to no more than three injections. Consider interventional ultrasound to guide injections. NSAIDs and corticosteroid injections are aimed at symptom relief; it is the rehabilitation exercises that seem to improve outcomes. Platelet-rich plasma injections, FAST (Focused Aspiration of Scar Tissue) technique by Tenex and percutaneous tenotomy or fenestrations of origin of flexor tendon are being used. It is hypothesized that these help initiate healing in damaged tendons but are not yet proven to be effective.[17] The goal with rehabilitation is to achieve pain reduction and improve strength to help prevent vulnerability to tension overload. If symptoms persist for greater than 1 year and the above-mentioned interventions have not been successful, consider a surgical consult for possible debridement of the degenerative proximal portion of the pronator teres and flexor carpi radialis with gentle curettage of the medial epicondyle.

Prognosis and return to play

The athlete may return to play when they are asymptomatic, which typically is after 6 to 12 weeks of treatment. Up to 90% have excellent recovery and do not need surgery. If surgery is needed, the patient will need to be immobilized in a splint, then receive flexibility and strengthening for 12 weeks. Once the patient returns to play it is important to identify any equipment or technique inadequacies to avoid recurrence.

Flexor-Pronator Strain

Mechanism of injury

The mechanism of injury of flexor-pronator strain is acute injury to the flexor-pronator distal to the common tendon origins at the medial epicondyle. This is due to valgus stress or sudden contraction to the elbow, which causes partial or microrupture of the flexor mass. This can occur during the late cocking or acceleration phase of throwing and often is a result of an inadequate warm-up or fatigue in throwers.

Physical examination

The complaints with flexor-pronator strain are similar to medial epicondylitis but the symptoms are more acute. Focal tenderness at the medial epicondyle or distally over the pronator muscle belly will be noted. Mild edema or ecchymosis may be visible and there is pain with resisted pronation or wrist flexion.

Imaging

Acute plain radiographs will be normal. Office ultrasound is helpful in ruling out hematoma, nerve entrapment, and partial torn flexor tendons. In severe cases consider MRI.

Differential diagnosis

Differential diagnosis should include UCL injury, hematoma, partially torn flexor tendon, and ulnar or median nerve entrapment.

Treatment

Rest, NSAIDs, ice, and PT that includes deep tissue techniques, modalities, and eccentrics are the mainstay of therapy. Therapy should be aimed at improving motion and strength with a gradual return to sport.

Prognosis and return to play

Many patients will be asymptomatic after 2 to 3 weeks of rest. They should gradually return to play and, if symptoms return, be prohibited from throwing until symptoms resolve.

UCL Sprain or Rupture

Mechanism of injury

The mechanism of injury for UCL sprain or rupture is microtears or complete rupture of the UCL. This occurs from repetitive valgus stress, which causes tensile loading of the UCL and results in microtears or complete rupture as often seen in pitching, other throwing, or racket sports.

Physical examination

Usually, throwing athletes will complain of a gradual onset of medial elbow pain that is made worse with valgus stress and improved with rest. The pain worsens when throwing exceeds 75% of normal velocity. Occasionally, the UCL can completely rupture in a single event in which a significant valgus force is applied to the UCL.[19,20] The UCL is tender to palpate just distal to the medical epicondyle over the anterior oblique ligament and may have visible swelling. Pain is increased with valgus stressing of the elbow in flexion or with a milking maneuver.

Imaging
Plain radiographs may show an avulsion fracture or a medial collateral ligament ossicle, loose bodies, or marginal osteophytes. Consider including manual or gravity valgus stress views to confirm diagnosis. A greater than 2 mm gap with valgus stress is considered abnormal. An MRI is useful for evaluations of tears and contrast increases the sensitivity. Office ultrasound is also very useful.

Differential diagnosis
Differential diagnosis should include ulnar neuritis, medial epicondylitis, and flexor pronator muscle rupture or strain.

Treatment
Conservative treatment includes rest, ice, NSAIDs, and PT to correct motion or strength limitations in the elbow, as well as scapular and core stabilization, correcting throwing mechanics, and limiting pitch count. PT should aim at regaining full ROM and maintaining strength. Consider a hinged elbow brace to protect the elbow from valgus stress. Complete tears may require surgical reconstruction (eg, the Tommy John procedure). Consider surgery in athletes with full tears who wish to return to play or in patients who have documented partial tears with instability or have a stable joint but have persistent medial pain with activity for 3 months of conservative treatment.[21]

Prognosis and return to play
Full-tear injuries are season-ending injuries and postsurgical rehabilitation lasts 12 to 18 months with 80% of patients achieving good results. There are variable outcomes with nonoperative management.

Ulnar Nerve Compression Syndrome

Mechanism of injury
Ulnar nerve compression syndrome is also known as cubital tunnel syndrome because of compression of the ulnar nerve as it crosses the elbow. Most often the onset is insidious and can be triggered by trauma, cubitus valgus deformity, or subluxation of the ulnar nerve at the medial epicondyle. This injury can be seen in strength athletes who excessively concentrate on triceps.

Physical examination
The onset is gradual. Patients complain of an aching medial elbow and forearm pain with numbness at the ring and small fingers, along with grip weakness and decreased ROM. Symptoms often awake patient at night. There may be a positive Tinel sign over the cubital tunnel along with a positive ulnar nerve compression test, Froment test, or subluxation of the ulnar nerve with elbow flexion. The Froment test assesses the ulnar nerve by testing the adductor pollicis muscle. The patient tries to grasp a piece of paper between their thumb and index finger while the examiner attempts to pull the paper away. If the patient is forced to flex the tip of the thumb to maintain their grip on the paper, then this is evidence of an ulnar nerve lesion and the Froment test is positive. The patient will also have a weak grip and flexor digitorum profundus to the small finger.

Imaging
Electromyogram or nerve conduction velocity tests show slowing conduction across the elbow in 20% to 25% of cases. Plain radiographs are typically normal

but may show osteophytes or cubitus valgus deformity. Ultrasound is also useful for diagnosis by looking for entrapment or increased cross-sectional area of the ulnar nerve.

Differential diagnosis

Differential diagnosis should include cervical radiculopathy, thoracic outlet syndrome, ulnar nerve compression at wrist at Guyon canal, and UCL injury.

Treatment

Conservative treatment includes NSAIDs, modifying training, nighttime splinting, and elbow pads. An anterior transposition could be considered if there is a poor response to conservative measures. Interventional ultrasound for guided injections and hydrodissection could also be considered.

Prognosis and return to play

Prognosis and return to play depends on severity and chronicity of neuropathy. If surgical intervention is needed, the patient can expect to return to full activity after 4 to 6 weeks.

LATERAL ELBOW INJURIES

Lateral Epicondylitis

Mechanism of injury

Lateral epicondylitis is thought to be a result of microtrauma and incomplete healing of the common extensor tendon (CET) at its origin on the lateral epicondyle. The CET is made up of fibers from four muscles implicated in wrist and finger extension, including the extensor carpi radialis brevis (ECRB), extensor digitorum ED, extensor digiti minimi, and extensor carpi ulnaris (ECU). Overuse of these muscles, possibly secondary to frequent concentric forces on the tendon, result in microtears and an initial inflammatory healing response. Although lateral epicondylitis was originally documented in tennis players, resulting in the term tennis elbow, only about 5% to 10% of people who suffer from lateral epicondylitis actually play tennis. Conversely, about 50% of tennis players will suffer from tennis elbow at some point in their career, which is thought to be mostly due to single backhand hits.[22]

Physical examination

Patients will complain of lateral elbow pain that localizes to the lateral epicondyle. Tenderness to palpation is isolated to the common extensor origin (CEO) on the lateral epicondyle or just distal to it, and may be extremely tender. Elbow ROM is generally unaffected. Patients will have pain with grasping while in elbow extension, pain with resisted wrist extension, and a positive Thomas test (pain with resisted extension of the long finger). They may or may not have decreased grip strength, which is usually secondary to pain.

Imaging

Plain radiographs may be done in the setting of an unclear clinical diagnosis to rule out intra-articular pathologic conditions. Ultrasound is the preferred imaging modality for diagnosis and treatment of lateral epicondylitis, especially if it has been refractory to an initial trial of conservative therapy. Because they are relatively superficial, the CEO and CET can be visualized easily with ultrasound. It may show hypoechoic swelling of the CET, loss of fibrillar pattern, calcifications within the tendon itself, and fluid within or around the tendon sheath. Advanced disease may show bone spurring or cortical erosions of the epicondyle.

Differential diagnosis
Differential diagnosis should include radiohumeral arthritis, radial nerve injury, and osteochondritis dissecans of the capitellum.

Treatment
The treatment of lateral epicondylitis has evolved to include several accepted, although not necessarily evidence-based treatments, ranging from noninvasive to semi-invasive to surgical. Initial treatment is generally rest, ice, compression and elevation with or without PT. Studies have shown that early initiation of structured PT can improve functional pain scores compared with standard watching and waiting. It is thought this is a result of increased stem cell production to promote healing as the muscle is used.[23] Other conservative approaches may include wrist splinting to limit wrist extension, a counterforce strap, or discontinuation of the causative activity. Interventions that are commonly used include corticosteroid injections and, less commonly, platelet-rich plasma injections with or without percutaneous tenotomy. Steroids may improve pain in the short term; however, they seem to lengthen the overall course of the injury. PRP preliminarily shows promise in refractory cases, but there are no randomized studies supporting its superiority over existing treatments. It may be more useful in chronic cases in which the initial inflammatory healing process has stopped and a chronic fibrosis is present. PRP or tenotomy in that case may revitalize the inflammatory process and allow for complete tendon healing.[24–26]

Referral
Most cases resolve within 1 year. Patients who are refractory to the treatments listed above may benefit from surgical treatment. Fewer than 10% of patients require referral for surgery.

Prognosis and return to play
Most patients return to normal function within 1 year of initial symptoms. The cause of lateral epicondylitis may be predictive of the response to therapy. If the overuse occurred due to activity the patient performs at work or on a daily basis, it may be more refractory to treatment.

RC Chondromalacia

Mechanism of injury
RC chondromalacia is the degeneration of the radiohumeral joint at the capitellar articulation. This is most likely caused by repetitive valgus stress, resulting in compression at the RC articularion.[27] This is an overuse injury.

Physical examination
Patients will complain of lateral elbow pain as well as mechanical symptoms. There may be localized tenderness and swelling in the joint. Catching and locking are associated with chondromalacia, whereas a snapping sensation may be related to synovial hypertrophy and plica band irritation. Pain may be reducible with palpation or compression of the RC joint with valgus stress, particularly with the elbow in extension.

Imaging
Plain radiographs may show joint space narrowing, osteophytes, or loose bodies.

Differential diagnosis
Differential diagnosis should include osteochondritis dissecans, lateral epicondylitis, and stress fracture.

Treatment
The goal of treatment is to reduce symptoms and prevent further damage. NSAIDs may be helpful, as is rest and ice. Reducing inflammation, particularly of the surrounding synovium, may be helpful in reducing mechanical symptoms.

Referral
If imaging reveals loose bodies or there are significant mechanical symptoms, patients may benefit from arthroscopic debridement and surgical referral is appropriate.

Prognosis and return to play
RC chondromalacia is a chronic condition and goals for return to play are improvement of symptoms and prevention of worsening the condition. Activities that specifically cause RC compression or valgus stress should be avoided. Return to play is mainly dictated by pain.

Posterior Interosseus Nerve Syndrome

Mechanism of injury
The mechanism of injury for posterior interosseus nerve (PIN) syndrome is compression of the PIN along the radial tunnel at one or more of five potential sites, resulting in denervation of ECRB, ECU, extensor digitorum communis, extensor digiti minimi, abductor pollicis longus, EPL (extensor pollicis longus), EPB (extensor pollicis brevis), and EIP (extensor indicis proprius).

1. Fibrous band anterior to RC joint between brachialis and brachioradialis
2. Recurrent radial vessels as they course across the PIN at radial neck (leash of Henry)
3. Leading edge of ECRB
4. Distal edge of supinator
5. Proximal edge of supinator, called the arcade of Fröhse and is a variant seen in 30% to 50% of population.[28]

PIN syndrome can also be a result of synovial hypertrophy secondary to rheumatoid arthritis.

Physical examination
The primary symptom of PIN compression is weakness. Patients are unable to extend their fingers or thumb. Extension of the wrist is intact; however, there is pronounced radial deviation because the ECR (extensor carpi radialis) is still functional. In contract, the primary complaint of radial tunnel syndrome, which is mechanistically similar, is pain.

Imaging
Nerve conduction studies are the most helpful diagnostic tool in PIN syndrome. If the ultrasound is skillfully done, the PIN can be imaged and an increased cross-sectional area will show at the area of compression. It generally shows normal radial sensory conduction and chronic denervation of affected muscles. MR can show abnormal signal intensity of the affected muscles.

Differential diagnosis
Differential diagnosis should include radial tunnel syndrome, radial nerve compression proximal to elbow (C8 nerve root compression), and extensor tendon rupture.

Treatment
Treatment should include avoidance of exacerbating movement. Steroid injections are difficult because localization of the site of compression is difficult. However, it

is generally reasonable to attempt one steroid injection. It is important to address functional weakness to prevent contractures. Hand therapy, as well as placement of a dynamic finger extension splint, is warranted. NSAIDs are useful in reducing inflammation and improving compression. Ultrasound-guided hydrodissection has shown to help release area of compression around nerve and alleviate symptoms. Splints that limit pronation and wrist flexion may also prevent worsening of impingement.

Referral

If there is no improvement after 3 months of conservative treatment, the patient may be referred to surgery for decompression.

Prognosis and return to play

Early treatment generally results in better outcomes. If therapy and treatment are initiated before atrophy of muscles or permanent nerve damage, function may return to normal. If PIN syndrome has been chronic before treatment, surgical tendon transfer may be necessary to regain functional use of hand.

Radial Head Fracture

Mechanism of injury

The most common mechanism of injury for radial head fracture is a fall on an outstretched hand, more likely with a pronated hand and elbow in slight flexion. It also may be the result of a direct blow to the lateral elbow.

Physical examination

The patient will complain of limited, painful forearm ROM and tenderness over the radial head. There may also be swelling or ecchymosis.

Imaging

Radiographs may clearly show fracture or may only have evidence of fracture with sail sign (elevated anterior fat pad) or a posterior fat pad. CT or MRI is sometimes used to better characterize the fracture for better treatment planning. Radial head fractures are classified using the Mason system.[29] Imaging results may include

i. Nondisplaced, no mechanical obstruction
ii. Less than 2 mm displacement or greater than 30° angulation
iii. Comminuted fracture
iv. Fracture with elbow dislocation.

Differential diagnosis

Differential diagnoses should include supracondylar fracture, olecranon fracture, elbow subluxation or dislocation and nursemaids elbow.

Treatment

Treatment based on Mason classification includes

i. Early mobilization, which has shown to have better outcomes than brief immobilization, a sling for comfort, repeat films in 1 to 2 weeks, and PT for motion and strength if needed
ii. If displacement is less than 2 mm and less than 30°, nonsurgical treatment may be considered. Otherwise, open reduction, internal fixation (ORIF) is indicated, with almost universal healing and excellent functional outcomes
iii. Repair with fixation versus radial head excision or prosthesis, depending on extent of injury; treatment similar for class III and IV.[30]

Referral
Most class II, and all class III and IV fractures require evaluation and fixation by a surgeon.

Prognosis and return to play
Return to play for class I is about 2 to 3 months. It is similar for class II depending on how quickly surgery was performed and how it was tolerated. Many people with class III and IV fractures have persistent pain, elbow instability, and may require further procedures. Those that do well may return to play in 4 to 6 months.

PEDIATRIC ELBOW INJURIES

Supracondylar Fracture

Mechanism of injury
Supracondylar fractures are the most common pediatric elbow fractures. The peak incidence is 6 to 7 years. These fractures usually occur from a fall on an outstretched hand with hyperextension at the elbow. They also may result from a direct blow or fall on a flexed elbow.

Physical examination
Patients will complain of posterior elbow pain, and may have swelling, ecchymosis, or deformity. A dimple or ecchymosis over the anterior distal humerus may suggest injury to the brachialis. An S-shaped deformity can be seen with 100% posterior displacement of the distal fragment. Care should be taken to do a complete neurovascular evaluation of the forearm and hand. Compartment syndrome and nerve palsies are not unusual, most commonly of the radial nerve or anterior interosseous nerve. It is also important to look for other injuries, including distal forearm fractures.

Imaging
Radiographs including AP and lateral views are useful for both identifying apparent and occult fractures. On the AP view, a Baumann angle can be calculated by drawing two lines, one perpendicular to the long axis of the humerus and one parallel through the capital physis. The lateral view can show the elevated anterior or posterior fat pad or sail sign, which indicates a hemarthrosis. Displacement can be detected by drawing a line along the anterior border of the humerus, which should go through the center of the capitellum. About 95% of supracondylar fractures will have some degree of posterior displacement. Classification of fractures based on the Gartland classification system include[31]

i. Nondisplaced
ii. Displaced with angulation, but the posterior cortex remains intact
iii. Complete displacement of distal fragment with no cortex intact.

Differential diagnosis
The differential diagnosis should include other traumatic fractures.

Treatment
Based on Gartland classification, treatment includes

i. A long arm cast for 4 weeks, then reimaging
ii. Attempt at closed reduction and casting; if fracture is not stable at 90° of flexion, fixation is required; casting in hyperflexion may result in Volkmann ischemia
iii. Always-required fixation.

If there is greater than 10° varus deformity when compared with contralateral elbow, fixation required despite level of posterior displacement.[32]

Referral

For above indications requiring surgery. About 20% of fractures ultimately require open reduction and fixation.[31]

Prognosis and return to play

In the absence of neurovascular compromise, children generally do well despite severity of fracture and return to play in 2 to 6 months. Those with compartment syndrome of nerve palsies may require prolonged treatment as a result of those injuries.

Radial Head Subluxation (aka Nursemaid's Elbow)

Mechanism of injury

The mechanism of injury for radial head subluxation is inferior displacement of the radial head with annular ligament tear and displacement into the RC joint, resulting is limited ROM and pain. It is seen almost exclusively in children less than 6 years old and is a result of poor attachment of the annular ligament to the radial head, as well as a relatively narrow radial head in comparison to the radial neck. Displacement most commonly occurs when axial traction is placed on a pronated forearm with elbow extension. An example is when an adult quickly lifts child up by wrist.

Physical examination

The patient will complain of elbow pain and likely splint his or her arm against the body. There will be limited elbow ROM with supination and flexion. A parent may only notice that their child is not using the arm normally, without complaint of pain.

Imaging

In general, imaging is not necessary if the clinical presentation is consistent with nursemaid's elbow. If there is a history of trauma or concern for other injury, plain films should be performed. Positioning for a plain film may result in reduction of the radial head.

Differential diagnosis

Differential diagnosis should include fracture.

Treatment

Historically, supination-flexion was the maneuver used to reduce a subluxed radial head. However, studies have shown that hyperpronation has a more successful initial reduction rate and causes less discomfort to the patient. One study reports a 95% reduction rate on first attempt with hyperpronation, compared with 77% with supination-flexion.[33,34]

Referral

Referral for surgical evaluation is rarely indicated or needed.

Prognosis and return to play

Children with nursemaid's elbow are often back to normal immediately after reduction. Rarely, an underlying anatomic variant which includes deformity of radial head may predispose a child to recurrent subluxations, in which case further imaging and evaluation may be warranted.

Medial Apophysitis (aka Little Leaguer's Elbow)

Mechanism of injury

This is one of many overuse injuries that can occur with valgus extension overload, most commonly in the overhead throwing athlete. It is common in adolescent baseball players with open medial epicondyle apophysis.

Physical examination

Presentation frequently is a result of decreased throwing velocity, poor accuracy, and decreased endurance. The patients also complain of progressive medial elbow pain. This usually occurs in the middle or end of a season. Examination will reveal tenderness over the medial epicondyle and pain with valgus stress. The patient will have pain with resisted wrist flexion, and may have a slight flexion contracture at the elbow.

Imaging

Bilateral AP films of the elbow should be obtained for comparison. The affected elbow may show fragmentation at the medial epicondyle, bony irregularity, or widening of the physis on the affected side.

Differential diagnosis

Differential diagnosis should include medial epicondyle avulsion fracture, UCL tear, and medial epicondylitis.

Treatment

The most important part of treatment of these athletes is rest. Pitchers should not throw for 4 to 6 weeks. During that time, rest, ice, and NSAIDs may be used for symptomatic improvement. After a period of rest and when the athlete is asymptomatic, she or he may begin strengthening and stretching.

Referral

Rarely, conservative treatment fails and surgical evaluation maybe appropriate.

Prognosis and return to play

Players may return to competitive pitching in about 12 weeks if they follow initial guidelines for rest. The most important part of return to play is preventing future injuries. A competitive pitcher with a history of medial apophysitis would benefit from professional evaluation of their pitching mechanics to prevent further overuse injuries. Most overseeing bodies of Little League and youth baseball have adopted pitch counts to prevent these injuries. The American Academy of Pediatrics recommends limiting pitches to 200 per week and 90 per outing. USA baseball is more conservative, with counts based on the pitcher's age and ranging from 75 to 125 per week and 50 to 75 per outing.[35]

Osteochondritis Dissecans Capitellum

Mechanism of injury

This overuse injury results from a combination of microtrauma to the RC joint in the setting of tenuous blood supply to the capitellum. It most commonly affects baseball pitchers and gymnasts. RC compression occurs late in the cocking phase of a pitch, and at full elbow extension during gymnastics, making these athletes prone to repetitive trauma to the capitellum. The radial head has been found to have stiffer cartilage than the capitellum, causing a stress mismatch and overloading the articular cartilage. Poor healing secondary to limited blood supply in the setting of microtrauma results in separation of the articular cartilage from the subchondral bone. It most commonly affects athletes ages 11 to 15 years.[36]

Physical examination
Patients will complain of several months of pain over the lateral elbow. It is improved with rest and rarely are there night symptoms. Patients may have decreased ROM, specifically loss of elbow extension. Mechanical symptoms may occur, especially if there is a loose body or fragmentation of cartilage. Usually, there is a positive RC compression test, done by pronation and supination of the forearm with the elbow at full extension.

Imaging
AP films done with 45° of flexion best isolate the RC joint and may show flattening of the subchondral bone or loose bodies in the joint. MRI or MR arthrography may show earlier signs of an osteochondritis dissecans capitellum and will be more helpful in determining fragment stability, which is helpful in treatment planning.

Differential diagnosis
Differential diagnosis should include RC chondromalacia, lateral epicondylitis, and Panner disease (usually in 7–12 year olds, avascular necrosis [AVN] of capitellum).

Treatment
Nonoperative treatment is indicated for early lesions with no loose bodies or fragmentation. This requires the athlete to completely stop the causative activity for at least 6 months. Pitchers are generally advised to not play that position again. Strengthening exercises may begin when symptoms have resolved. NSAIDs can be helpful and PT may be useful to regain any lost ROM. About 50% of lesions that initially are treated nonoperatively will heal.

Referral
Surgery is indicated in any patient with fragmentation or loose bodies, or who has failed conservative treatment with no improvement in 6 months. Arthroscopic debridement, microfracture, and occasionally osteo-articular transfer system (OATS) procedures are indicated.

Prognosis and return to play
Osteochondritis dissecans requires a significant amount of complete rest and abstinence from causative activity for healing to occur. Compliant patients may return to play in 6 months to a year if they are symptom free.

SUMMARY

The reader of this article should now be familiar with elbow injuries that occur at the medial, lateral, anterior, and posterior aspects, including pediatric elbow injuries. The reader should be able to understand the description, imaging, anatomy, mechanism of injury, physical examination, diagnostics, differential diagnosis, management, cause for referral to an orthopedic surgeon, controversies, and advancements in management for each type of injuries included in the anterior, posterior, lateral and medical elbow.

REFERENCES

1. Tsai WC, Yang YM. Fluoroquinolone-associated tendinopathy. Chang Gung Med J 2011;34(5):461–7.
2. Miyamoto RG, Elser F, Millett PJ. Distal biceps tendon injuries. J Bone Joint Surg Am 2010;92(11):2128–38.

3. Quach T, Jazayeri R, Sherman OH, et al. Distal biceps tendon injuries – current treatment options. Bull NYU Hosp Jt Dis 2012;68(2):103–11.
4. Thatte MR, Mansukhani KA. Compressive neuropathy in the upper limb. Indian J Plast Surg 2011;44(2):283–97.
5. Bridgeman C, Naidu S, Kothari MJ. Clinical and electrophysiological presentation of pronator syndrome. Electromyogr Clin Neurophysiol 2007;47(2):89–92.
6. Mulvaney SW. Ultrasound guided percutaneous neuroplasty of the lateral femoral cutaneous nerve for the treatment of meralgia paresthetica: a case report and description of a new ultrasound-guided technique. Curr Sports Med Rep 2011; 10(2):99–104.
7. Benjamin HJ, Briner WW. Little League elbow. Clin J Sport Med 2005;15:37–40.
8. Taylor DW, Petrera M, Hendry M, et al. A systemic review of the use of platelet-rich plasma in sports medicine as a new treatment for tendon and ligament injuries. Clin J Sport Med 2011;21:344–52.
9. Chang HY, Wang CH, Chou KY, et al. Could forearm Kinesio Taping improve strength, force sense, and pain in baseball pitchers with medical epicondylitis? Clin J Sport Med 2012;0:1–7.
10. Weng PW, Wang SH, Wu SS. Misdiagnosed avulsion fracture of the triceps tendon from the olecranon insertion: case report. Clin J Sport Med 2006;16:364–5.
11. Vidal AF, Drakos MC, Allen AA. Biceps tendon and triceps tendon injuries. Clin Sports Med 2004;23:707–22.
12. Radunovic G, Vlad V, Micu MC, et al. Ultrasound assessment of the elbow. Med Ultrason 2012;12(2):141–6.
13. Mair SD, Isbel WM, Gill TJ, et al. Triceps tendon ruptures in football players. Am J Sports Med 2004;32:431–4.
14. Kooima CL, Anderson K, Craig JV, et al. Evidence of subclinical medial collateral ligament injury and posteromedial impingement in professional baseball players. Am J Sports Med 2004;32:1602–6.
15. Mehta JA, Bain GI. Elbow dislocations in adults and children. Clin Sports Med 2004;23:609–27.
16. Ciccotti MC, Schwartz MA, Ciccotti MG. Diagnosis and treatment of medial epicondylitis. Clin Sports Med 2004;23:693–705.
17. Mishra A, Pavelko T. Treatment of chronic elbow tendinosis with buffered platelet rich plasma. Am J Sports Med 2006;34:1774–8.
18. Hang DW, Chao CM, Hang YS. A clinical and roentgenographic study of Little League elbow. Am J Sports Med 2004;32:79–84.
19. Safran MR. Elbow injuries in athletes. Clin Sports Med 2004;23.
20. Carlisle JC, Gerlach DJ, Wright RW. Netter's Sports Medicine. Philadelphia: Saunders Elsevier; 2010. p. 360–7.
21. Rudzki JR, Paletta GA. Juvenile and adolescent elbow injuries in sports. Clin Sports Med 2004;23:581–609.
22. Behrens SB, Deren ME, Matson AP, et al. A review of modern management of lateral epicondylitis. Phys Sportsmed 2012;40(2):34–40.
23. Peterson M, Butler S, Eriksson M, et al. A randomized controlled trial of exercise versus wait-list in chronic tennis elbow (lateral epicondylitis). Ups J Med Sci 2011;116(4):269–79.
24. Saccomanni B. Corticosteroid injection for tennis elbow or lateral epicondylitis: a review of the literature. Curr Rev Musculoskelet Med 2010;3(1–4):38–40.
25. Park JY, Park HK, Choi JH, et al. Prospective evaluation of the effectiveness of a home-based program of isometric strengthening exercises: 12 month follow-up. Clin Orthop Surg 2010;2(3):173–8.

26. Rayan F, Rao V, Purushothamdas S, et al. Common extensor origin release in recalcitrant lateral epicondylitis—role justified? J Orthop Surg Res 2010;5:31.
27. Chumbley EM, O'Connor FG, Nirschl RP. Evaluation of overuse elbow injuries. Am Fam Physician 2000;61(3):691–700.
28. Andreisek G, Crook DW, Burg D, et al. Peripheral neuropathies of the median, radial, and ulnar nerves: MR imaging features. Radiographics 2006;26: 1267–87.
29. Black WS, Becker JA. Common forearm fractures in adults. Am Fam Physician 2009;80(10):1096–102.
30. Erturer E, Seckin F, Akman S, et al. The results of open reduction and screw or K-wire fixation for isolated type II radial head fractures. Acta Orthop Traumatol Turc 2010;44(1):20–6.
31. Kraus R, Wessel L. The treatment of upper limb fractures in children and adolescents. Dtsch Arztebl Int 2010;107(51–52):903–10.
32. Brubacher JW, Dodds SD. Pediatric supracondylar fractures of the distal humerus. Curr Rev Musculoskelet Med 2008;1(3–4):190–6.
33. Crowther M. Elbow pain in pediatrics. Curr Rev Musculoskelet Med 2009;2(2): 83–7.
34. Karasick D. Nursemaid elbow revisited and a review of congenital radioulnar synestosis. Radiographics 2004;24:1608–10.
35. Cassas KJ, Cassettari-Wyhas A. Childhood and adolescent sports-related overuse injuries. Am Fam Physician 2006;73(6):1014–22.
36. Bojanic I, Smoljanovic T, Dokuzovic S. Osteochondritis dissecans of the elbow: excellent mid-term follow-up results in teenage athletes treated by arthroscopic debridement and microfractures. Croat Med J 2012;53(1):40–7.

Treatment of Hand and Wrist Injuries

Kenneth M. Bielak, MD, MBA*, Julie Kafka, MD,
Tom Terrell, MD, MPhil

KEYWORDS

- Hand injury • Wrist injury • Dislocations • Tendinitis
- Triangular fibrocartilage complex tear • Mallet finger • Boutonnière deformity
- Scaphoid fracture

KEY POINTS

- Fracture of the distal radius and/or ulna is a common clinical problem, comprising approximately 0.66% of United States emergency room visits.
- Plain radiographs are the mainstay of the diagnosis of distal radius fractures.
- Because fractures to the carpal bones typically are the result of high-energy impact, the clinician must keep a high index of suspicion for associated soft-tissue and ligamentous injury.
- The sports medicine clinician must decide early on definitive treatment after discussing various options with patients.
- Fractures of the metacarpals are the second most common type of upper extremity fracture.

ANATOMY OF THE WRIST

The carpal bones are 8 bones in 2 rows emanating off the radius and ulna terminus, which comprise approximately 3 cm of the proximal hand: the proximal row consists of the scaphoid, lunate, triquetrum, and pisiform, and the distal row contains the trapezium, trapezoid, capitate, and hamate (**Fig. 1**).

Attention to surface anatomy can assist in identifying and palpating individual carpal bones. The scaphoid bone bridges the proximal and distal rows and can be palpated within the "snuff box" (between the tendons of the extensor pollicis brevis and extensor pollicis longus). The lunate can be palpated just ulnar to the sulcus created by the base of the scaphoid off the distal radius and is in line with the third phalanx, and is more prominent with flexion of the wrist. The triquetrum is palpated distal to

Department of Family Medicine, University of Tennessee Health Science Center, Graduate School of Medicine, University of Tennessee, 1924 Alcoa Highway, Knoxville, TN 37920, USA
* Corresponding author.
E-mail address: kbielak@utmck.edu

Prim Care Clin Office Pract 40 (2013) 431–451
http://dx.doi.org/10.1016/j.pop.2013.02.006 primarycare.theclinics.com
0095-4543/13/$ – see front matter

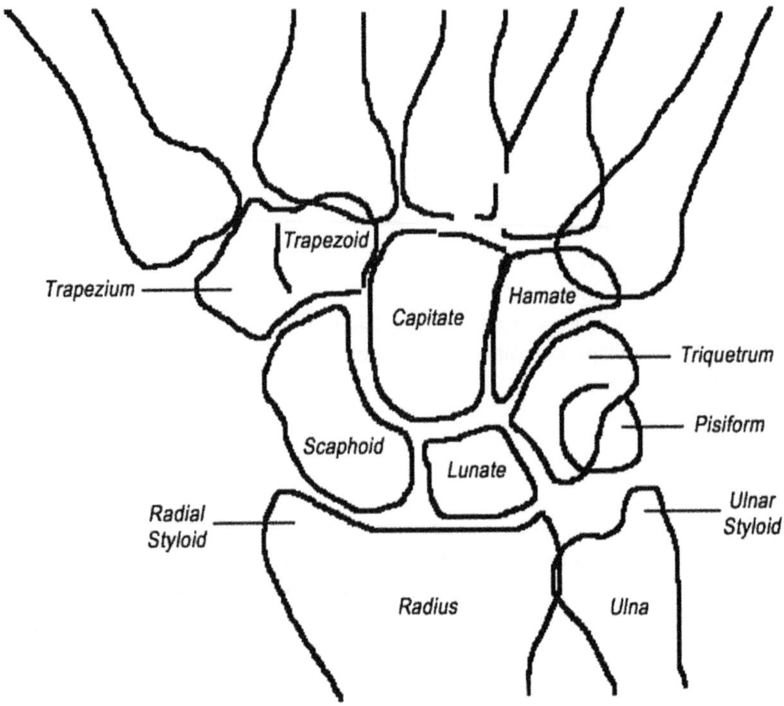

Fig. 1. Anatomy of the wrist.

the ulnar bone. The pisiform is palpated on the volar aspect of the distal wrist in line with the fifth phalanx. It is actually considered a sesamoid bone associated with the flexor carpi ulnaris tendon. The radial side of the distal carpal bones begins with the trapezium, which can be palpated just proximal of the first metacarpal. The trapezoid, though difficult to palpate, is found just proximal to the dorsal index metacarpal. The capitate is proximal to the third dorsal metacarpal. The hamate is just proximal to the dorsal fifth metacarpal. The hook of the hamate can be palpated deep in the hypothenar eminence by rolling the opposite thumb off the pisiform toward the second metacarpophalangeal (MCP) joint.

There are intrinsic ligaments (intercarpal) and extrinsic ligaments from the radius, ulna, and metacarpal ligaments that attach to the carpal bones. (The reader is directed to any anatomy text for the labeling of volar and dorsal intercarpal and extrinsic ligaments of the hand and wrist.)

FRACTURES

Distal Radius Fractures

Epidemiology

Fracture of the distal radius and/or ulna is a common clinical problem, occurring in roughly 0.66% of United States emergency room (ER) visits.[1] These fractures occur in 2 different populations: children who sustain high-energy trauma and the osteoporotic elderly whose fractures are caused by much less impact. In women older than 50 years the lifetime risk has been estimated to be 15%.[2–4] In children younger than 16 years, distal radial fractures occur more frequently than any other fracture.[5] There has been a statistically significant increase in the incidence of distal radial fractures in children, thought to be due to changing patterns of physical activity[6,7] and increasing obesity rates (leading to increased impact with falls).[8]

Mechanism of injury

The mechanism of injury for distal radial fractures often is different between the younger and the older population. In general, young adults will sustain the injury from high-energy trauma and the older population usually experiences a low-impact injury, such as a simple fall on an outstretched hand. Because of the significant forces that may lead to a fracture, especially in high-velocity sports, an injury to the wrist requires a thorough assessment to rule out further complex injuries beyond that of a fracture. Fractures to the distal ulna may occur in similar fashion to fractures of the distal radius and are typically associated with such fractures. Stress fractures, typically associated with overuse, may also occur in either bone.

Physical evaluation

Initially on physical examination one should assess for swelling, pain, and limited range of motion. The classic deformity seen in a distal radius fracture, first described by Colles, is a "silver fork" deformity. Because other concomitant injuries can occur in conjunction with distal radius fractures, the wrist should be thoroughly examined for injury to the carpal bones, carpal ligaments, the triangular fibrocartilage complex (TFCC), and the distal radioulnar joint. In addition, the more dorsal the displacement of the distil fracture fragment, the greater the chance of injury to the median nerve. Thus a thorough assessment of the area is necessary to both prevent further injury during fracture manipulation and assess for concomitant injuries.

Radiologic evaluation

Plain radiographs are the mainstay of the diagnosis of distal radius fractures (**Fig. 2**). Posteroanterior (PA) and lateral plain radiographs are assessed for angulation and displacement of the fracture, specifically noting radial height, radial inclination, and volar tilt.[9] The images determine the palmar tilt angle on lateral radiographs (normally around 11°) and radial height on anteroposterior (AP) view. Any shortening of the radial height on the AP radiograph by 50% (5 mm) or more is considered to lead to long-term functional impairment.

Further imaging, such as computed tomography (CT) scans, may be necessary for surgical planning involving intra-articular displacements. When assessing for stress fractures, plain radiographs may be beneficial if they show periosteal reactions. Otherwise, a bone scan or magnetic resonance imaging (MRI) is necessary to confirm the diagnosis.

Treatment

Stress fractures are typically treated with splinting and rest, with gradual progression toward resuming full activity. Physical therapy may also be recommended to correct biomechanical issues that may have contributed to the problem. Four to 6 weeks of rest and rehabilitation may be required.

For stable minimally displaced fractures of the distal radius, cast immobilization for 4 to 6 weeks remains standard.

Controversy regarding optimal treatment exists when the fractures become angulated or shortened, and there have been multiple studies assessing the amount of displacement (shortening and angulation) that is acceptable. Some investigators[10] recommend referral and appropriate reduction (either closed or surgical) for any fracture that is likely to be unstable. Several factors, including a dorsal angulation of greater than 20° (normal angulation is a palmar angulation of around 11°) and greater

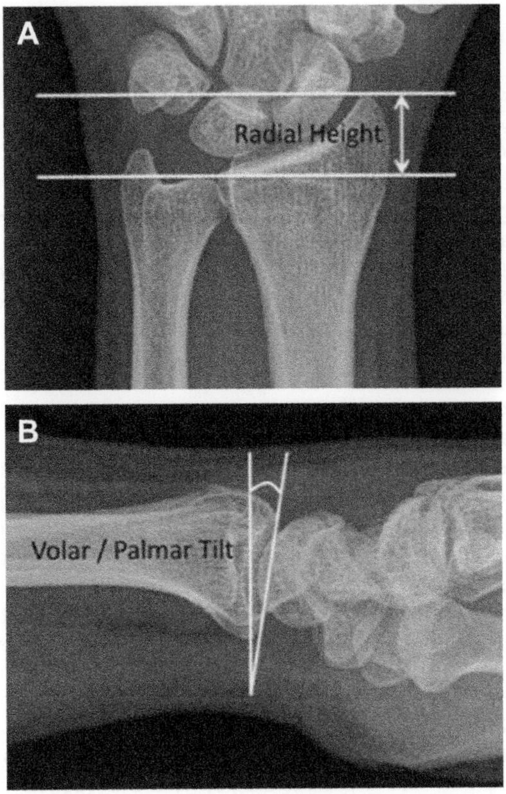

Fig. 2. Radiographs of distal radius fractures. (*A*) determines the palmar tilt angle on lateral radiographs (normally around 11 degrees) and (*B*) radial height on anteroposterior (AP) view. (*From* Ang SH, Lee SW, Lam KY. Ultrasound-guided reduction of distal radius fractures. Am J Emerg Med 2010;28(9):1002–8; with permission.)

than 5 mm of radial shortening, are presumed to lead to instability or long-term disability,[10–12] Many surgeons will opt for surgical treatment for shortened, angulated fractures; however, recently a systematic review concluded that cast immobilization provided functional outcomes similar to those for surgical intervention in patients older than 60 years, despite residual angulation and shortening.[13]

In a recent article, Henry[14] insists that from a clinical-decision standpoint only 2 questions need to be answered: (1) Has the articular surface been disrupted to the point of instability? (2) Is the metaphysis incompetent to bear load? If the answer to either of these questions is yes, then some type of surgical fixation will be required. A wide variety of surgical treatments for unstable distal radial fractures is available, including closed reduction and percutaneous pinning, external fixation, individual fragment fixation, dorsal plates, and volar locking plates.

Issues in operative treatment

Bone graft The recommendation for bone grafting is usually apparent in cases aimed at preventing radial shortening by providing additional structural support.[15] There are primarily 3 types of bone grafting options: autogenous, allograft, and bone graft substitutes. Each option has its advantages and disadvantages. The often cited disadvantages of autograft substitution are donor-site morbidity and increased surgical time. The primary disadvantage for allograft and bone graft substitutes is that they are expensive.[16] In a recent review, Handoll and Watts[17] focused on the treatment of dorsal metaphyseal voids with bone grafts or bone graft substitutes; they concluded that bone graft and substitutes may improve final radiographic alignment but do not alter functional outcomes.

Internal versus external fixation There has been a slow shift in operative management from external fixation toward open reduction and internal fixation (ORIF). This trend has occurred without strong evidence to support the change.[18] External fixation with Kirschner (K)-wires requires the wrist to be immobilized in a cast for 6 weeks before the flexible wires can be removed.[19] ORIF with locking plates, on the other hand, allows the patient to move their wrist more quickly because of the rigid nature of the hardware.[19] A recent meta-analysis comparing operative treatments for displaced unstable radius fractures found that ORIF using volar plates yielded greater forearm supination, better maintenance of volar tilt, and improved subjective and functional outcomes when compared with external fixation. External fixation was been found to lead to greater recovery of grip strength.[20]

A recent German review,[21] however, concluded that either technique was suitable and that long-term results were similar. The investigators noted that plates were more expensive, required longer surgical times, and had a higher risk of injury to nerves or blood vessels during the procedure.[22]

Rehabilitation

With nondisplaced distal radius fractures, cast immobilization is maintained for 4 to 6 weeks before rehabilitation. In patients aged 60 years or older, the immobilization time should be minimized to limit stiffness. Depending on the stability of the fracture, it may be appropriate to transition to a wrist splint and early rehabilitation. The wrist splint has been shown to minimize postimmobilization stiffness in comparison with a cast.[23]

Long-term complications

Fractures with displacement have been associated with the development of radiocarpal osteoarthritis; however, these radiographic changes did not necessarily demonstrate poor long-term functional outcome.[24]

Scaphoid Fractures

Epidemiology

The scaphoid bone is the most common carpal bone fracture, whereby the usual mechanism of injury is a fall on the outstretched hand.

Physical evaluation

Because fractures to the carpal bones typically are the result of high-energy impact, the clinician must maintain a high index of suspicion for associated soft-tissue and ligamentous injury.

Snuffbox tenderness should be sought for scaphoid fractures, and complete hand examination must be done to search for any concomitant injuries.

Radiologic evaluation

Scaphoid fractures are often difficult to diagnose on plain films, with a wide range of sensitivities reported in the literature (roughly between 70% and 86%).[25] Nondisplaced fractures are notoriously more difficult to visualize. Scaphoid fractures are typically grouped into proximal third (usually defined as the proximal one-quarter to one-fifth of the bone),[26] middle third, and distal third fractures, as this classification helps the clinician decide on optimal treatment. Because plain radiographs are limited in their ability to diagnose these fractures (sensitivity of roughly 75%) especially in the acute setting, CT or MRI may be needed to make the diagnosis of subtle fractures or stress fractures.

Treatment: operative versus nonoperative

Distal and middle one-third scaphoid fractures have the best chance of healing without operative intervention because they have a good vascular supply and are often nondisplaced. These fractures may be treated with a short arm thumb spica cast for 10 to 12 weeks, with an expected healing rate of 95%.[27,28]

Proximal (or displaced) scaphoid fractures often require surgery because they have a more precarious blood supply and, hence, a higher incidence of nonunion. One recent meta-analysis[26] documented a 34% nonunion rate in proximal fractures treated conservatively. Some investigators,[28] however, still see nonoperative treatment as a viable option for these fractures, noting similar healing rates when all nondisplaced scaphoid fractures are grouped together and reviewed. Their comparison of surgical versus conservative treatment, however, did not perform subgroup analysis on proximal fractures in isolation, making their work of little use in resolving the question of optimal treatment for proximal fractures. Of note, they did find a greater incidence of late (12 years after treatment) radiographic scaphoid-trapezial arthritis in patients treated surgically, although subjective symptoms did not differ.

Recent advances in operative techniques have reduced surgical morbidity by decreasing manipulation of tissue by arthroscopic repair and by using small compression screws that minimize interruption of vascular supply. These techniques can accelerate healing and rehabilitation.[29]

Expected return to sport participation

The sports medicine clinician must decide early on definitive treatment after discussing various options with patients.[30] Patients returning to noncontact sports who have been treated conservatively with casting are allowed to return to sport immediately once casting is in place. In patients treated surgically, returning to noncontact sports can be allowed with protective padding once wounds have healed and the patient is comfortable. Of course, treatments should be individualized, and patients with proximal third fractures may be treated more gingerly than those with middle and distal fractures.

In patients returning to contact sports, most investigators[31] favor the following protocol, In patients treated with casting, a full 6-week period of "no play" is mandated to allow initial healing before competition is allowed in a "playing cast" for the final 6 weeks of casting. Often a CT of the scaphoid will be obtained at 6 weeks to ensure that healing has begun before return to play is allowed. In patients with surgically treated scaphoid fractures, return to play will usually be allowed after 3 to 6 weeks with appropriate playing-cast protection. Thus, surgical treatment may result in an earlier return to play (in a playing cast) in these athletes. Usually, a CT to document healing is recommended before allowing the player to discard the protective cast. Other investigators[32] allow immediate return to contact sports with protective casting after surgery.

Future trends

Wrist arthroscopy can provide quicker recovery and rehabilitation time by using minimally invasive techniques such as pin fixation, intramedullary fixation, and transcutaneous pin stabilization of various carpal fractures and dissociations.[33] In the hands of the skilled surgeon this approach may allow return to play in a shorter time.

Metacarpal Fractures

Epidemiology

Fractures of the metacarpals are the second most common type of upper extremity fracture, usually classified by the anatomic location of the factures: head, neck, shaft, and base. The most common fracture site of the first metacarpal is at the base, and the neck and shaft are the most common sites for the second through fifth metacarpals. The most common fracture of the hand is a fracture of the fifth metacarpal, accounting for approximately 50% of all metacarpal fractures and 20% of all hand fractures.[34]

Mechanism of injury

Metacarpal base fractures most commonly occur as a result of a direct blow with a hard object or a torsional force to the finger. It is common to see involvement of the carpometacarpal (CMC) joint with these fractures. Specifically, the Bennett fracture involves the first CMC joint. Fractures of the second and third metacarpals rarely displace, owing to their fixed position at the CMC joint. With injuries to the fourth or fifth metacarpal, the motor branch of the ulnar nerve may be affected.

Metacarpal shaft fractures are more common on the ulnar side of the hand and occur most frequently at the fifth metacarpal.[29] Fractures to the shaft can present as transverse, oblique, or comminuted. The injury mechanism that causes a transverse fracture is usually a direct blow to the metacarpal. Oblique fractures are caused by a twisting force, and comminuted injuries result from significant trauma.

The mechanism that causes a metacarpal neck fracture involves direct trauma to a clenched fist, such as punching a wall. The location of injury is most commonly the fourth or fifth metacarpal bone and is termed a boxer's fracture. The trauma causes the metacarpal head to displace with volar angulation, leading to significant tenderness on the bony palmar surface of the hand.

The rarest of the metacarpal fractures is an injury to the metacarpal head. The mechanism is usually crush injuries or a direct blow, which can have associated avulsion of the collateral ligaments. The second metacarpal is most commonly involved.

Physical evaluation

On examination, the metacarpal will appear swollen with pain at the area of fracture. Often, pain is exacerbated with axial compression of the affected finger. There will be limited range of motion. Abduction and adduction of the fourth and fifth fingers should be tested to ensure integrity of the ulnar nerve. Assessment for a potential rotational deformity should include slight flexion of the fingers toward the volar aspect of the hand, with note taken of any overlap of the digits or rotation of the nail plate.

Radiographic evaluation

All suspected hand fractures should be evaluated with PA, lateral, and oblique films. Because of the overlap of the metacarpals, the lateral view and oblique view are important in identifying certain metacarpal fractures.[35] The radiographs should be examined for shortening, angulation, malrotation, and comminution. Some fractures may be subtle to identify and may require CT or MRI to confirm the diagnosis.

Operative versus nonoperative treatment

The majority of metacarpal fractures do not require surgery. The anatomic location of the injury tends to dictate the intervention required. Specifically, limited angulation of metacarpal neck fractures is well tolerated. As long as there is little rotation deformity, the fourth and fifth metacarpals can tolerate up to 30° of angulation, and the second and third metacarpals can tolerate up to 10°. The exact amount of acceptable degrees of angulation for closed treatment has been a controversial topic in the past. One cadaveric study suggested that any fifth metacarpal fracture angle greater than 30° impaired motor function.[36] For nonoperative treatment the patient is placed in an ulnar gutter splint for 3 to 4 weeks with the MCP joints in 70° to 90° of flexion. This splint is recommended to prevent collateral ligament shortening and loss of joint mobility.

Metacarpal shaft fractures can be immobilized in a radial or ulnar gutter splint if they are nondisplaced. As with neck fractures, some angulation is tolerated with this injury. At the second and third metacarpal shafts, 10° of angulation is tolerated, whereas 20° is acceptable for the fourth and fifth metacarpals. If the metacarpal is shortened by more than 5 mm, orthopedic referral should be made. Percutaneous pinning, intramedullary fixation, or ORIF can be used to treat this injury. With percutaneous fixation techniques complications have been noted to occur in 16% to 18% of patients. These complications include pin loosening, pin-tract infections, osteomyelitis, nonunion, and injury to nerve, tendon, or artery.[37,38]

Fractures to the base of the second, third, and fourth metacarpals tend to be stable because of their fixed position at the CMC joints and to the neighboring metacarpals, whereas fifth metacarpal base fractures are unstable and nearly always require surgical fixation. Fixation is commonly through ORIF with plates and screws. Most metacarpal head fractures are referred to an orthopedist because they are intra-articular and usually comminuted.[39] Small avulsion fractures can be treated nonoperatively if the fragment is small and displaced no more than 3 mm.

Issues in operative treatment

One of the disadvantages of plating systems is the need to remove the plate in the future. Studies have reported that bioabsorbable miniplate and screw osteofixation systems have proven efficacy and utility in craniomaxillofacial surgery.[40] Bioabsorbable screws and plates designed for use in the hand have recently become more commonplace and have shown promising results in case studies. Adequate stability has been demonstrated without plate failure or cases of nonunion.[41] However, bioabsorbable implants have a potential complication of inducing a foreign-body reaction, requiring removal of the hardware. One recent case series found that 4 of 9 patients treated with absorbable hardware experienced such a reaction and required hardware removal.[42] More studies are needed to further address this possible fixation technique.

Phalangeal Fractures

Epidemiology

Distal phalanx fractures are the most common, followed by proximal phalanx and middle phalanx fractures. One can extrapolate from data presented by the Centers for Disease Control and Prevention in the National Hospital Ambulatory Medical Care Survey of Emergency Departments that 3.6% of ER visits concerned fractures and 1.2% of visits involved hand and finger injuries.[43] One study found sports to be the main cause of fracture in the 10- to 29-year-old age group, and accidental falls to be the leading cause in those aged 70 years or older.[44]

Mechanism of injury

The most frequent cause of injury to the distal phalanx is a crush injury or axial load injury.[44] Often there will be associated soft-tissue injury to the fingertip or nail bed. Fractures of the middle and proximal phalanx are usually caused by a blow to the dorsum of the hand.

Physical evaluation

Swelling, pain, erythema, deformity, and tenderness to palpation are all common signs of injury. The assessment should also include finger alignment, ligament integrity, neurovascular status, and flexion and extension of the joints.[45] Stability should also be evaluated to ensure appropriate management of dislocated joints.

Radiographic evaluation

Three views on plain radiographs are obtained to better evaluate phalangeal fractures: AP, lateral, and oblique. The lateral view requires isolation from the remaining digits. Radiographs are carefully examined for rotation, shortening, and angulation.[34]

Operative versus nonoperative treatment

Most phalangeal fractures can be treated nonoperatively. Specifically, distal phalanx fractures heal well when splinted for 3 to 4 weeks. It is recommended that the splint be used until the finger is no longer painful. Follow-up radiographs are usually not necessary. Both middle and proximal phalanx fractures that are nondisplaced can be treated by buddy taping for 3 to 4 weeks. A repeat radiograph should be completed at 7 to 10 days after injury to assess alignment. Patients with these fractures should be seen regularly, to evaluate joint motion and return to normal function. ORIF with plate fixation is most often chosen for unstable phalangeal shaft fractures in high-demand athletes to provide rigid internal fixation, and allow immediate range of motion and more rapid return to sport. In addition, percutaneous headless compression screws are used in elite athletes with unicondylar fractures.[46]

Consultation from an orthopedic surgeon should be requested for any open injury, malrotated fractures, displaced fractures that cannot maintain their reduction, and fractures associated with vascular injury.[47] Specifically, K-wires can be used to immobilize distal fractures, and closed reduction and internal fixation with percutaneous screws or K-wires can be used to manage middle and proximal phalanx fractures. ORIF is usually used when the former fails.[48]

METACARPOPHALANGEAL JOINT DISLOCATION

Mechanism of Injury

MCP joint dislocations can occur from hyperextension injury at the involved joint. CMC dislocations can occur with high-energy axial load on the metacarpals. More than 1 metacarpal can be involved with high-energy loads.

Physical Evaluation

The dislocated segment is obvious on examination. It is imperative to ascertain the neurovascular status of the digits, as there may be compromise to the skin with pressure necrosis. A simple dislocation is one that can be easily manually reduced. A complex dislocation, involving interposition of the volar plate within the joint, is impossible to manually reduce. Such injuries can often be identified by dimpling on the volar surface, and usually require open reduction.

Radiographic Evaluation

If the effort to manually reduce fails on the field, it is necessary to obtain radiographic imaging to assess the extent of injury before proceeding with further reduction. Radiographic analysis can be used to rule out associated fractures both prereduction and postreduction.

Operative Versus Nonoperative Treatment

Proper closed reduction involves a firm grip on the proximal phalanx while applying axial traction and restorative pressure over the dislocated phalangeal head. Inability to accomplish a closed reduction is likely the result of the volar plate insertion, which will require open reduction with careful dissection to prevent iatrogenic injury to the supporting structures.[49]

Rehabilitation

A dorsal blocking splint can be used, with early rehabilitation concentrating on active motion.

PROXIMAL INTERPHALANGEAL JOINT DISLOCATION

Dorsal dislocation of the proximal interphalangeal joint (PIP) is the most common type of finger dislocation.[45] Radiographs are recommended before reduction (to exclude any associated fracture) by some investigators, but practically speaking close reduction is done immediately on the field. Closed reduction is accomplished by longitudinal traction with slight extension while the other hand is providing relocating pressure over the dorsal aspect of the displaced digit. Bracing that allows full flexion and blocks the terminal 30° of extension is necessary for at least 3 weeks, but buddy taping with the adjacent finger can be accomplished to allow motion as long as the joint aligns well. Referral to a hand specialist is needed if a dislocation cannot be reduced; is unstable following reduction; or involves significant ligament, tendon, or soft-tissue injury.

DISTAL INTERPHALANGEAL JOINT DISLOCATION

Dislocations of the distal interphalangeal joint (DIP) usually occur dorsally and can be associated with a volar skin laceration. This injury typically occurs with a longitudinal compressive force such as a ball hitting directly, causing hyperextension of the joint. Treatment is usually by closed reduction, with the DIP joint then splinted in 10° of flexion for a minimum of 3 weeks.

SCAPHOLUNATE INSTABILITY/DORSAL INTERCALATED SEGMENTAL INSTABILITY

The scapholunate ligament is important in supporting the namesake structures of the proximal radial carpal bones, and may easily be dismissed as a "simple wrist sprain" if a high index of suspicion is not maintained. Left untreated, the scapholunate ligament dissociation can lead to dorsal intercalated segment instability (DISI), chronic pain, weakness, and long-term degenerative changes.

Epidemiology

Scapholunate injuries may be more common than appreciated, and may occur in up to 5% of patients who present to emergency departments with acute wrist pain.[50] The incidence of scapholunate ligament disruption or instability may be even higher in patients with fractures of the scaphoid or other carpal bones.[51,52]

Clinical Picture

The usual mechanism of injury is a fall on an outstretched hand. Clinically patients can complain of ether acute or chronic wrist pain.

Radiographic Evaluation

With scapholunate disruption, clenched-fist radiographs, with compressive force transmitted across the scapholunate junction, usually reveal an increased gap between the scaphoid and lunate (typically 2–3 mm or less). On lateral films, the angle subserved by the longitudinal axes of the scaphoid and lunate on lateral films ranges from 30° to 60°. A scapholunate angle of greater than 60° indicates scapholunate dissociation and a DISI pattern.

Static scapholunate gaps on radiographs are usually only present in cases of more chronic scapholunate instability. It is important to obtain dynamically loaded images of the wrist such as AP, supinated, and clenched-fist views, to appropriately evaluate acute tears of the scapholunate ligament.

Treatment

There is no consensus on the appropriate treatment of scapholunate instability. For partial tears of the scapholunate ligament, an initial trial of splinting and/or casting is recommended.[33,53] Arthroscopic debridement with or without pinning can be an option in patients in whom initial conservative treatment is unsuccessful.[54,55]

Complete tears require surgical intervention, often with intraoperative assessment of carpal instability directing the specific surgical procedure to be used.[56] Acute injuries have better outcomes, and chronic tears over 3 months old may pose some difficulty in obtaining the best reduction and best chances of healing. Ultimately, referral to a hand orthopedic specialist with extensive experience will be necessary to make the right decision for treatment.

Scapholunate injuries have shown good improvement in realignment after surgery, but long-term follow-up (range 4–12 years) shows return to preoperative deformity, with more than 80% having posttraumatic arthritis. The search for an optimal solution continues.[57]

BOXER'S KNUCKLE

Clinical Picture

Boxer's knuckle, usually occurring at the second or third MCP joint, is usually due to a direct blow or repeated blows to the knuckle, such as with boxing or martial arts. With these injuries, a tear of the tissues that hold the central extensor tendon in place (extensor hood), results in the extensor tendon subluxing to the ulnar side (usually) of the MCP joint during flexion. Patients have difficulty actively extending at the MCP joint. The examiner often can manually extend the finger and relocate the tendon,[58] but once it is flexed it cannot be reextended, which gives the appearance of a trigger finger.[59]

Physical Evaluation

Characteristic physical examination features of MCP joint extensor hood disruption include swelling and tenderness at the site of injury and decreased joint motion, often with an extensor lag. The central tendon subluxation is accentuated by flexion of the joint, and a palpable, markedly tender gap at the site of extensor hood rupture may be present.

Treatment: Operative Versus Nonoperative

For extensor hood disruption and its resultant tendon displacement, the consensus of opinion is that surgical repair is necessary[59,60] to restore extensor integrity and to maintain optimal joint function. Although the authors could find no controlled trials comparing conservative with surgical treatment for this injury, several case series have shown a near 100% success with surgical repair.[58,60,61] Many of these studies included patients who had failed conservative treatment (exact treatment not specified), contributing to the consensus that surgical treatment is optimal.

Expected Return to High-Level Competition Following Operative Treatment

A period of rest for complete postoperative healing, in combination with adequate protection of the boxer's hand when the athlete returns to activity, is critical for recovery. The patients in the case series reported above returned to activity with full range of motion 5 months postoperatively.[58] The taping and wrapping for boxers should be precisely contoured to the anatomic configurations of the hand so as to diffuse potentially traumatic forces and protect the hand from this injury. State boxing commissions have guidelines for taping.

TRIANGULAR FIBROCARTILAGE COMPLEX TEAR

Epidemiology

The precise incidence of TFCC tears is unknown,[62] but are reported as "fairly common" in gymnasts, athletes who plant their hands during athletic activity, and athletes who use their fists or a stick, bat, racquet, or pole.[63,64]

Mechanism of Injury

The most common mechanism of injury is a severe torsion, distraction, or impact that overwhelms the innate tensile strength of the ligament or tendon.

History and Physical Evaluation

There is often a history of injury that involves axial load on a pronated wrist, and symptoms are generally provoked by activities that involve wrist rotation. Patients generally present with ulnar-sided wrist pain that is usually associated with painful snaps, clicks, or pops. Examination findings include pain with palpation over the TFCC at the area between the ulna styloid and pisiform bone. Pain is often also found over the extensor carpi ulnaris because tendinosis of this tendon commonly coexists. Several provocative maneuvers, such as the supination lift test, have been described to help diagnose this problem.[65]

Radiologic Evaluation

The imaging literature contains an abundance of data showing excellent accuracy of MRI of the triangular fibrocartilage.[66] However, the type of TFCC tear substantially influences the accuracy of MRI. Although excellent results have been reported for central and radial-side tears (up to 97% accuracy),[67] MRI has not been proved to be accurate in the detection of peripheral tears of the ulnar attachment of the triangular fibrocartilage.[68] These tears often appear as noncommunicating tears extending from the distal radioulnar joint into the triangular fibrocartilage. A recent study showed that peripheral tears were detected by high-resolution MRI arthrography with sensitivity of 85%, specificity of 76%, and accuracy of 80%.[69] Another study found TFCC tears to have 90% sensitivity and 75% specificity by MRI arthrography.[70] One additional study downplays the role of routine MRI and provides a caveat: an MRI study of 103 wrists in asymptomatic volunteers revealed 39 abnormalities, thus calling in to question the clinical meaning of various findings on MRI examinations. To make the MRI evaluation useful, imaging results must be viewed in the context of the history and examination.[62]

Treatment: Operative Versus Nonoperative

Tears are graded with treatments directed to the different grades of injury. The reader is referred to a review that highlights the Palmer grading system.[71]

Clinical management may include splinting, as minor tears can resolve with splints and/or cortisone injections. In cases where initial imaging studies are negative but symptoms persist despite rest and splinting, wrist arthroscopy is recommended. For larger tears, arthroscopic intervention is the treatment of choice, enabling the surgeon to carefully remove torn TFCC while sparing other important elements of the fibrocartilage complex and restoring normal anatomic relationships.[72]

Issues in Operative Treatment

Hermansdorfer and Kleinman[73] reported the largest series of open repairs for chronic tears. Patients in this study had a 73% satisfaction rate. Corso and colleagues,[74] in a multicenter study, showed a 93% satisfaction rate with arthroscopic repairs and a return to activity at 3 months.

Expected Return to High-Level Competition Following Operative Treatment

The physician treating high-level athletes may consider a more aggressive approach to the patient with suspected TFCC/distal radioulnar joint injury. If distal radioulnar joint instability is demonstrated, early intervention with arthroscopy and peripheral TFCC repair is recommended. If the distal radioulnar joint is stable and symptoms are present for 2 to 3 weeks, arthroscopy is also indicated.[63]

A high-performance athlete may return to sport as soon as 3 weeks after surgery if he or she is able to wear a sugar-tong splint while playing. Otherwise, it is generally advisable to wait until motion and strength are at least at 80% of the contralateral side at 5 to 6 weeks.[75]

GAMEKEEPER'S THUMB: ULNAR COLLATERAL LIGAMENT TEAR

This injury was first described among Scottish gamekeepers who broke the necks of their prized birds with vigorous thumb motion, causing thumb abduction and injury to the ulnar collateral ligament (UCL). Skiers sustain "skier's thumb" injuries from the stress of ski poles on the UCL with the thumb receiving a valgus stress, exacerbated by grip and the restrained strap position.[76] Falling on the outstretched hand may also cause significant UCL stress. One study indicates that UCL sprains accounted for 7% of skiing injuries over an 11-year period at a ski resort in Wyoming.[77]

Physical Examination

The ulnar aspect of the MCP joint of the thumb has localized swelling, bruising, and tenderness.

The diagnosis of a complete UCL rupture can be confirmed by performing a valgus stress test with the thumb held in 30° of MCP flexion. If no solid end point is felt on valgus stress then a complete tear is likely. Local injection of 1 mL of plain lidocaine into the MCP joint may be helpful in assessing the acutely injured patient. A Stener lesion, which occurs when the distal portion of the ruptured UCL becomes trapped superficial to the intact adductor aponeurosis, is unlikely to be caused by provocative testing.[78]

Radiologic Evaluation

Plain radiographs are recommended in patients with tenderness over the ulnar aspect of the MCP joint. Radiographs may reveal an avulsion fracture of the proximal phalanx of the thumb. Stress radiographs are no longer recommended. MRI may be necessary to confirm a Stener lesion. Ultrasonography, with appropriate training and thorough knowledge of the anatomy, can be a useful adjunct to the clinical examination owing to its dynamic imaging, ease of use, and timeliness.[79] In one study, MRI was more useful than ultrasonography when differentiating displaced from nondisplaced tears because on T2-weighted sequence the normal UCL is rarely homogeneously hypointense, as it can be with ultrasonography.[80] In this same study, sensitivity and specificity were both 100% for MRI, whereas sensitivity was 88% for ultrasonography, with specificity 83% for displaced ruptures and 91% for nondisplaced ruptures.

Treatment

Patients with a firm end point to valgus stress testing may be diagnosed with a partial UCL tear, and nonoperative treatment is favored.[81] Incomplete tears may be treated in a short arm thumb spica cast for 4 to 6 weeks followed by the use of an Orthoplast splint for sport activities. Patients who have no discernible end point on UCL stress testing typically need surgery. If the patient has a Stener lesion (this may be difficult to differentiate on physical examination and may require MRI), surgical intervention is also necessary. In addition, more significant laxity (greater than 20°) may also require surgical intervention. Of special note, delayed reconstruction of the ligament has outcomes similar to those of acute reconstruction, making immediate diagnosis less critical.[82]

BOUTONNIÈRE DEFORMITY OR ACUTE CENTRAL SLIP INJURIES

The boutonnière deformity (BD) refers to a chronic deformity related to an acute disruption of the central slip of the extensor tendon at the PIP joint, followed by eventual volar displacement of the lateral bands.[83] The resulting deformity exhibits loss of extension at the PIP joint and a compensatory hyperextension of the DIP joint.

Physical Examination

Central slip injuries are often missed in the acute setting. In one series of 47 patients presenting with a boutonnière deformity, 23 had an initial missed diagnosis.[84] Careful initial examination is therefore critical, and will usually reveal tenderness over the dorsum of the PIP joint and lack of active extension at the PIP. The Elson test is a reliable test for central slip injury. The PIP joint is bent 90° over the edge of a table and the middle phalanx is extended against resistance. With a central slip injury there will be weak PIP extension and the DIP will go rigid. In the absence of a central slip injury, the DIP remains "floppy."[85]

Radiologic Evaluation

Plain radiographs are usually normal but may show an avulsion fracture (which may require surgery if the bony fragment is displaced more than 3 mm from the joint surface).

Treatment

For an acute central slip injury or an early boutonnière deformity without significant subluxation of the lateral bands, the central slip injury can be splinted for 4 to 6 weeks, with good results expected.[86] In the chronic boutonnière injury there may be a PIP flexion contracture, and serial splinting may be needed to achieve full active extension. Surgical interventions are typically used if there is significant subluxation or development of a chronic deformity. If therapy and splinting are not successful there are several surgical options available, including terminal tenotomy, extensor reconstruction, and salvage surgery such as arthrodesis and arthroplasty.[87]

Rehabilitation

Splinting and close observation with physical therapy is recommended to prevent the chronic boutonnière deformity.

MALLET FINGER

Mallet injuries are the most common closed tendon injury in athletes,[88] and are caused by disruption of the extensor digitorum communis tendon at its DIP insertion. These injuries are usually caused by an axial and volarly directed force applied to the tip of the finger while the DIP is in neutral position. Acute mallet deformities are those presenting within 4 weeks of injury, whereas chronic deformities present later than 4 weeks after injury.[89]

Physical Evaluation

Mallet injuries are usually easily diagnosed by simple observation of the deformity, because most patients develop an extensor lag at the DIP joint immediately after injury. However, it is important to perform a careful examination in the acute setting (to assess DIP extension against resistance) because the deformity may be delayed by a few hours or even days.[90] If this injury is missed, the DIP heals in a flexed "mallet-like" position.

Radiologic Evaluation

Radiographs help to differentiate between tendinous and bony mallet-type injuries.[91]

Operative Versus Nonoperative Treatment

In closed injuries without fracture splinting, placing the DIP in slight hyperextension leads to healing within 6 to 8 weeks. The splint must be worn 24 hours a day, and if the patient removes it and flexes the joint (possibly disrupting the tendon again), the timing must start over. There is no consensus on the type of splint or the precise duration of use.[92,93]

Most investigators agree that closed mallet fracture injuries involving less than one-third of the articular surface can be reliably treated with extension splinting alone.[90] In addition, several investigators[94–96] recommend closed treatment of nearly all mallet fractures regardless of fracture size, noting no difference in surgical versus conservative treatment in their reviews of significant fractures involving greater than 30% of articular surfaces or displaced bony fragments.

Issues in Operative Treatment

Surgical fixation is still indicated in certain conditions such as open injuries, palmar subluxation of the distal phalanx, or failed conservative treatment.[92] Some investigators still recommend surgery for fractures that involve more than 50% of the articular surface, although this continues to be controversial.[97]

Expected Return to Play at High Level of Competition

Gripping, throwing, and catching would be restricted or impossible with the injured finger immobilized,[88] and return to play must be individualized because many factors (eg, specific type of sport participation, age, hand dominance, chronicity of injury) are among the many issues that must be considered when developing a treatment and strategy for a particular athlete to return to play.[31]

JERSEY FINGER

Jersey finger is one of the few acute tendon injuries that requires surgical fixation immediately after injury. The timing of presentation has major implications for repair.[98] The typical mechanism of injury involves the passively flexed finger being violently forced into an extended position, causing a disruption of the flexor digitorum profundus (FDP) tendon. Football players commonly grab onto an opponent's jersey with a flexed DIP joint, resulting in disruption of the tendon and leading to the term "jersey finger." The fourth or fifth fingers are most commonly affected. The acute physical examination of this injury reveals a painful swollen flexor aspect of the distal phalanx and DIP joint, and the absence of normal active DIP flexion. Swelling may make it difficult to assess active flexion, so a high index of suspicion must be maintained and DIP flexion deficits must be carefully sought.[99] The proper clinical evaluation and management of this injury is absolutely essential in achieving a good functional outcome.

Radiography and Imaging

Radiographs may reveal an avulsion injury to the FDP tendon. Ultrasonography may be helpful in visualizing the FDP and avulsed bony fragments during passive and dynamic motion,[100] but is limited by the ability to visualize deep structures.[101]

Treatment

Depending on the level of FDP retraction, fully functional outcome is best achieved with early surgical intervention. Surgical management of type I and type II injuries (type I injuries retract to the palm, type II retract to the PIP joint) needs to be completed within 7 to 10 days of injury, whereas type III injuries (bony fragment is distal to the A4 pulley) may be treated more than 10 days after injury.[102]

Return to Play

Protocols emphasize early motion after surgery leading to full use of the finger between 3 and 6 months postoperatively. Each case should be evaluated individually with respect to rehabilitation and return to play.[98]

Future Trends

Delayed repair of jersey finger continues to be a difficult surgical problem. Recently several newer techniques,[103] including a "Z-step" lengthening of the FDP tendon, have been described.[104] The optimal reparative procedure has yet to be definitively elucidated.

REFERENCES

1. Chung KC, Spilson SV. The frequency and epidemiology of hand and forearm fractures in the United States. J Hand Surg Am 2001;26:908.
2. Cummings SR, Black DM, Rubin SM. Lifetime risks of hip, Colles', or vertebral fracture and coronary heart disease among white postmenopausal women. Arch Intern Med 1989;149:2445–8.
3. Mallmin H, Ljunghall S, Persson I, et al. Risk factors for fractures of the distal forearm: a population-based case-control study. Osteoporos Int 1994;4:298–304.
4. Oyen J, Brudvik C, Gjesdal CG, et al. Osteoporosis as a risk factor for distal radial fractures: a case-control study. J Bone Joint Surg Am 2011;93:348–56.
5. Cheng JC, Ng BK, Ying SY, et al. A 10-year study of the changes in the pattern and treatment of 6493 fractures. J Pediatr Orthop 1999;19:344–50.

6. Khosla S, Melton LJ 3rd, Dekutoski MB, et al. Incidence of childhood distal forearm fractures over 30 years: a population-based study. JAMA 2003;290:1479–85.
7. Sinikumpu JJ, Lautamo A, Pokka T, et al. The increasing incidence of paediatric diaphyseal both-bone forearm fractures and their internal fixation during the last decade. Injury 2012;43:362–6.
8. Wetzsteon RJ, Petit MA, Macdonald HM, et al. Bone structure and volumetric BMD in overweight children: a longitudinal study. J Bone Miner Res 2008;23:1946–53.
9. Medoff RJ. Essential radiographic evaluation for distal radius fractures. Hand Clin 2005;21:279–88.
10. Altissimi M, Mancini GB, Azzarà A, et al. Early and late displacement of fractures of the distal radius. The prediction of instability. Int Orthop 1994;18:6.
11. Slutsky DJ. Predicting the outcome of distal radius fractures. Hand Clin 2005;21(3):289–94.
12. Rodríguez-Merchán EC. Management of comminuted fractures of the distal radius in the adult. Conservative or surgical? Clin Orthop Relat Res 1998;(353):53–62.
13. Diaz-Garcia RJ, Oda T, Shauver MJ, et al. A systematic review of outcomes and complications of treating unstable distal radius fractures in the elderly. J Hand Surg Am 2011;36:824–35.
14. Henry MH. Distal radius fractures: current concepts. J Hand Surg 2008;33:1215–27.
15. Leung KS, Shen WY, Leung PC. Ligamentotaxis and bone grafting for comminuted fractures of the distal radius. J Bone Joint Surg Am 1989;71:838–42.
16. Tosti R, Ilyas AM. The role of bone grafting in distal radius fractures. J Hand Surg 2010;35:2082–4.
17. Handoll HG, Watts AC. Bone grafts and bone substitutes for treating distal radial fractures in adults. Cochrane Database Syst Rev 2008;(2):CD006836.
18. Koval KJ, Harrast JJ, Anglen JO, et al. Fractures of the distal part of the radius. The evolution of practice over time. Where's the evidence? J Bone Joint Surg Am 2008;90:1855–61.
19. Costa ML, Achten J, Parsons NR, et al. A randomised controlled trial of percutaneous fixation with Kirschner wires versus volar locking-plate fixation in the treatment of adult patients with a dorsally displaced fracture of the distal radius. BMC Musculoskelet Disord 2011;12:201.
20. Wei DH, Poolman RW, Bhandari M, et al. External fixation versus internal fixation for unstable distal radius fractures: a systematic review and meta-analysis of comparative clinical trials. J Orthop Trauma 2012;26:386–94.
21. Meier R, Krettek C, Probst C. Treatment of distal radius fractures: percutaneous Kirschner-wires or palmar locking plates? Unfallchirurg 2012;115:598–605 [in German].
22. Willis AA, Kutsumi K, Zobitz ME, et al. Internal fixation of dorsally displaced fractures of the distal part of the radius. A biomechanical analysis of volar plate fracture stability. J Bone Joint Surg Am 2006;88:2411–7.
23. O'Connor D, Mullett H, Doyle M, et al. Minimally displaced Colles' fractures: a prospective randomized trial of treatment with a wrist splint or a plaster cast. J Hand Surg Br 2003;28:50–3.
24. Giannoudis PV, Tzioupis C, Papathanassopoulos A, et al. Articular step-off and risk of post-traumatic osteoarthritis. Evidence today. Injury 2010;41:986–95.

25. Tiel-van Buul MM, van Beek EJ, Borm JJ, et al. The value of radiographs and bone scintigraphy in suspected scaphoid fracture. A statistical analysis. J Hand Surg Br 1993;18:403–6.
26. Eastley N, Singh H, Dias JJ, et al. Union rates after proximal scaphoid fractures; meta-analyses and review of available evidence. J Hand Surg Eur Vol 2012. Published online before print. Available at: http://jhs.sagepub.com/content/early/2012/06/25/1753193412451424.abstract. Accessed February 12, 2012.
27. Cooney WP 3rd, Dobyns JH, Linscheid RL. Nonunion of the scaphoid: analysis of the results from bone grafting. J Hand Surg Am 1980;5:343–54.
28. Saeden B, Törnkvist H, Ponzer S, et al. Fracture of the carpal scaphoid: a prospective, randomised 12-year follow-up comparing operative and conservative treatment. J Bone Joint Surg Br 2001;83:230–4.
29. Geissler WB. Carpal fractures in athletes. Clin Sports Med 2001;20:167–88.
30. Marchessault J, Conti M, Baratz ME. Carpal fractures in athletes excluding the scaphoid. Hand Clin 2009;25:371–88.
31. Kovacic J, Bergfeld J. Return to play issues in upper extremity injuries. Clin J Sport Med 2005;15:448–52.
32. Gaston RG. Scaphoid fractures in professional football players. Hand Clin 2012; 28:283–4.
33. Whipple TL. The role of arthroscopy in the treatment of wrist injuries in the athlete. Clin Sports Med 1998;17:623–34.
34. Peterson JJ, Bancroft LW. Injuries of the fingers and thumb in the athlete. Clin Sports Med 2006;25:527–42, vii–viii.
35. Chin SH, Vedder NB. MOC-PSSM CME article: metacarpal fractures. Plast Reconstr Surg 2008;121(Suppl 1):1–13.
36. Birndorf MS, Daley R, Greenwald DP. Metacarpal fracture angulation decreases flexor mechanical efficiency in human hands. Plast Reconstr Surg 1997;99: 1079–83 [discussion: 1084–5].
37. Stahl S, Schwartz O. Complications of K-wire fixation of fractures and dislocations in the hand and wrist. Arch Orthop Trauma Surg 2001;121:527–30.
38. Botte MJ. Complications of smooth pin fixation of fractures and dislocations in the hand and wrist. Clin Orthop Relat Res 1992;276:194–201.
39. Light TR, Bednar MS. Management of intra-articular fractures of the metacarpophalangeal joint. Hand Clin 1994;10:303–14.
40. Ashammakhi N, Peltoniemi H, Waris E, et al. Developments in craniomaxillofacial surgery: use of self-reinforced bioabsorbable osteofixation devices. Plast Reconstr Surg 2001;108:167–80.
41. Waris E, Ninkovic M, Harpf C, et al. Self-reinforced bioabsorbable miniplates for skeletal fixation in complex hand injury: three case reports. J Hand Surg Am 2004;29:452–7.
42. Givissis PK, Stavridis SI, Papagelopoulos PJ, et al. Delayed foreign-body reaction to absorbable implants in metacarpal fracture treatment. Clin Orthop Relat Res 2010;468:3377–83.
43. McCaig LF, Burt CW. National Hospital Ambulatory Medical Care Survey: 2000 emergency department summary. Adv Data 2001;(320):1–34.
44. De Jonge JJ, Kingma J, van der Lei B, et al. Phalangeal fractures of the hand. An analysis of gender and age-related incidence and aetiology. J Hand Surg Br 1994;19:168–70.
45. Borchers JR, Best TM. Common finger fractures and dislocations. Am Fam Physician 2012;85:805–10.

46. Gaston RG, Chadderdon C. Phalangeal fractures: displaced/nondisplaced. Hand Clin 2012;28:395–401, x.
47. Jones NF, Jupiter JB, Lalonde DH. Common fractures and dislocations of the hand. Plast Reconstr Surg 2012;130:722e–36e.
48. Geissler WB. Operative fixation of metacarpal and phalangeal fractures in athletes. Hand Clin 2009;25:409–21.
49. Afifi AM, Medoro A, Salas C, et al. A cadaver model that investigates irreducible metacarpophalangeal joint dislocation. J Hand Surg Am 2009;34:1506–11.
50. Jones WA. Beware the sprained wrist. The incidence and diagnosis of scapholunate instability. J Bone Joint Surg Br 1988;70:293–7.
51. Tang JB. Carpal instability associated with fracture of the distal radius. Incidence, influencing factors and pathomechanics. Chin Med J (Engl) 1992;105:758–65.
52. Weber ER. Biomechanical implications of scaphoid waist fractures. Clin Orthop 1980;149:83–9.
53. Wolfe SW. Scapholunate instability. J Am Soc Surg Hand 2001;1:45–60.
54. Kozin SH. The role of arthroscopy in scapholunate instability. Hand Clin 1999;15:435–44, viii.
55. Ruch DS, Poehling GG. Arthroscopic management of partial scapholunate and lunotriquetral injuries of the wrist. J Hand Surg Am 1996;21:412–7.
56. Mitsuyasu H, Patterson RM, Shah MA, et al. The role of the dorsal intercarpal ligament in dynamic and static scapholunate instability. J Hand Surg Am 2004;29:279–88.
57. Amadio PC. Specialty update: what's new in hand surgery. J Bone Joint Surg Am 2012;94:569–73.
58. Hame S, Melone C. Boxer's knuckle in the professional athlete. Am J Sports Med 2000;28:879–82.
59. Melone CP Jr, Polatsch DB, Beldner S. Disabling hand injuries in boxing: boxer's knuckle and traumatic carpal boss. Clin Sports Med 2009;28:609–21, vii.
60. Arai K, Toh S, Nakahara K, et al. Treatment of soft tissue injuries to the dorsum of the metacarpophalangeal joint (boxer's knuckle). J Hand Surg Br 2002;27:90–5.
61. Hame SL, Melone CP Jr. Boxer's knuckle. Traumatic disruption of the extensor hood. Hand Clin 2000;16:375–80, viii.
62. Iordache SD, Rowan R, Garvin GJ, et al. Prevalence of triangular fibrocartilage complex abnormalities on MRI scans of asymptomatic wrists. J Hand Surg Am 2012;37:98–103.
63. Rettig AC. Athletic injuries of the wrist and hand: part II: overuse injuries of the wrist and traumatic injuries to the hand. Am J Sports Med 2004;32:262–73.
64. Rettig AC. Athletic injuries of the wrist and hand. Part I: traumatic injuries of the wrist. Am J Sports Med 2003;31:1038–48.
65. Buterbaugh GA, Brown TR, Horn PC. Ulnar-sided wrist pain in athletes. Clin Sports Med 1998;17:567–83.
66. Potter HG, Asnis-Ernberg L, Weiland AJ, et al. The utility of high-resolution magnetic resonance imaging in the evaluation of the triangular fibrocartilage complex of the wrist. J Bone Joint Surg Am 1997;79:1675–84.
67. Schmitt R, Christopoulos G, Meier R, et al. Direct MR arthrography of the wrist in comparison with arthroscopy: a prospective study on 125 patients. Rofo 2003;175:911–9.
68. Haims AH, Schweitzer ME, Morrison WB, et al. Limitations of MR imaging in the diagnosis of peripheral tears of the triangular fibrocartilage of the wrist. AJR Am J Roentgenol 2002;178:419–22.

69. Rüegger C, Schmid MR, Pfirrmann CW, et al. Peripheral tear of the triangular fibrocartilage: depiction with MR arthrography of the distal radioulnar joint. AJR Am J Roentgenol 2007;188:187–92.
70. Mahmood A, Fountain J, Vasireddy N, et al. Wrist MRI Arthrogram v wrist arthroscopy: what are we finding? Open Orthop J 2012;6:194–8.
71. Ahn AK, Chang D, Plate AM. Triangular fibrocartilage complex tears: a review. Bull NYU Hosp Jt Dis 2006;64:114–8.
72. Geissler WB. Arthroscopic knotless peripheral ulnar-sided TFCC repair. Hand Clin 2011;27:273–9.
73. Hermansdorfer JD, Kleinman WB. Management of chronic peripheral tears of the triangular fibrocartilage complex. J Hand Surg Am 1991;16:340–6.
74. Corso SJ, Savoie FH, Geissler WB, et al. Arthroscopic repair of peripheral avulsions of the triangular fibrocartilage complex of the wrist: a multicenter study. Arthroscopy 1997;13:78–84.
75. Zlatkin MB, Rosner J. MR imaging of ligaments and triangular fibrocartilage complex of the wrist. Radiol Clin North Am 2006;44:595–623, ix.
76. Campbell JD, Feagin JA, King P, et al. Ulnar collateral ligament injury of the thumb. Treatment with glove spica cast. Am J Sports Med 1992;20:29–30.
77. Warme WJ, Feagin JA Jr, King P, et al. Ski injury statistics, 1982 to 1993, Jackson Hole Ski Resort. Am J Sports Med 1995;23:597–600.
78. Adler T, Eisenbarth I, Hirschmann MT, et al. Can clinical examination cause a Stener lesion in patients with skier's thumb?: a cadaveric study. Clin Anat 2012;25:762–6.
79. Ebrahim FS, De Maeseneer M, Jager T, et al. US diagnosis of UCL tears of the thumb and Stener lesions: technique, pattern-based approach, and differential diagnosis. Radiographics 2006;26:1007–20.
80. Hergan K, Mittler D, Oser W. Ulnar collateral ligament: differentiation of displaced and nondisplaced tears with US and MR imaging. Radiology 1995;194:65–71.
81. Ritting AW, Baldwin PC, Rodner CM. Ulnar collateral ligament injury of the thumb metacarpophalangeal joint. Clin J Sport Med 2010;20:106–12.
82. Fairhurst M, Hansen L. Treatment of "Gamekeeper's Thumb" by reconstruction of the ulnar collateral ligament. J Hand Surg Br 2002;27:542–5.
83. Nugent N, O'Shaughnessy M. Closed central slip injuries—a missed diagnosis? Ir Med J 2011;104:248–50.
84. Le Bellec Y, Loy S, Touam C, et al. Surgical treatment for boutonnière deformity of the fingers. Retrospective study of 47 patients. Chir Main 2001;20:362–7.
85. Elson RA. Rupture of the central slip of the extensor hood of the finger: a test for early diagnosis. J Bone Joint Surg Br 1986;68:229–31.
86. Williams MS, Fair J, Wilckens J. Quick splint for acute boutonnière injuries. Phys Sportsmed 2001;29:69–70.
87. Williams K, Terrono AL. Treatment of boutonnière finger deformity in rheumatoid arthritis. J Hand Surg Am 2011;36:1388–93.
88. Yeh PC, Shin SS. Tendon ruptures: mallet, flexor digitorum profundus. Hand Clin 2012;28:425–30, xi.
89. Garberman SF, Diao E, Peimer CA. Mallet finger: results of early versus delayed closed treatment. J Hand Surg Am 1994;19:850–2.
90. Bendre AA, Hartigan BJ, Kalainov DM. Mallet finger. J Am Acad Orthop Surg 2005;13:336–44.
91. Wang QC, Johnson BA. Fingertip injuries. Am Fam Physician 2001;63:1961–6.
92. Cheung JP, Fung B, Ip WY. Review on mallet finger treatment. Hand Surg 2012;17:439–47.

93. O'Brien LJ, Bailey MJ. Single blind, prospective, randomized controlled trial comparing dorsal aluminum and custom thermoplastic splints to stack splint for acute mallet finger. Arch Phys Med Rehabil 2011;92:191–8.
94. Wehbé MA, Schneider LH. Mallet fractures. J Bone Joint Surg Am 1984;66:658–69.
95. Schneider LH. Fractures of the distal interphalangeal joint. Hand Clin 1994;10:277–85.
96. Kalainov DM, Hoepfner PE, Hartigan BJ, et al. Nonsurgical treatment of closed mallet finger fractures. J Hand Surg Am 2005;30:580–6.
97. Smit JM, Beets MR, Zeebregts CJ, et al. Treatment options for mallet finger: a review. Plast Reconstr Surg 2010;126:1624–9.
98. Shippert BW. A "complex jersey finger": case report and literature review. Clin J Sport Med 2007;17:319–20.
99. Tuttle HG, Olvey SP, Stern PJ. Tendon avulsion injuries of the distal phalanx. Clin Orthop Relat Res 2006;445:157–68.
100. de Gautard G, de Gautard R, Celi J, et al. Sonography of jersey finger. J Ultrasound Med 2009;28:389–92.
101. Goodson A, Morgan M, Rajeswaran G, et al. Current management of jersey finger in rugby players: case series and literature review. Hand Surg 2010;15:103–7.
102. Lubahn JD, Hood JM. Fractures of the distal interphalangeal joint. Clin Orthop Relat Res 1996;(327):12–20.
103. Stewart DA, Smitham PJ, Nicklin S, et al. A new technique for distal fixation of flexor digitorum profundus tendon. J Plast Reconstr Aesthet Surg 2008;61:475–7.
104. Sawaya ET, Choughri H, Pelissier P. One-stage treatment of delayed 'jersey finger' by Z-step lengthening of the flexor digitorum profundus tendon at the wrist. J Plast Reconstr Aesthet Surg 2012;65:264–6.

Overuse Injuries

Richard E. Rodenberg, MD[a,*], Eric Bowman, DO[b],
Reno Ravindran, MD[c]

KEYWORDS

- Tendinopathy • Tendinosis • Nitric oxide • Eccentric strengthening
- Sound assisted soft tissue massage (SASTM)
- Augmented soft tissue mobilization (ASTM) • Nitric oxide therapy
- Platelet-rich plasma (PRP)

KEY POINTS

- The term *tendinopathy* should be thought of as a broad spectrum of tendon disorders and used to describe any abnormal conditions of the tendon.
- Tendinosis refers to tendon degeneration without the clinical or histologic signs of an inflammatory response that is thought to develop over a prolonged time frame.
- Tendinitis can occur over a short period of time and refers to incomplete tendon degeneration resulting in vascular disruption with bleeding and an inflammatory repair response.
- Conservative treatment of tendinosis starting with a sound rehabilitation program seems to be the best place to start while reserving surgical approaches as a last resort for recalcitrant cases that have failed conservative management.

INTRODUCTION

Tendinosis is a condition that frustrates patients and clinicians alike. An active individual's quality of life often suffers because of chronic pain and the inability to perform athletic and occupation-related activities. In severe cases, the pain and dysfunction associated with tendinosis can affect activities of daily living. The condition is not easily treated with usual methods, such as physical therapy and nonsteroidal antiinflammatory drugs (NSAIDs). In fact, based on an evolving understanding of the pathophysiology of tendon injury, certain treatments may not serve any role at all in the treatment of tendinosis. This article reviews the epidemiology, pathophysiology, and emerging treatments related to chronic tendon injury.

[a] NCH Sports Medicine Fellowship Program, Division of Sports Medicine, Department of Pediatrics, Nationwide Children's Hospital, The Ohio State University College of Medicine, 5680 Venture Drive, Dublin, OH 43017, USA; [b] Division of Sports Medicine, Department of Pediatrics, Nationwide Children's Hospital, 5680 Venture Drive, Dublin, OH 43017, USA; [c] Division of Sports Medicine, Department of Pediatrics and Family Medicine, Nationwide Children's Hospital, The Ohio State University College of Medicine, 5680 Venture Drive, Dublin, OH 43017, USA
* Corresponding author.
E-mail address: Richard.Rodenberg@nationwidechildrens.org

Prim Care Clin Office Pract 40 (2013) 453–473
http://dx.doi.org/10.1016/j.pop.2013.02.007 primarycare.theclinics.com
0095-4543/13/$ – see front matter

EPIDEMIOLOGY

Over the course of history, athletes have placed high demands on their bodies. In the past several decades, we have seen an increased activity level in these athletes and find that they are putting more demands on their bodies than ever before. The increased incidence and prevalence of overuse injuries becomes more apparent as these athletes spend more time training year round. The recreational athletes, the so-called weekend warriors, have continued to experience overuse injuries as they have in the past, but there has also been an increase in the level of overuse injuries among young athletes as they participate in the early specialization of their sport.[1,2]

Physical activity and exercise induces tremendous levels of stress on the muscles and tendons, thus increasing the risk of potential injury. The tendon plays a very important role as an active element of the muscle tendon unit in physical activity and, therefore, is subject to overuse injury.[3,4] It has been reported that approximately 50% of all sports injuries are secondary to overuse. The frequency of overuse injuries evaluated in the primary clinic setting is greater, proportionately, comprising twice the frequency of acute injuries.[1] Additional data report that overuse injuries account for approximately 7% of all physician office visits in the United States.[2]

Sports Injuries from an Epidemiologic Approach

Looking at the epidemiology of sports injuries can be quite different than that of other types of disease processes. The epidemiology of sports looks to quantify the occurrence of sports injuries in relation to who is affected by injuries, where and when the injuries occur, and what the outcomes are.[3] By understanding these details, there can be strategies and methods in place that will allow for better prevention and management of sports-related injuries. By prevention of these injuries, there can be a reduction in the short- and long-term social and economic costs associated with them.[5]

Age can also be a determining factor for different types of overuse injuries. It is a well-known fact that in the pediatric and adolescent population, tendons and ligaments are stronger than the epiphyseal plate. Because of this relative imbalance of strength, after acute trauma, a growing child is more apt to injure the epiphyseal plate before injuring a tendon or ligament. With regard to tendinous injuries seen in children, they are more likely to suffer injuries to the insertion sites of tendon at the apophyses rather than to the main body of the tendon as is commonly seen in the adult population.[6] According to Jarvinen,[7] older patients or athletes presenting to a musculoskeletal clinic are more likely to present with more traditional overuse injuries, including rotator cuff injuries (18%), Achilles tendon and calf injuries (20%), and medial and lateral epicondylitis, from sport- and work-related activity.

Another epidemiologic consideration is gender. Most tendon injuries have historically occurred in males, but the incidence in females, especially those younger than 30 years, is steadily increasing. One possible reason for this includes the dramatic increase in female participation in sports over the past several decades. These young women are not only participating in more sports but are also participating in more high-risk sports that can lead to both acute and overuse injuries.[8]

Achilles Tendinopathy/Overuse Injuries

There have been several studies that have looked at the cause, location, and types of tendon injuries in the Achilles. Several of these studies have revealed that most Achilles problems occur in men, with running being the main sport (53%). More than two-thirds of the injuries in competitive athletes involve the paratenon and

20% involve the tendon insertion site (refer to **Fig. 1**). Although malalignment of the lower extremity is found in 60% of individuals with an Achilles overuse injury, there does not seem to be a direct cause-effect relationship between them.[3,9]

Patellar Tendinopathy/Overuse Injuries

Knee complaints are one of the most common musculoskeletal injuries prompting treatment. It has been reported that about one-third of sports injuries involve the knee. The most common knee disorders reported to present in the sports clinic include jumper's knee (20%), Osgood-Schlatter disease (10%), patellar paratendinopathy (6%), hamstring tendinopathy (3%), and iliotibial band (ITB) syndrome (2%).[10]

ITB Syndrome

ITB syndrome results from chronic friction between the ITB and the lateral femoral condyle. It is often seen in distance runners, military recruits, and cyclists but can occur in any activity that requires repetitive flexion of the knee.[3] When the knee is in about 20° to 30° of flexion, the ITB rubs against the lateral femoral condyle. It has been reported that approximately 14% of patients with overuse injuries of the knee had ITB syndrome.[10] Data indicate this issue to be more common in long distance runners/joggers and skiers.[3] Other contributing factors to ITB syndrome include genu varum, excessive pronation, lateral condyle spur, leg length discrepancy, abrupt increase in running load, or changing terrain (ie, started training on hills).[11]

Quadriceps Tendinopathy

Although quadriceps tendinopathy is a cause of knee pain from overuse, it is far less common than patellar tendinopathy given its increased strength, mechanical advantage, and better vascularity compared with the patella tendon.[3] In older people with quadriceps tendinopathy, there are often degenerative changes present consisting of calcification of the tendon or spur formation at the superior pole of the patella.[3]

Hamstring syndrome presents with pain that occurs over the ischial tuberosity and radiates into the posterior aspect of the thigh. It often occurs from the thick tendinous structures at the origin of the hamstrings becoming scarred and fibrotic. Most athletic

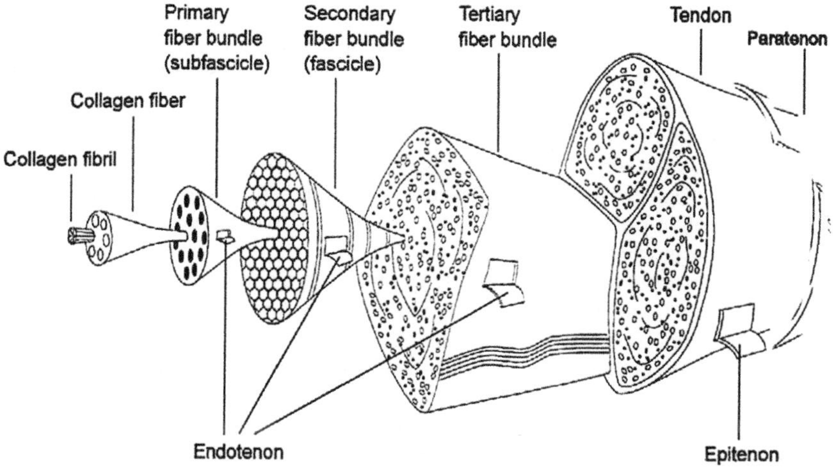

Fig. 1. Tendon structure. (*From* Fecorczyk JM. Tendinopathies of the elbow, wrist, and hand: histopathology and clinical considerations. J Hand Ther 2012;25:191–201; with permission.)

patients that this affects include those who are active in sprinting, hurdling, or jumping, and soccer.[3]

Lateral and Medial Epicondylitis

Lateral epicondylitis occurs with excessive use of the wrist extensors and forearm supinators. It has been reported that up to 40% of tennis players will suffer from this condition, and it will generally affect 1% to 2% of the population. Lateral epicondylitis is 5 to 9 times more likely to occur than medial epicondylitis.[12] The incidence of lateral epicondylitis is 2.0 to 3.5 times higher in individuals aged older than 40 years compared with individuals aged younger than 40 years. Also, it is higher among those who play sports more than 2 hours a day compared with those who play less than 2 hours daily.[13] Medial epicondylitis is common in throwing and golf athletes as a result of overuse of the forearm, wrist, and finger flexor muscles, especially the pronator teres and flexor carpi radialis.[12]

Although not addressed in the epidemiology section of this article, it is important to remember that overuse injuries and tendinopathies happen elsewhere throughout the body. Some of the common additional areas and injuries include rotator cuff and biceps tendonitis, patellofemoral syndrome, and medial tibial stress syndrome.

HEALTHY TENDON: STRUCTURE AND FUNCTION

To understand clinical issues related to the painful tendon, the practitioner must understand normal tendon function and anatomy as well as the proposed causes for the pathology related to tendinopathy.

The tendon's job is to transmit the force of muscle contraction to bone, across joints, to produce body movement and promote joint stabilization.[14–16] Basic components of normal healthy tendon consist of a fibrous connective tissue made up of a complex arrangement of cells, collagen bundles, and ground substance (extracellular matrix). The ground substance is a viscous substance rich in proteoglycans.[14,15,17,18] Tenocytes (fibroblastlike cells) are the cellular component of the tendon and are able to proliferate, produce collagen, elastin, and proteoglycans, thereby maintaining the normal structure and homeostasis of the ground substance.[14,19] Collagen provides the tendon tensile strength, with type 1 collagen representing greater than 90% of the total collagen in a normal tendon. Elastin helps to provide compliance and elasticity. The ground substance or extracellular matrix provides structural support for the tenocytes and collagen fibers (fibers). Proper maintenance of a healthy matrix allows the tendon the ability to resist mechanical forces and repair itself in response to injury. There is a complex communication between the tenocytes and extracellular matrix that allows the tenocytes to initiate alteration of the matrix and the matrix can elicit changes in cell proliferation, migration, apoptosis, and morphogenesis. Proteoglycans are protein/polysaccharide complexes that serve to help the tissue resist compressive forces placed on the tendon.[14,19]

The tendon is arranged in a hierarchy of increasing complexity starting with the collagen fibril and moving upward to the collagen fiber (fiber), primary bundle, secondary fiber (fiber) bundle, tertiary fiber (fiber) bundle, and lastly the tendon (please see **Fig. 1**).[17,18] This hierarchy is separated by layers as the structure of the tendon begins to take shape. The epitenon consists of a fine connective tissue sheath that is like a synovial membrane. On gross inspection, the epitenon appears white and glistening. It is continuous on its inner surface and extends deeper into the tendon between the tertiary bundles as the endotenon. The epitenon/endotenon layer contains the vascular, lymphatic, and nerve supplies for the tendon. In some tendons, there is a more superficial layer of loose areolar connective tissue called the *paratenon* that may surround the epitenon. This paratenon is comprised mainly of type I and II collagen fibrils, elastic fibrils, and an inner lining of synovial cells. The paratenon covers tendons that move in a straight line and are capable of great elongation and functions as an elastic sheath that permits free movement of the tendon against the surrounding tissue. If present, the combination of epitenon and paratenon is called the *peritendon*. The classic double-layered synovial sheath may replace the paratenon but is only present in tendons at areas of increased mechanical stress. This double-layered sheath is lined by synovium and termed the *tenosynovium*.[14,17,18]

TENDON INJURY

Tendon healing occurs through 3 overlapping phases including inflammation, repair with collagen production, and remodeling. This healing process becomes defective in an overuse tendon–type injury resulting in inadequate repair.[14,15]

The term *tendinopathy* should be thought of as a broad spectrum of tendon disorders and used to describe any abnormal conditions of the tendon. The terminology of tendon injury is best characterized by Bonar's modification of Clancy's classification of tendinopathies including tendinosis, tendinitis, paratenonitis, and paratenonitis with tendinosis. Tendinosis refers to tendon degeneration without the clinical or histologic signs of an inflammatory response that is thought to develop over a prolonged time frame. Tendinitis can occur over a short period of time and refers to incomplete tendon degeneration resulting in vascular disruption with bleeding and an inflammatory repair response. Paratenonitis also develops over a brief time frame but is confined to the superficial outer layer of the tendon involving the paratenon alone. If the tendon is enclosed in a sheath, this would include synovitis. Pathology related to the paratenonitis would also involve an inflammatory response.[14,15,17,18] Paratenonitis with tendinosis refers to a combination of paratenon inflammation and intratendinous degeneration.[14,17,18]

The histologic appearance of a normal tendon under light microscopy is strikingly different when compared with a tendon suffering from an overuse-type tendinopathy injury and is what defines Bonar's modification of Clancy's classification of tendinosis. Healthy tendon is made up of dense parallel bundles of clearly defined, slightly wavy collagen oriented along the long axis of the tendon. The tenocytes are evenly distributed between the collagen bundles. The ground substance matrix is not readily apparent, and there is an absence of fibroblasts and myofibroblasts.[14,15,18] Tendinosis reveals distinct histologic changes compared with normal tendon, resulting in collagen disarray with a loss of the parallel and longitudinal alignment of the collagen bundles interspersed with increased ground substance. The tenocytes become more apparent and take on a more chondroid-type appearance. There is an increase in type III collagen compared with type I collagen. There is an increase in cellularity marked by an increase in the number of myofibroblasts and fibroblasts. However, there is an absence of inflammatory cells indicating no significant inflammatory response in tendinosis compared with an acute injury or tendinitis. Also significant in the histology is the presence of an increased infiltration of new blood vessels and nerves marking neovascularization.[15,18,20] This histologic response seems to represent an insufficient repair process that leads to tendon degeneration.[20]

The exact pathologic processes that cause tendinosis have yet to be elucidated, but tendinosis seems to be the response to an overuse injury resulting in a pathologic cascade of changes in the normal tendon reparative process described as a cycle of degeneration and attempted failed regeneration.[2] It is not clear whether the initial pathologic event in the cascade is caused by a loss in the integrity of the extracellular matrix or the cells within the tendon matrix.[15,19] Possibly, fatigued tendons lose their innate reparative ability with intensive repetitive activity, which leads to cumulative microtrauma leading to the weakening of the collagen cross-linking and the extracellular matrix.[20] It has been postulated that even though histologic samples of biopsy specimens reveal no inflammatory infiltration in the tendinopathic tendons, studies indicate an inflammatory cascade may play a role in the pathology early on in tendinopathy. This inflammatory cascade is mediated by macrophages, mast cells, B and T lymphocytes; which are speculated to appear early on in the tendinopathy, producing proinflammatory cytokines (ie, interleukins).[20,21] Repetitive mechanical stress in combination with the proinflammatory cytokines and transforming growth factor β (TGF-β) can stimulate tenocytes to transform into myofibroblasts. The myofibroblasts are important for tendon healing; but if they do not undergo apoptosis, the myofibroblasts will propagate leading to fibrosis.[21] Also, an increase in apoptosis in healthy tenocytes may be related to oxidative stress, leading to the breakdown in the reparative process.[19] Tissue hypoxia probably plays an important role in the cascade leading to tendon degeneration. The hypoxia may play a role in upregulating matrix metalloproteinases (MMPs), which are enzymes that degrade tendon matrix components. An increase in MMPs activity can cause degradation of the extracellular matrix. A balance between the MMPs and their inhibitors probably plays a role in the maintenance of a healthy extracellular matrix.[15,19–21] Hypoxia is also tied to upregulation of vascular endothelial growth factor, which stimulates angiogenesis in the tendon.[21] Angiogenesis in combination with local noxious stimuli and enhanced nociceptive fibers leads to an ingrowth of sensory nerve fibers alongside of blood vessels, which is thought to be the causative factor of pain in tendinosis.[15,20,21] The end state of this pathologic cascade is thought to be tendon rupture manifesting from a series of partial macroscopic tears.[20]

TREATMENT OPTIONS

The optimal treatment of tendinosis is debated. As our understanding of the science behind the pathology of tendinosis increases, advances in treatment can be made based at the molecular level. This section focuses on the evidence behind the treatment modalities used in the care of tendinosis. Nonoperative treatment is still the mainstay in the treatment of this disorder and is the focus of this review.

Physical Therapy and Other Modalities

Eccentric strengthening

Eccentric strengthening has been around for many years and is one of the mainstays of the treatment of tendinopathy. It is regularly used in Achilles and patellar tendinopathies but also can be used for hamstring tendinopathy. It involves the application of load and muscle exertion to a lengthening muscle. There are many randomized and observational studies that have found eccentric exercises to be an effective treatment (see later discussion). Eccentric strengthening seems to stimulate tissue remodeling and normalization of tendon structure. This treatment is typically done under the watchful eye of a licensed physical therapist because it is important that eccentric strengthening is done with proper technique. Overloading the musculotendinous junction can lead to further injury. Clinical research supports the efficacy of eccentric strengthening, although the evidence of the mechanism is unclear. Shalabi and colleagues[22] found that eccentric training of the gastrocnemius-soleus complex in chronic Achilles tendinopathy resulted in decreased tendon volume and decreased intratendinous signal as seen on an magnetic resonance imaging. Some investigators suggest there is neovascularization, which resolves after 12 weeks of eccentric training.[23] A systematic review by Kingma and colleagues[24] examined the efficacy of eccentric strengthening on outcome measures of pain and physical functioning in patients with chronic Achilles tendinopathy. The study included 3 randomized controlled trials and 6 controlled trials. Six of the studies used protocol by Alfredson and colleagues,[25] whereas the other 3 used eccentric exercises along with stretching and cryotherapy. The duration of eccentric training was 6 to 12 weeks and was compared with concentric training, surgery, and use of a night splint. The results showed a mean reduction in pain of 60% with eccentric training compared with 33% in control groups.[24] Similarly, another study looked at patients through a 12-week course of eccentric training and showed that it was more effective than a traditional concentric strengthening program for treating Achilles and patellar tendinopathy in recreational athletes.[26,27] Another systematic review done by Larsson and colleagues[28] reviewed 13 articles comparing various treatment methods for patellar tendinopathy and found strong evidence for the use of eccentric training for patellar tendinopathy. Eccentric strengthening should be used in the treatment of tendinopathies either alone or in conjunction with other modalities. There are no absolute contraindications to eccentric strengthening.

Sound-assisted soft tissue massage/friction-based massage

Sound-assisted soft tissue massage (SASTM) or augmented soft tissue mobilization (ASTM), also known as a form of friction massage, refers to the application of a friction-directed force onto a tendon or ligament to promote or induce physiologic and structural tissue changes. This treatment is accomplished with the use of an instrument. The exact mechanism of how soft tissue mobilization improves healing is unclear, but there are theories. According to Norris,[29] the purpose of frictional massage is to promote a local hyperemia, massage analgesia, and reduce adherent scar tissue. Prentice[30] hypothesized that frictional massage may facilitate tendon healing by enhancing the inflammatory process to completion so that the later stages of healing can occur. Davidson and colleagues'[31] findings supported Prentice and found that augmented soft tissue mobilization promotes healing via increased fibroblast recruitment. In a study done by Gehlsen and colleagues,[32] 30 male white rats were randomly assigned to one of 5 groups. A tendonitis, tendonitis plus light ASTM, tendonitis plus medium ASTM, tendonitis plus extreme ASTM, and a control with surgery. The Achilles tendons of each group were then harvested 1 week after the last ASTM treatment. Fibroblast numbers were assessed by light microscopy. The results showed an increase number of fibroblasts in the extreme ASTM group. ASTM has been used in the clinical setting with variable success. There are no true randomized controlled studies in the current literature, but there are no absolute contraindications to ASTM.

Cryotherapy

Cryotherapy is one of the most commonly used modalities in sports medicine. This therapy involves the application of cold to an injured area for therapeutic purposes to reduce inflammation and pain. Cryotherapy results in vasoconstriction and decreased blood flow to the area, which in turn reduces inflammation and swelling. It also has an effect on pain through the gate control theory and temporary inhibiting effects to the neuromuscular system causing an analgesic effect. Cryotherapy is widely used for acute injuries but has also been used in chronic or overuse injuries. There are various methods of cryotherapy, which include ice bags, ice massages, chemical cold packs, ice water immersion, ice circulating units, and vapocoolant sprays. There have been numerous studies that show the beneficial effects of cryotherapy on acute injuries; there have not been many studies that have studied the effects of cryotherapy in chronic conditions. In the authors' experience, cryotherapy is most beneficial when used as an adjunct to eccentric strengthening. Contraindications to cryotherapy include cold hypersensitivity, cold intolerance, and Raynaud disease.[33]

Low-level laser therapy

Low-level laser therapy (LLLT) makes the use of light energy delivered to the body's tissue for therapeutic purposes. The laser sources are at powers too low to cause measurable temperature increases. This therapy has been used in various musculoskeletal conditions, including tendinopathies. The biologic effects include ATP production, enhanced cell function, and increased protein synthesis. LLLT has also been shown to have positive effects on the reduction of inflammation, increase of collagen synthesis, and angiogenesis.[34] A systematic review with meta-analysis done on LLLT showed there to be conflicting evidence. Twenty-five controlled trials met the inclusion criteria. There was conflicting evidence from multiple trials. Twelve trials showed a positive effect, and 13 trials were inconclusive or showed no effect. The conclusion of the systematic review was that LLLT can potentially be effective in treating tendinopathy when recommended doses are used.[34] Similarly, a systematic review of the literature in 2008 reviewed 14 randomized clinical trials evaluating LLLT; 2 were discarded because of inadequate controls. Five studies showed improvement treating tendinopathy with LLLT compared with placebo, whereas 7 studies showed no difference.[35] Four systematic reviews have addressed LLLT and all agreed the best current level of evidence does not support its use in the treatment of tendinopathy.[36–39] Contraindications include use over cancerous areas, eyes, open wounds, pregnancy, and over epiphysis.

Ultrasound therapy

Therapeutic ultrasound is used for 2 purposes: nonthermal tissue healing effects and thermal effects. Nonthermal effects are achieved by low-frequency intensity and cause movement of fluids along cell membranes and the formation of gas-filled bubbles. This is thought to promote tissue repair. Thermal effects increase tissue temperature and increase cellular activity, which in turn increases blood flow, tissue extensibility, reduces muscle spasm, and reduces pain.[40] This is achieved at higher intensity and should be used with caution as to not cause patients added discomfort. Ultrasound therapy can be used for various tendinopathies, including Achilles and patellar tendons. A study published in 1998 compared the use of phonophoresis versus ultrasound in the treatment of common musculoskeletal conditions and concluded that both treatments decreased pain and increased pressure tolerance and the use of phonophoresis did not augment the benefits.[41] A systematic review identified 8 well-controlled trials of which 3 trials demonstrated benefits with therapeutic ultrasound used in the treatment of lateral epicondylitis and calcific supraspinatus tendonitis. The other 5 studies showed no real benefit.[35] Contraindications include ischemic areas, deep vein thrombosis; anesthetic areas; actively infected areas; and application to injury of the eyes, heart, skull, and genitals. It should be avoided in pregnancy over the trunk or abdomen and in stress fractures or osteoporotic areas.

Iontophoresis/phonophoresis

Phonophoresis involves the use of ultrasound energy to assist the diffusion of medication through the skin and into affected areas. Iontophoresis involves the use of electrical pulse waves to transport medication to an injured area. The most common medications used are corticosteroids, lidocaine, salicylates, and acetic acid.[33] Iontophoresis and phonophoresis can be used safely for all tendinopathies. There are conflicting studies in the literature regarding the efficacy of these modalities. A systematic review identified 6 adequately controlled studies and 4 of them reported no improvement compared with controls.[35] Contraindications for use are similar to those of therapeutic ultrasound.

Extracorporeal Shock-Wave Therapy

Extracorporeal shock-wave therapy (ESWT) is a single-impulse acoustic wave generated by 3 main techniques, which are electromagnetic, electrohydraulic, or a piezoelectric source. Each of these represents a different technique of generating shock waves. The electrohydraulic principle represents the first generation of shock waves. This consists of high-energy acoustic waves generated by underwater explosion with high-voltage electrode spark discharge. The electromagnetic technique involves an electric current passing through a coil to produce a strong magnetic field. The piezoelectric technique involves many piezocrystals mounted in a sphere that receives a rapid electrical discharge that induces a pressure pulse surrounding water steepening to a shock wave. The arrangements of the crystals cause self-focusing of the waves toward the target center and lead to an extremely precise focusing and high energy within a defined focal volume. When comparing different shockwave devices, the important parameters include distribution, energy density, and the total of the second focal point in addition to the principle of shock-wave generation of each device. A shock-wave pattern differs from ultrasound wave in that ultrasound waves are typically biphasic and have a peak pressure of 0.5 bars. Shock-wave therapy is uni-phasic, with a peak pressure as high as 500 bars.[42] In other words, the peak pressure of a shock wave is approximately 1000 times that of an ultrasound wave. The energy at the focal point is recorded in millijoules per area (mJ/mm^2); based on this value, shock waves are classified as low, medium, or high energy.[43]

The mechanism by which ESWT works is not well understood. Recent animal studies have stated that ESWT may stimulate the production of angiogenic markers and neovascularization as well as reduce calcitonin gene relayed peptide expression in dorsal root ganglions. This induces tissue repair and regeneration.[44]

There have been several studies that have reported favorable results of ESWT in athletes with various tendinopathies, including patellar, Achilles, supraspinatus, and lateral epicondylitis of the elbow. A study done by Peers and colleagues[45] compared 13 knees treated surgically with 15 knees treated with ESWT and reported comparable functional outcome in patients with patellar tendinopathy resistant to conservative treatments.

A study looking at Achilles tendinopathy compared 25 patients treated by eccentric strengthening with 25 patients treated with repetitive ESWT, and the results showed ESWT to be superior to treating recalcitrant Achilles tendinopathy.[46] A randomized controlled study took 40 patients with chronic proximal hamstring tendinopathy and assigned them to either receive ESWT or traditional NSAID, physiotherapy, and an exercise program for hamstring muscles. They were followed at 1 week, 3, 6, and 12 months after the end of treatment. At the 3-month follow up, results showed a significant reduction in pain by 50% in 17 out of 20 of the shock-wave group and 2 out of 20 in the traditional treatment group.[47]

A newer therapeutic modality, ESWT seems to be safe, effective, and noninvasive. Early studies seem promising; however, longer prospective randomized studies and long-term assessment are needed to further document clinical improvement and associated structural changes before ESWT becomes a mainstream treatment of tendinopathy.

MEDICATION-BASED THERAPY

NSAIDSs

NSAIDs work on pain by inhibiting the cyclooxygenase (COX) pathway, which transforms arachidonic acid to prostaglandins, prostacyclins, and thromboxanes with of the goal of reducing the inflammatory response to injury. COX-2 provides the main contribution to the inflammatory response and is responsible for sensitizing pain receptors, elevating body temperature, and recruiting inflammatory cells to the area of injured tissue.[48,49] NSAIDs are used extensively in the treatment of musculoskeletal injury and probably deserve a place in the treatment of shorter-term muscle and tendon injury (ie, tendinitis or tenosynovitis). However, based on NSAIDs' mechanism of action and what is known about the histologic makeup of a tendinosis injury, NSAIDs should provide little benefit in the treatment of this issue.[15,17,18,35,48–50] Andres and Murrell[35] did a systematic review of the literature and identified 37 randomized clinical trials evaluating NSAID use in the treatment of tendinopathy. Seventeen of these studies were placebo controlled. Andres and Murrell's review indicated that oral and local NSAID use was effective in relieving pain associated with tendinopathy in the short term (7–14 days). Three of the 17 placebo-controlled studies revealed no improvement with NSAIDs. Patients who presented with a longer duration and greater severity of symptoms were more likely to have a poor response to any form of NSAID use.[35] However, even if NSAIDs do provide some pain relief in chronic tendinosis injury, they do not result in changes beneficial to the healing process and may in fact be detrimental. In the initial stages of tendon injury, an inflammatory response is required for normal repair. NSAID inhibition may be deleterious to the fine balance of tendon repair initiated early on in the injury through the inflammatory cascade.[49] In addition, pain control through the use of NSAIDs may also be a double-edged sword, allowing patients to ignore early symptoms, leading to further tendon damage and ultimately a delay in definitive healing.[17,18,48,49] Care must also be taken when using NSAIDs with regard to the high risk of side effects related to the renal system, the cardiovascular system (ie, worsening of hypertension and cardiovascular disease), asthma exacerbation, and gastrointestinal bleeding. This point is especially true in our older athletes and patients because many of these individuals are likely to have the aforementioned medical comorbidities.[48,50] At best, a short course of NSAIDs may be reasonable in the treatment of acute pain in a tendon condition associated with inflammation (tendinitis/tenosynovitis) or possibly early on in a tendon overuse injury but not in the chronic treatment of symptoms related to tendinosis. The debate around the use of NSAIDs in tendon injury continues with investigators indicating care and judicious use of NSAIDs for these conditions.[2,35,48,50]

Nitric Oxide Therapy

Nitric oxide (NO) is a soluble gas synthesized by 3 NO synthetase enzymes (NOSs). The 3 forms of NOSs include inducible, endothelial, and neuronal. All 3 forms seem to be expressed in fibroblastlike cells.[51,52] Increases in NOSs have been shown to be upregulated in response to tendon injury in animal models including a rat exercise overuse model. Increased NOSs enzyme activity has also been correlated in human tissue samples of torn rotator cuff samples seen at surgery. NO seems to have 2 functions revolving around cell signaling and in a nonspecific immune response similar to superoxide.[52]

With regard to tendon healing, it seems that NO synthesis as processed through the NOSs enzymes is important to tendon healing.[15,52] Rats fed a competitive NOS inhibitor were found to have significantly reduced healing of their Achilles tendons compared with rats drinking an inactive enantiomer.[52] In addition to the experiments indicating NOSs upregulation in animal tendon injury models, other studies have indicated that exogenous NO can enhance tendon collagen synthesis, tendon healing, and that inhibition of NO synthesis results in a smaller cross-sectional area and mechanical strength of healing Achilles tendons in rats.[15,52]

The aforementioned basic science evidence has fueled research using exogenous NO in the form of glyceryl trinitrate patches in the treatment of tendinosis. Most of the studies using exogenous NO in human tendinosis have been accomplished by Paoloni and colleagues[53–56] through 3 studies looking at the use of glyceryl trinitrate patches in chronic extensor tendinosis of the elbow, noninsertional Achilles tendinosis, and supraspinatus tendinosis. These studies were randomized, controlled, and double blinded and designed to see if exogenous topical NO would enhance tendon healing and reduce pain in humans. Through the use of topical glyceryl trinitrate patches, Paoloni and colleagues[53] were able to show improvement in pain, increased power, and improved function at the aforementioned studied areas. In the chronic extensor tendinosis at the elbow study group, at 6 months, 81% of patients treated with topical glyceryltrinitrate were asymptomatic during activities of daily living (ADLs) compared with 60% of patients who had tendon rehabilitation alone. The noninsertional Achilles tendinopathy study group revealed that 78% of patients in the study group were asymptomatic with ADLs compared with 49% in the placebo group at 6 months.[54] The supraspinatus tendinopathy study group revealed 46% of the study group compared with 24% of the placebo group was asymptomatic with ADLs at 6 months.[55] All 3 studies revealed improvement in pain-free ADLs, with the studies involving the Achilles and supraspinatus tendinosis revealing decrease in pain with activity in general.[51–55] In a 3-year follow-up study of topical glyceryl trinitrate treatment in chronic noninsertional Achilles tendinopathy, Paoloni and colleagues[35,56] were able to show persistent improvement in the NO-treated group compared with the control group. Even though there is no histologic confirmation, these results suggest that treatment with exogenous NO not only has an effect on pain control but also in tendon healing. In 2010, Gambito and colleagues[57] published a meta-analysis identifying 7 randomized clinical trials looking at the effects of topical nitroglycerin in the treatment of tendinopathies. The analysis revealed that topical nitroglycerin provides short-term pain relief to a maximum of 6 months in ADLs in acute and chronic tendinopathies. Also, there was strong evidence to suggest that topical nitroglycerin (NTG) is effective in enhancing tendon forces in the chronic phase.

When used in the treatment of tendinopathy, topical glyceryl trinitrate is considered an Food and Drug Administration (FDA) off-label use. The dose used in studies revolves around using a 5-mg/24-h delivery glyceryl trinitrate patch divided into quarters and placed directly over the point of maximal tenderness (delivery of 1.25 mg/24 h of medication).[2,35] The patch is changed daily and left in place until symptom resolution, with most studies maintaining patch placement anywhere from 8 weeks to 6 months.[57] Most side effects related to treatment with topical NTG revolve around contact dermatitis, dizziness, and headaches. The headaches and dizziness are related to vasodilation-induced hypotension, and headaches can be severe enough to cause cessation of treatment.[35,51,57] In addition to the use of topical NTG, most investigators would encourage its use in conjunction with a comprehensive physical therapy program.

INJECTION-BASED TREATMENT

Corticosteroids

Corticosteroid treatment of tendinopathies has been a mainstay of treatment for decades. The choice to use corticosteroid injections was initially caused by their anti-inflammatory effects, and their use still continues despite sufficient evidence that demonstrates that inflammation does not play a significant role in tendinosis. They are still a first-line therapy in a short-term tendinitis. One of the proposed methods for the benefit that steroid injections provide revolves around their effects on the surrounding tissue. It has been postulated that the degenerative changes found in a tendon lead to inflammation of the surrounding soft tissues that lead to pain and swelling. In this situation, the antiinflammatory effects of the steroid would provide symptomatic relief, but the underlying degenerative changes causing the problem still remain.[2,58]

Although the treatment of tendinopathies with steroid injections has been a first-line approach, there is considerable evidence published that demonstrates that the efficacy of these injections should be questioned. Studies have shown that there may be initial pain relief but that there is often recurrence of pain in the long term.[2,15,16,18,21] Newcomer and colleagues[59] demonstrated in their study of lateral epicondylitis that there were no significant differences between corticosteroid injection and rehabilitation and that all patients, regardless of treatment modality, had equal improvement of pain scores at 6 months. Their conclusion was that a rehabilitation program should be the first-line treatment. Coombes and colleagues[60] did a systematic review looking at injections in the management of tendinopathies and found that for lateral epicondylitis and rotator cuff pain, the corticosteroid injection helped with pain initially but offered no intermediate or long-term benefit. Alvarez and colleagues[61] also showed consistent data in regard to chronic rotator cuff tendinosis. Their study demonstrated that a subacromial injection of betamethasone was no more effective than anesthetic alone in improving disease-specific quality of life, range of motion, or impingement signs in chronic rotator cuff tendinosis. Finally, in a systematic review, van Ark and colleagues[62] discovered that corticosteroid injection had the worst relapse pain rate of all when compared with eccentric and resistance groups and other injection therapies when reevaluated long term at 6 months and beyond.

Although corticosteroid injections are used as a first-line treatment, they are not without risks or complications. Shrier and colleagues[63] via a systematic review identified several side effects of corticosteroid injections. The overall incidence of side effects with locally injected steroid is approximately 1% and can include skin atrophy and depigmentation (which can be permanent). Nichols[64] reported that of the 43 studies that they reviewed, 15% to 23% experienced complications associated with corticosteroid injection therapy. The most common side effects reported were postinjection pain (9.7%), skin atrophy (2.4%), skin depigmentation (0.8%), localized erythema and warmth (0.7%), and facial flushing (0.6%).[64] There have been several studies to come forth and report concerns of tendon rupture, primarily in the weight-bearing tendons (Achilles and patellar). Gill has reported that there is a safe and efficacious peritendinous Achilles injection that can be completed under fluoroscopic guidance to confirm delivery around the tendon rather than within it, supposedly minimizing the risk of tendon rupture.[65]

Given the evidence in the literature at this time, it seems that corticosteroid injections for the treatment of short-term symptoms associated with tendinopathy provide pain relief but offer little in long-term management of tendinosis.

Platelet-Rich Plasma

Platelet-rich plasma (PRP) can be used to treat a variety of chronic overuse conditions, including Achilles tendinopathy, patellar tendinopathy, rotator cuff tendinopathy, and medial and lateral epicondylitis of the elbow. There have been investigational studies to look at its application to chronic muscle strains, fibrosis, and joint capsular laxity for the past couple of decades. The purpose of PRP is to help augment the natural healing process to allow a quicker return to sport or work.[2]

PRP is a concentrate of platelets that are obtained from the patients' own blood that is centrifuged down into its various components. The layer PRP, with its increased concentration of platelets and growth factors, is then selectively drawn off, activated via exogenous or endogenous methods, and reinjected at the site of injury. The potential to modify the natural healing pathway of tendons and ligaments is related to the increased concentration of growth factors and bioactive proteins released by activated platelets (**Table 1**).[66] Through the action of these growth factors, there is the theoretical goal of minimizing inflammation and fibrosis while maximizing myofiber regeneration.[67] Specifically, the goal of therapy is to increase the expression of procollagen types I and III, thereby improving the mechanical properties, promoting tendon cell proliferation, and tendon healing.[62]

Until recently, there was minimal research placed on the efficacy and outcomes of PRP. Over the past few years, the amount of research on PRP has increased considerably, but there still needs to be more well-controlled randomized studies conducted. Currently, the research available on PRP has conflicting results. de Vos and his colleagues[68] conducted a study that showed PRP injection did not improve pain or functional outcomes for patients with chronic Achilles tendinopathy who were all treated with a concurrent eccentric exercise program. At the 1-year follow-up, there was no evidence for the use of PRP based on pain scores and ultrasound tendon structure. Expanding on this study, de Vos and colleagues[68,69] also determined that injecting PRP for the treatment of chronic midportion Achilles tendinopathy does not contribute to an increased tendon structure or alter the degree of neovascularization, based on ultrasound, compared with placebo.[70] Paoloni and colleagues[71] conducted a systematic review and concluded there is currently no significant evidence in human clinical trials for the efficacy of PRP in treating ligament and tendon injuries that is superior to that of any other injection treatment to date. Conversely, Taylor and colleagues[66] discovered in their systematic review of in vivo studies that there was

Table 1
Growth factors released by activated platelets

Growth Factor	Function
Transforming growth factor-β1	Matrix synthesis
Platelet-derived growth factor	Stimulate angiogenesis, cell proliferation, mitogen for fibroblasts
Basic fibroblast growth factor	Proliferation of fibroblasts and myoblasts, angiogenesis
Vascular endothelial growth factor	Angiogenesis
Epidermal growth factor	Proliferation of epithelial and mesenchymal cells
Insulinlike growth factor	Stimulate fibroblast and myoblasts
Hepatocyte growth factor	Angiogenesis

From Taylor D, Petrera M, Hendry, M, et al. A systematic review of the use of platelet-rich plasma in sports medicine as a new treatment for tendon and ligament injuries. Clin J Sports Med 2011;21(4):344–52; with permission.

some improvement noted with PRP. There have been several other studies that have shown significant improvement with the use of PRP. Specifically, Peerbooms and colleagues[72] looked at PRP versus corticosteroid injection for lateral epicondylitis and found that there were significant improvements in the PRP group in both pain and function at the 1-year follow-up, with the PRP group having a success rate of 73% compared with 49% in the steroid group. Gaweda and colleagues[73] reported a significant improvement in clinical scores for pain and ultrasound parameters for Achilles tendinopathy.[66] However, Filardo and colleagues[74] looked at PRP with physical therapy versus physical therapy alone and concluded that there was no significant improvement with the addition of PRP, leading to their conclusion that for patellar tendinopathy, the more important treatment is the physical therapy and not the PRP.[2]

At this time, there are few side effects of PRP noted in the literature, but overall there is little known about its safety. The most common side effects listed include a marked pain response, local inflammation, and stiffness.[71] Bovine thrombin used in early trials of PRP has been recognized to cause an immune response resulting in life-threatening coagulopathies and is no longer used.[67] The use of calcium chloride as an activating agent has mitigated this risk. There have been several theoretical risks postulated regarding PRP injection, including acting as a promoter of carcinogenesis secondary to the promotion of the division and proliferation of mutated cells, but there has never been a reported case.[66]

Of final note on PRP, Deren and his colleagues[75] did a Web-based study through an Internet search engine to evaluate the data available to patients regarding PRP. Their study concluded that some Web-based references to PRP therapy are biased and inaccurate. Their concern is that some readers will misinterpret such easily available but poorly controlled information, potentially leading to the use of unproven therapies. Based on the data that is currently available in quality randomized controlled trials, there is still conflicting evidence as to the efficacy of PRP in overuse tendon injuries.

Autologous Blood

The concept of using whole autologous blood as an injection-based management for tendinopathies is a comparatively new method of treatment. Studies to this point have examined its use in Achilles and patellar tendinopathies, medial and lateral epicondylitis of the elbow, and plantar fasciitis. James and his group[76] hypothesize that autologous blood injections have a similar mechanism of action to PRP. The autologous blood preparations, rich in growth factors, induce cell proliferation and promote the synthesis of angiogenic factors during the healing process, which lead to subsequent collagen regeneration.[62,76] Some of the more specific growth factors that seem to play a role are TGF-β and fibroblast growth factor, specifically acting as humeral mediators, triggering the healing cascade.[2,77]

There are very limited studies that have been done on autologous blood injection to this point. Published material consists of mostly prospective case series regarding outcomes of its use. These series are limited by small sample sizes and lack of controls. Three of these case series showed statistically significant improvements in their outcomes compared with baseline. Edwards and colleagues[78] had an 88% improvement from baseline, Gani and colleagues[79] reported 64% improvement from baseline, and Connell and colleagues[80] reported a median pain score of 0 at the follow-up.[77] Kazemi and colleagues[81] conducted a randomized controlled study for lateral epicondylitis of autologous whole blood injection versus a corticosteroid injection and found that at the follow-up, the autologous blood group did significantly better in all outcome measures.[2] Finally, Creaney and his colleagues[82] did a study on lateral epicondylitis that continued to be painful following conservative treatment with physical therapy. In their study, they randomized patients into a PRP group and an autologous blood group. Their results demonstrated that 70% of these patients improved with either PRP or autologous blood injections.

With the current evidence reported in the literature, autologous blood injection seems to be a potentially promising treatment method for tendinopathy, but more controlled research is needed to determine its efficacy and potential side effects.

Prolotherapy

The use of prolotherapy has dated back to the 1930s since its time of treatment of pain associated with presumed ligament laxity.[77] It has recently become a topic of more interest as a treatment option for tendinopathy, back pain, and other overuse injuries. It currently is being studied primarily for use in lateral epicondylitis, Achilles and patellar tendinopathies, back pain, and medial tibial stress syndrome. The process of prolotherapy involves injecting proliferating agents at several sites on a painful ligament or tendon insertion to induce an inflammatory response and lead to healing. This inflammatory response reportedly results in hypertrophy and strengthening of collagenous structures.[83] There are 3 commonly used agents in prolotherapy and all have different mechanisms of action. Dextrose, the most commonly used agent, causes osmotic cellular rupture, phenol-glycerin-glucose causes local cellular irritation, and sodium morrhuate causes chemotactic attraction of inflammatory mediators.[2,84]

In a systematic review, Rabago and colleagues[84] determined that there is limited high-quality data supporting the use of prolotherapy. In regard to the pain associated with lateral epicondylitis, Scarpone and colleagues[85] reported a statistically significant improvement of 90% of patients receiving prolotherapy at 16 weeks (controls had 22% improvement). In a prospective case series without a placebo group, Lyftogt[86] demonstrated 94% improvement compared with baseline with prolotherapy. Holmes and his colleagues[87] looked at prolotherapy for anterior knee pain and found that those who received prolotherapy improved in all of their outcome categories, leading to their conclusion that dextrose prolotherapy seems to be an effective treatment option for anterior knee pain in a select group of patients. Finally, Ryan and colleagues[88] found that in their study of prolotherapy for overuse patellar tendinopathy, there was a reduction of pain and an improvement in ultrasound appearance following ultrasound-guided dextrose injections for refractory cases. These findings led them to suggest that dextrose prolotherapy may modify patellar tendinopathy at the tissue level and that fibrillar changes may play a role in tendon nociception.

Given the limited research that is available at this time, it is difficult to be sure of the true efficacy of prolotherapy. It seems to be a relatively safe, potential way of treating tendinopathy. There needs to be more randomized controlled trials to evaluate its true efficacy.

Skin-Derived Tenocytelike Cells

It is understood that there are several factors that contribute to the inflammatory process involved in overuse tendon injuries. Some of the new literature being published is beginning to investigate the use of tendonlike tenocytes to alter the pathology and ultimately help lead to healing. It is understood that stem cells are able to self-renew or develop into multiple different lineages of cell lines. In a 2009 published study, de Mos[89] and his group showed that human tendon cells have an intrinsic differentiation potential and suggested a plausible role for altered tendon-cell differentiation in the pathophysiology of tendinosis.[89,90] Several animal models have also previously demonstrated that regeneration of tendon tissue can be achieved by the implantation of tenocyte cells that have the ability to lay down collagen matrix.[91,92] In a more recent prospective clinical pilot study, Connell and colleagues[90] used autologous skin-derived tenocytelike cells and, under ultrasound guidance, injected patients with refractory lateral epicondylitis. These patients subsequently had a follow-up at 6 weeks, 3 months, and 6 months and demonstrated self-reported symptom improvement. They also monitored the healing response by ultrasound that showed statistically significant changes in the number of tears, number of new vessels, and tendon thickness. Their results led to the conclusion that skin-derived tenocytelike cells can be cultured in the laboratory to yield a preparation of collagen-producing cells that lead to clinical improvement of refractory lateral epicondylitis.

To this point, there have been no placebo-controlled trials involving tenocyte treatment of overuse tendinopathy. This treatment modality could offer another option for patients suffering from tendinosis, but better-designed studies are needed to help elucidate a clear treatment benefit.

SURGICAL OPTIONS

Although surgical options are not the focus of this review, it should be mentioned as an option in recalcitrant cases of tendinosis that fail the aforementioned conservative approaches. The goal of the surgical procedure in relation to the pathology associated with tendinosis is to excise areas of failed healing and fibrosis as well as pathologic nerve and vascular ingrowth related to angiogenesis. Through this process, it is hypothesized that bleeding will initiate the healing process thereby restoring vascularity and initiate stem cell ingrowth and protein synthesis that will promote healing.[2,21,93] Based on the hypothesized effect of surgical treatment on the tendon tissue, it probably is not only the debridement of tissue that leads to tendon healing but the overall stimulation of a new healing process in correlation with careful progression of rehabilitation that leads to tendon healing.[2,18]

Surgical procedures are divided among open procedures, arthroscopic, and percutaneous tenotomies. Percutaneous tenotomy has evolved out of a desire to develop less-invasive surgical techniques. The procedure is effective in cases of isolated tendinosis with a well-defined nodular lesion less than 2.5 cm in length and no involvement of the paratenon.[2,93] The procedure can be performed in the ambulatory setting, under local anesthesia, using ultrasound guidance to confirm the precise location of the tendinosis.[2,93]

Comparison of surgical techniques is difficult because of the limited randomized controlled studies. It seems that the success of surgical procedures is related to the site of tendinosis, the associated pathologic condition (ie, tendon tear), and the method used.[2,35] The best success seems to be seen in surgery for lateral epicondylitis, with success rates in the 65% to 95% range based on retrospective or prospective case series.[35]

Even when successful, surgery for tendinosis is not a quick fix allowing immediate return to sport or previously aggravating activities. Prospective outcome studies have noted return to sport time frames of 4 to 6 months, 6 to 9 months, and 9 to 12 months for elbow, Achilles, and patella tendon surgery, respectively.[18] This delayed return to full activity probably reflects the complex reparative healing process induced by the surgical procedure that must have adequate time to fully blossom and transpire to fruition to allow for complete healing.

Despite the evidence of successful treatment with regard to surgical intervention, the procedures are not without morbidity. Treatment failure rates can be as high as 20% to 30%, with difficulty predicting who will not respond well to the procedure.

Because of the high morbidity and failure rates, it is suggested that surgery be reserved as a last resort for patients who have failed maximum conservative management for tendinopathy.[2,35]

SUMMARY

Tendinopathy and, more precisely, chronic tendon issues related to tendinosis are conditions difficult to treat. This condition often leads to the patients' quality of life declining because of the inability to participate in exercise, athletic activity, occupation-related activities, and even ADLs. By better understanding the pathophysiology related to the development of tendinosis, we as clinicians will be better able to understand the treatments options available and their limitations while at the same time allowing for novel therapies to be developed. Based on the aforementioned review, conservative treatment of tendinosis starting with a sound rehabilitation program seems to be the best place to start while reserving surgical approaches as a last resort for recalcitrant cases that have failed conservative management.

REFERENCES

1. Wilder R, Sethi S. Overuse injuries: tendinopathies, stress fractures, compartment syndrome, and shin splints. Clin Sports Med 2004;23:55–81.
2. Skjong C, Meininger A, Ho S. Tendinopathy treatment: where is the evidence? Clin Sports Med 2012;31:329–50.
3. Maffulli N, Wong J. Types and epidemiology of tendinopathy. Clin Sports Med 2003;22:675–92.
4. Maffulli N, Benazzo F. Basic sciences of tendons. Sports Med Arthrosc 2000;8: 1–5.
5. Tursz A, Crost M. Sports related injuries in children. A study of their characteristics, frequency and severity, with comparison to other types of accidental injuries. Am J Sports Med 1986;14(4):294–9.
6. Bruns W, Maffulli N. Lower limb injuries in children in sports. Clin Sports Med 2000;19(4):637–62.
7. Jarvinen M. Epidemiology of tendon injuries in sports. Clin Sports Med 1992; 11(3):493–504.
8. Smith FW, Smith BA. Musculoskeletal differences between males and female. Sports Med Arthrosc 2002;10:98–100.
9. Kvist M. Achilles tendon overuse injuries: a clinical and pathophysiological study in athletes [dissertation]. Finland: Turku University; 1991.
10. Newell SG, Bramwell S. Overuse injuries to the knee in runners. Phys Sportsmed 1984;12:81–6.
11. Messier SP, Edwards DG, Martin DF, et al. Etiology of iliotibial band friction syndrome in distance runners. Med Sci Sports Exerc 1995;27:951–60.
12. Gabel GT. Acute and chronic tendinopathies at the elbow. Curr Opin Rheumatol 1999;11:138–43.
13. Kannus P, Aho H, Jarvinen M, et al. Computerised recording of visits to an outpatients sports clinic. Am J Sports Med 1987;15:79–85.
14. Brinker MR, O'Connor DP, Almekinders LC, et al. Chapter 1 section A basic science and injury of muscle, tendon, and ligament. In: DeLee J, Drez D, Miller M, editors. DeLee & Drez's orthopaedic sports medicine principles and practice. 3rd edition. Philadelphia: Saunders Elsevier; 2010. p. 20–31.
15. Kaeding C, Best TM. Tendinosis: pathophysiology and nonoperative treatment. Sports Health 2009;1:284–92.

16. Magnaris CN, Narici MV, Almedkinders LC, et al. Biomechanics and pathophysiology of overuse tendon injuries. Ideas on insertional tendinopathy. Sports Med 2004;34(14):1005–17.
17. Khan KM, Cook JL, Bonar F, et al. Histopathology of common tendinopathies. updates and implications for clinical management. Sports Med 1999;27(6): 393–408.
18. Khan K, Cook J. The painful nonruptured tendon: clinical aspects. Clin Sports Med 2003;22:711–25.
19. Xu Y, Murrell GA. The basic science of tendinopathy. Clin Orthop Relat Res 2008; 466:1528–38.
20. Choi L. Chapter 14 Overuse injuries. In: DeLee J, Drez D, Miller M, editors. DeLee & Drez's orthopaedic sports medicine principles and practice. 3rd edition. Philadelphia: Saunders Elsevier; 2010. p. 611–4.
21. Ackermann PW, Renstrom P. Tendinopathy in sport. Sports Health 2012;4(3): 193–201.
22. Shalabi A, Kristofferson-Wilberg M, Svenson L, et al. Eccentric training of the gastrocnemius-soleus complex in chronic Achilles tendinopathy results in decreased tendon volume and intratendinous signal as evaluated by MRI. Am J Sports Med 2004;32(5):1286–96.
23. Ohberg L, Alfredson H. Effects on neovascularization behind the good results with eccentric training in chronic mid-portion Achilles tendinosis? Knee Surg Sports Traumatol Arthrosc 2004;12(5):465–70.
24. Kingma JJ, de Knikker R, Wittink HM, et al. Eccentric overloading training in patients with chronic Achilles tendinopathy: a systematic review. Br J Sports Med 2007;41(6):e3.
25. Alfredson H, Pietilä T, Jonsson P, et al. Heavy load eccentric calf muscle training for the treatment of chronic Achilles tendinosis. Am J Sports Med 1998;26:360–6.
26. Jonsson P, Alfredson H. Superior results with eccentric compared to concentric quadriceps training in patients with jumper's knee: a prospective randomized study. Br J Sports Med 2005;39:847–50.
27. Mafi N, Lorentzon R, Alfredson H. Superior short term results with eccentric calf muscle training compared to concentric training in a randomized prospective multicenter study on patients with chronic Achilles tendinosis. Knee Surg Sports Traumatol Arthrosc 2001;9:42–7.
28. Larsson M, Käll I, Nilsson-Helander K. Treatment of patellar tendinopathy-a systematic review of randomized controlled trials. Knee Surg Sports Traumatol Arthrosc 2012;20:1632–46.
29. Norris CM. Sports injuries. New York: Butterworth-Heinermann; 1993. p. 109–11.
30. Prentice W. Therapeutic modalities in sports medicine. 3rd edition. St Louis (MO): Mosby; 1994. p. 336–49.
31. Davidson C, Ganion L, Gehlsen G, et al. Rat tendon morphological and functional changes resulting from soft tissue mobilization. Med Sci Sports Exerc 1997;29: 313–9.
32. Gehlsen G, Ganion L, Helfst R. Fibroblast responses to variation in soft tissue mobilization pressure. Med Sci Sports Exerc 1999;31(4):531–5.
33. Mangine R, Eifert-Mangine M, Middendorf WA. Chapter 5 section B use of modalities in sports. In: DeLee J, Drez D, Miller M, editors. DeLee & Drez's orthopaedic sports medicine principles and practice. 3rd edition. Philadelphia: Saunders Elsevier; 2010. p. 233–6.
34. Tumity S, Munn J, McDonough S, et al. Low level laser treatment of tendinopathy: a systematic review with meta-analysis. Photomed Laser Surg 2010;28:3–16.

35. Andres BM, Murrell GA. Treatment of tendinopathy. what works, what does not, and what is on the horizon. Clin Orthop Relat Res 2008;466:1539–54.
36. Green S, Buchbinder R, Hetrick S. Physiotherapy interventions for shoulder pain. Cochrane Database Syst Rev 2003;(2):CD004258.
37. Mclaughlin GJ, Handoll HH. Interventions for treating acute and chronic Achilles tendonitis. Cochrane Database Syst Rev 2001;(2):CD000232.
38. Stasinopoulos D, Johnson MI. Effectiveness of low level laser therapy for lateral elbow tendinopathy. Photomed Laser Surg 2005;23:425–30.
39. Trudel D, Duley J, Zastrow I, et al. Rehabilitation for patients with lateral epicondylitis: a systematic review. J Hand Ther 2004;17:243–66.
40. Steves RG. Physical modalities in sports medicine in Madden C. In: Putukian M, Young CC, McCarty EC, editors. Netter's sports medicine. Philadelphia: Saunders Elsevier; 2010. p. 313–4.
41. Klaiman M, Shrader J, Danoff J, et al. Phonophoresis versus ultrasound in the treatment of common musculoskeletal conditions. Med Sci Sports Exerc 1998; 30(9):1349–55.
42. Wang C. Extracorporeal shockwave therapy in musculoskeletal disorders. J Orthop Surg Res 2012;7:11.
43. Galasso O, Amelio E, Riccelli D, et al. Short term outcomes of extracorporeal shock wave therapy for the treatment of chronic non-calcific tendinopathy of the supraspinatus: a double blind randomized, placebo controlled trial. BMC Musculoskelet Disord 2012;13:86.
44. Chung B, Wiley P. Effectiveness of extracorporeal shock wave therapy in the treatment of previously untreated lateral epicondylitis. Am J Sports Med 2004;32:7.
45. Peers KH, Lysens RJ, Brys P, et al. Cross-sectional outcome analysis of athletes with chronic patellar tendinopathy treated surgically and by extracorporeal shock wave therapy. Clin J Sport Med 2003;13(2):79–83.
46. Rompe JD, Furia J, Maffuli N. Eccentric loading compared with shock wave treatment for chronic insertional Achilles tendinopathy. A randomized controlled trial. J Bone Joint Surg Am 2008;90(1):52–61.
47. Cacchio A, Rompe J, Furia J, et al. Shockwave therapy for the treatment of chronic proximal hamstring tendinopathy in professional athletes. Am J Sports Med 2011;39(1):146–53.
48. Mehallo CJ, Drezner JA, Bytomski JR. Practical management: nonsteroidal antiinflammatory drug (NSAID) use in athletic injuries. Clin J Sport Med 2006;16(2): 170–4.
49. Magra M, Maffulli N. Nonsteroidal antiinflammatory drugs in tendinopathy friend or foe. Clin J Sport Med 2006;16(1):1–3.
50. Paoloni JA, Milne C, Orchard J, et al. Non-steroidal anti-inflammatory drugs in sports medicine: guidelines for practical but sensible use. Br J Sports Med 2009;43:863–5.
51. Hauk JM, Hosey RG. Nitric oxide therapy: fact or fiction? Curr Sports Med Rep 2006;5:199–202.
52. Murrell GAC. Using nitric oxide to treat tendinopathy. Br J Sports Med 2007;41: 227–31.
53. Paoloni JA, Appleyard RC, Nelson J, et al. Topical nitric oxide application in the treatment of chronic extensor tendinosis at the elbow. Am J Sports Med 2003; 31(6):915–20.
54. Paoloni JA, Appleyard RC, Nelson J, et al. Topical glyceryl trinitrate treatment of chronic noninsertional Achilles tendinopathy. J Bone Joint Surg Am 2004;86(5): 916–22.

55. Paoloni JA, Appleyard RC, Nelson J, et al. Topical glyceryl trinitrate application in the treatment of chronic supraspinatus tendinopathy. Am J Sports Med 2005;33(6):806–13.
56. Paoloni JA, Murrell GA. Three-year follow-up study of topical glyceryl trinitrate treatment of chronic noninsertional Achilles tendinopathy. Foot Ankle Int 2007;28(10):1064–8.
57. Gambito ED, Gonzalez-Suarez CB, Oquinena TI, et al. Evidence on the effectiveness of topical nitroglycerin in the treatment of tendinopathies: a systematic review and meta-analysis. Arch Phys Med Rehabil 2010;91:1291–305.
58. Kongsgaard M, Kovanen V, Aagaard P, et al. Corticosteroid injections, eccentric decline squat training and heavy slow resistance training in patellar tendinopathy. Scand J Med Sci Sports 2009;19(6):790–802.
59. Newcomer K, Laskowski E, Idank D, et al. Corticosteroid injection in early treatment of lateral epicondylitis. Clin J Sport Med 2001;11:214–22.
60. Coombes BK, Bisset L, Vicenzino B. Efficacy and safety of corticosteroid injections and other injections for management of tendinopathy: a systematic review of randomized controlled trials. Lancet 2010;376:1751–67.
61. Alvarez CM, Litchfield R, Jackowski D, et al. A prospective, double blind, randomized clinical trial comparing subacromial injection of betamethasone and Xylocaine to Xylocaine alone in chronic rotator cuff tendinosis. Am J Sports Med 2005;33:255–62.
62. van Ark M, Zwerver J, Akker-Scheek I. Injection treatments for patellar tendinopathy. Br J Sports Med 2011;45:1068–76.
63. Shrier I, Matheson G, Kohl H. Achilles tendonitis: are corticosteroid injections useful or harmful? Clin J Sport Med 1996;6:245–50.
64. Nichols AW. Complications associated with the use of corticosteroids in the treatment of athletic injuries. Clin J Sport Med 2005;15:370–5.
65. Gill SS, Gelbke MK, Mattson SL, et al. Fluoroscopically guided low-volume peritendinous corticosteroid injection for Achilles tendinopathy. A safety study. J Bone Joint Surg Am 2004;86(4):802–6.
66. Taylor D, Petrera M, Hendry M, et al. A systematic review of the use of platelet-rich plasma in sports medicine as a new treatment for tendon and ligament injuries. Clin J Sport Med 2011;21:344–52.
67. Hamilton B, Best T. Platelet-enriched plasma and muscle strain injuries: challenges imposed by the burden of proof. Clin J Sport Med 2011;21:31–6.
68. de Vos RJ, Weir A, van Schie HT, et al. Platelet-rich plasma injection for chronic Achilles tendinopathy: a randomized controlled trial. JAMA 2010;303:144–9.
69. de Jonge S, de Vos R, Weir A, et al. Platelet-rich plasma for chronic Achilles tendinopathy: a double-blind randomized controlled trial with one year follow-up. Br J Sports Med 2011;45:e1.
70. de Vos RJ, Weir A, Verhaar J, et al. No effect of PRP on ultrasonographic tendon structure and neovascularization in chronic midportion Achilles tendinopathy. Br J Sports Med 2011;45:387–92.
71. Paoloni J, de Vos R, Hamilton B, et al. Platelet-rich plasma treatment for ligament and tendon injuries. Clin J Sport Med 2011;21:37–45.
72. Peerbooms JC, Sluimer J, Bruijn DJ, et al. Positive effect of an autologous platelet concentrate in lateral epicondylitis in a double-blind randomized controlled trial: platelet-rich plasma versus corticosteroid injection with a 1-year follow-up. Am J Sports Med 2010;38(2):255–62.
73. Gaweda K, Tarczynska M, Krzyzanowski W. Treatment of Achilles tendinopathy with platelet-rich plasma. Int J Sports Med 2010;31:577–83.

74. Filardo G, Kon E, Della Villa S, et al. Use of platelet-rich plasma for the treatment of refractory jumper's knee. Int Orthop 2010;34(6):909–15.
75. Deren M, DiGiovanni C, Feller E. Web-based portrayal of platelet-rich plasma injections for orthopedic therapy. Clin J Sport Med 2011;21:428–32.
76. James S, Ali K, Pocock C, et al. Ultrasound guided dry needling and autologous blood injection for patellar tendinosis. Br J Sports Med 2007;41:518–22.
77. Rabago D, Best T, Zgierska A, et al. A systematic review of four injection therapies for lateral epicondylitis: prolotherapy, polidocanol, whole blood and platelet-rich plasma. Br J Sports Med 2009;43:471–81.
78. Edwards SG, Calandruccio JH. Autologous blood injections for refractory lateral epicondylitis. J Hand Surg Am 2003;28:272–8.
79. Gani NU, Butt MF, Dhar SA, et al. Autologous blood injection in the treatment of refractory tennis elbow. Internet J Orthop Surg 2007;5. Available at: http://www.ispub.com/ostia/index.php?xmlFilePath=journals/ijos/vol5n1.tennis.xml. Accessed November 19, 2012.
80. Connell DA, Ali KE, Ahmad M, et al. Ultrasound-guided autologous blood injection for tennis elbow. Skeletal Radiol 2006;35:371–7.
81. Kazemi M, Azma K, Tavana B, et al. Autologous blood versus corticosteroid local injection in the short-term treatment of lateral elbow tendinopathy: a randomized clinical trial of efficacy. Am J Phys Med Rehabil 2010;89(8):660–7.
82. Creaney L, Wallace A, Curtis M, et al. Growth factor-based therapies provide additional benefit beyond physical therapy in resistant elbow tendinopathy: a prospective, single-blind, randomized trial of autologous blood injections versus platelet-rich plasma injections. Br J Sports Med 2011;45:966–71.
83. Rabago D, Best T, Beamsley M, et al. A systematic review of prolotherapy for chronic musculoskeletal pain. Clin J Sport Med 2005;15:376.
84. Banks A. A rationale for prolotherapy. J Orthop Med 1991;13(3):54–9.
85. Scarpone M, Rabago D, Zgierska A, et al. The efficacy of prolotherapy for lateral epicondylitis: a pilot study. Clin J Sport Med 2008;18:248–54.
86. Lyftogt J. Subcutaneous prolotherapy treatment of refractory knee, shoulder, and lateral elbow pain. Australasian Musculoskeletal Med 2007;12:110–2.
87. Holmes F, Sevier T. Dextrose prolotherapy for anterior knee pain: a randomized prospective double-blind placebo-controlled study. Clin J Sport Med 2004; 14(5):311.
88. Ryan M, Wong A, Rabago D, et al. Ultrasound-guided injections of hyperosmolar dextrose for overuse patellar tendinopathy: a pilot study. Br J Sports Med 2011; 45:972–7.
89. de Mos M, Koevoet WJ, Jahr H, et al. Intrinsic differentiation potential of adolescent human tendon tissue: an in-vitro cell differentiation study. BMC Musculoskelet Disord 2007;23:8–16.
90. Connell D, Datir A, Alyas F, et al. Treatment of lateral epicondylitis using skin-derived tenocyte-like cells. Br J Sports Med 2009;43:293–8.
91. Kryger GS, Chong AK, Costa M, et al. A comparison of tenocytes and mesenchymal stem cells for use in flexor tendon tissue engineering. J Hand Surg Am 2007;32:597–605.
92. Cao Y, Liu Y, Liu W, et al. Bridging tendon defects using autologous tenocyte engineered tendon in a hen model. Plast Reconstr Surg 2002;110:1280–9.
93. Maffulli N, Longo UG, Denaro V. Novel approaches for the management of tendinopathy. J Bone Joint Surg Am 2010;92:2604–13.

Sports Nutrition Needs

Before, During, and After Exercise

Roger Zoorob, MD, MPH[a,*], Mari-Etta E. Parrish, RD, LDN, CSSD[b], Heather O'Hara, MD, MPH[a], Medhat Kalliny, MD, PhD[a]

KEYWORDS

- Sports nutrition • Protein • Hydration • Carbohydrates • Fat metabolism
- Nutrition and performance

KEY POINTS

- Maintaining proper hydration by drinking during exercise has the largest beneficial effect on performance of any single nutritional intervention.
- Sufficient hydration with water alone is fine for mild to moderate activity for less than 1 hour and does not lead to significant dehydration.
- Pre-exercise carbohydrate ingestion improves performance when carbohydrate ingestion is maintained throughout exercise and high plasma glucose concentrations maintained.
- Moderate to intense physical activity lasting longer than 1 hour may require carbohydrate or electrolyte supplementation drinks as an appropriate source of hydration.
- Replacing fluids lost through sweat is top priority for recovery. A total of 16 to 24 oz of fluid should be consumed for every 1 lb lost.

INTRODUCTION

Nutrition before, during, and after exercise can make the difference between exercise improvement and injury. It can determine if it will be the worst or best performance for an athlete. A major cause of poor performance during competition is improper nutrition.[1] The athlete's nutrition outside of these times certainly affects performance. However, even if an athlete aces their nutrition at those times, but fails to mind proper fueling needs before, during, and after exercise it can still undermine their performance. Any athlete that desires to maximize their exercise gains and competition performance must focus on proper fueling for their sport, which includes taking in the proper type and amount of nutrients before, during, and immediately after their practice or competition.

[a] Department of Family and Community Medicine, Meharry Medical College, 1005 Dr D.B. Todd Boulevard, Nashville, TN 37208, USA; [b] Baptist Sports Medicine, Sports Nutrition Liaison, 3613 Doge Court, Nashville, TN 37204, USA
* Corresponding author.
E-mail address: rzoorob@mmc.edu

Prim Care Clin Office Pract 40 (2013) 475–486
http://dx.doi.org/10.1016/j.pop.2013.02.013
primarycare.theclinics.com
0095-4543/13/$ – see front matter

FUELING BEFORE SPORT

Eating and then exercising can cause many athletes to experience stomach cramping and indigestion during sport exertion. This may lead some to think they should avoid eating before practice or very close to game time. Such a decision can inhibit stamina if their sport is long in duration and exhaustive exercise. Kirwin and colleagues[2] found that providing 75 g of moderate glycemic carbohydrate 45 minutes before exhaustive exercise lasting longer than 1 hour can improve endurance capacity by 10% to 16% compared with providing only water. It is important to begin a practice or competition with nutritional stores maximized, especially glycogen stores and hydration stores. It is well established that a lack of adequate fuel, specifically glycogen, or fluid before exercise can negatively impact performance.[3–5]

How much an athlete needs to eat and what food choices they should make when fueling before practice or a competition depend on how much time they have before commencing exercise, how much they weigh, and what type of sport they will be performing (**Table 1**). Eating or drinking too great of volume before exercise can have opposite the desired effect: gastrointestinal problems and performance impairment.[6] The less they weigh and the less time they have prior, the smaller the quantity of food and the more important that the food choice is something that digests quickly, such as juice, sport drink, fruit, or plain crackers. Choosing a liquid fuel choice especially shortens gastric emptying time and lowers the residual intestinal load, which may be beneficial for nervous athletes or athletes who need to "make weight" before completion. These food choices should be high in carbohydrate, but low in fat, fiber, and protein because the latter nutrients delay gastric emptying, increasing the chances of gastrointestinal upset and delaying availability of energy availability from carbohydrates.

Although studies conflict regarding the importance of choosing high- or low-glycemic carbohydrates before exercise, it seems that one does not provide any

Table 1
Pre-exercise fuel needs

Hours Before Exercise Start	Amount of Nutrient Required	Sample Fuel Choices (150-lb Athlete)
4	4 g CHO/kg body weight, 16–24 oz fluid	(273 g CHO) 3 oz grilled chicken, 1 C brown rice, 1 C mixed vegetables, 16 oz apple juice followed in 1.5 h with 1 large bagel with 1 Tbsp peanut butter, 1 Tbsp honey, 16 oz chocolate milk, and then 1 h later with 4 fig-filled cookies, 1 large banana, and 16 oz water
3	3 g CHO/kg body weight, 16–24 oz fluid	(205 g CHO) 6-in turkey sub sandwich, low-fat condiments, 1 oz baked chips, 1 C mixed fruit, 16 oz grape juice, 2 fig cookies
2	2 g CHO/kg body weight, 16–24 oz fluid	(136 g CHO) 1 peanut butter and jelly sandwich, 1.5 C cherries with pits, 16 oz vanilla almond milk
1	1 g CHO/kg body weight, 16–24 oz fluid	(68 g CHO) 1 large banana, 12 oz chocolate soy milk, 12 oz water
<1	30 g CHO, 8–12 oz fluid	1.5 C grapes, 12 oz water

Abbreviation: CHO, carbohydrate.

performance enhancement over the other. Febbraio and colleagues[7] studied the effect of varied glycemic pre-exercise meals on eight trained cyclists. Each of the male athletes either received a high-glycemic index meal (mashed potatoes), low-glycemic index meal (muesli), or placebo meal (diet gelatin) 30 minutes before a 120-minute cycling bout at 70% Vo_2 max. This was followed by a 30-minute performance ride where total work was recorded. This test was repeated on each cyclist on three different occasions, at least a week apart, to allow for every subject to be tested with each of the varied glycemic pre-exercise meals. Although glucose and insulin levels varied in each test group before, during, and after exercise, no differences in work output was measured during the 30-minute performance cycle. Choosing low-glycemic over high-glycemic foods before exercise may affect substrate use, but neither seems to offer a clear performance benefit over the other.

Exceptions to these guidelines include the importance of ingesting protein before strength-building exercise. Before weight lifting, a strength athlete is likely to choose more protein and less carbohydrates, but still low fiber and fat, and ample fluids. Consuming amino acids before strength training may have an anticatabolic effect.[8] However, strength athletes need very little protein to achieve this effect. As little as 6 g of amino acids, combined with 35 g carbohydrate, just before resistance exercise improves protein muscle accretion.[9,10]

A full-size meal 3 to 4 hours before exercise start is ideal, and enhances endurance capacity.[11,12] Such amount of time safely allows for full digestion and absorption of nutrients. Food choices should be high in carbohydrate, low in fiber, and low in fat. A moderate amount of lean protein is encouraged. Ample fluids should also be included (5–7 mL/kg) to promote optimal hydration.[13] The goal of the precompetition meal is not to load up with large portions and multiple plates of food. The body more easily digest small amounts of food that are ingested at various intervals over time: one plate full of food for a meal and a small snack each of the hours leading up to exercise time (eg, banana an hour after, mini sport bar 1 h before, and sport drink just before beginning). Small amounts of fluid (6–12 oz) should be included along with all snacks or meals.

FUELING DURING SPORT

Hydration

Maintaining proper hydration by drinking during exercise has the largest beneficial effect on performance of any single nutritional intervention. Dehydration compromises cardiovascular function by decreasing blood flow to muscles and cardiac output.[14] The resulting increase in heart rate causes a decrease in stroke volume. Hypovolemia hampers an athlete's thermoregulation. The more hyperthermic an athlete is, the greater their work capacity decreases.[15] Low blood volume, from dehydration, also thwarts oxygen and glucose transport to muscle cells. At just a 2% loss in body fluids, an athlete's performance is impaired.[16,17] Fatigue and performance impairment caused by dehydration can cause athletes to compromise their physical mechanics. Therefore, not only does dehydration impair performance, it indirectly raises an athlete's risk of injury and directly raises their risk for heat-related illnesses.[18] Equally important to performance and hydration is ensuring an athlete does not drink in excess of their fluid and electrolyte losses. When serum sodium levels are diluted less than 130 mEq/L, intracellular swelling occurs and alters central nervous system function. This is labeled symptomatic hyponatremia and can occur when athletes drink in excess of their fluid losses, deplete their extracellular fluid sodium by heavy sweat loss, or a combination of high fluid intake and excessive sweating. Hyperhydration has no beneficial exercise performance effects.[19] Symptomatic hyponatremia and dehydration are negatively associated with exercise performance.

To optimize sport performance and minimize risk of injury, the hydration goal for every athlete should be to match their rate of losses, specifically fluid and electrolytes.[20] When an athlete does not have access to a formal sweat test to calculate their loss of fluids and electrolytes, they can attempt to calculate their own. By weighing before and immediately after exercise, subtracting any fluids lost by urination, and by adding any fluids consumed, an athlete can guesstimate the amount of individualized sweat rate (see **Table 2** for an example of a sweat rate tracking form). Electrolyte losses cannot be as easily measured, but sodium needs still can be estimated based on these same results. Average human sweat contains 920 to 1150 mg sodium per liter.[21] Because some athletes cannot always drink as much fluid as they are losing, it is necessary to increase the amount of sodium intake, along with maximal fluid intake, until the rate of sweat loss is kept at least less than a 2% loss. If sweat loss is high, including electrolytes in fluids consumed encourages greater fluid intake, aids in maintaining plasma volume, and reduces urine production.[21] When an athlete cannot tolerate greater fluid intake, increasing the amount of sodium ingested may help encourage hydration.[22] The American Dietetic Association and the American College of Sports Medicine and Dietitians of Canada recommend the individualized approach of matching fluid intake with sweat losses, but also generally advise athletes to drink 6 to 12 oz of fluid every 15 to 20 minutes as tolerated and to include sodium.[13] In general, the greater the loss of sweat, the more fluid and electrolytes are required to achieve euhydration.

It seems that minimizing dehydration may be part of the solution to aiding athletes in avoiding gastrointestinal issues while staying fueled during exercise.[23] The gut has become known as an important athletic organ, particularly in the case of endurance athletes who must consume the most fluid and fuel while exercising. Certain adaptations occur in the stomach and intestines of well-trained athlete's that allow them to better tolerate larger volumes of fluid or fuel. The average stomach volume is 50 to 100 mL, but it can expand up to 1000 mL with no increase in abdominal pressure. If some athletes are to match their fluid intake equal to their amount of sweat lost, their ingested fluid volume may exceed the comfort of the stomach's approximately 1000 mL expansion.[24] However, the higher the fluid volume, the higher is the gastric emptying rate. The addition of glucose greatly slows the gastric emptying rate, but can increase the rate of absorption by the intestines. The gastric emptying rate is not affected by exercise at a 25% to 75% $\dot{V}O_2$ max. More intense exercise ($\dot{V}O_2$ max >80%) delays gastric emptying.[25] In well-trained athletes there is an increase in intestinal transit and capacity to absorb food and fluid. In a study of marathon runners by Carrio and colleagues,[26] 10 runners and 10 sedentary individuals of similar age and gender were fed an egg sandwich injected with an isotope marker after an 8-hour fast. Each of the subjects was measured for radioactivity retention in their stomach at three intervals of 30-minutes while at rest. The 10 runners in the group returned a week later to repeat this procedure. However, as soon as they finished consuming their egg sandwich and were initially measured for radioactivity in their stomachs, they ran 4 to 4.5 miles during a 30-minute interval. Each runner had their gastric contents measured after the interval and then repeated the run interval and test two more times (90 minutes running total with <1 minute pause for gastric testing). The runner's basal gastric emptying rates were significantly faster than the sedentary test subjects at rest and while exercising. This suggests that with practice, athletes can improve gastric motility, but further minimize their risk of dehydration and associated gastrointestinal upset.

Table 2
Sweat rate tracker

Date	Temperature Index	Type of Training	Duration in Minutes	Weight Before Start (lb)	Weight at Event End (lb)	Amount of Fluid Consumed (oz)	Amount of Fluid Lost by Urine (oz)	Amount of Sodium Consumed by Food or Fluids	Sweat Rate per Hour	Fluids Required for Rehydration

Conversion: 16 oz fluid = 1 lb.
Sweat rate calculations = (wt before − end wt) + (lb fluids consumed − lb urine loss)/(minutes of exercise/60).
Rehydration needs calculation = (wt before − end wt) × 16–24 oz.

Carbohydrate Replacement

Taking in glucose while exercising spares muscle glycogen and increases an athlete's endurance capacity. It is not necessary to consume carbohydrates unless the exercised performed is at 75% $\dot{V}O_2$ max for less than an hour or unless the exercise duration will total more than 2 hours.[27] The amount of carbohydrate needed to sustain energy stores during prolonged exercise is 30 to 60 g of carbohydrate per hour. Carbohydrate from a single source, such as glucose, can only be oxidized at rates of approximately 60 g/h. However, when more than one type of carbohydrate is ingested (eg, combination of dextrose and fructose) the oxidation rate can increase slightly to 75 to 90 g/h.[27] Athletes should attempt the higher rate of carbohydrate oxidation with caution. Large amounts of carbohydrate intake during exercise may increase the incidence of gastrointestinal symptoms because of the decreased mesenteric blood flow to the intestines during high-intensity exercise, and especially in the presence of dehydration. Exercise performance and endurance capacity may be greatly enhanced with the increased oxidation of carbohydrate when exercise duration is high (>2.5 h).[28] For most athletes, it is recommended that they aim for 30 to 60 g of carbohydrate intake from varying sources during each hour of exercise.[13] To further minimize risk of gastrointestinal distress and to minimize the risk of energy deficits, it may be helpful to divide the 30 to 60 g of carbohydrate intake into smaller amounts (eg, 10–15 g carbohydrate every 15 minutes) to be ingested throughout the hour of activity.

When exercise is expected to last more than an hour, carbohydrate replacement should begin well before glycogen stores are emptied. McConell and colleagues[29] demonstrated that waiting until late in exercise (post 90 minutes cycling) to ingest carbohydrates impairs performance, compared with providing the same amount of carbohydrates at 15-minute intervals throughout exercise. Many factors affect how quickly glycogen stores are depleted, including amount of glycogen stores before exercise commencement, how well trained the athlete is, and the intensity of the exercise.[30] Athletes can increase their glycogen storage capacity with proper supercompensation strategies (carbohydrate loading) before exercise, which prolongs the necessity of carbohydrate intake.[31] Less-trained athletes use carbohydrate at a quicker rate than well-trained athletes. The more intense (higher $\dot{V}O_2$ max required for sport performance) the exercise, the more rapidly carbohydrate stores are recruited. Because of the varying rates of carbohydrate use and glycogen storage capacities of each individual athlete, it is generally advised that for long durations or exercise, carbohydrate replacement should begin before a full hour of exercise being completed.

Practical Considerations for Achieving Nutrient Needs During Sport

Many athletes get little time during competition to pause for eating and drinking. Using a sport drink is an all inclusive way to meet the nutrient demands of an athlete during practice or competition. Sport drink can provide not only the necessary fluids and electrolytes for adequate hydration, they also supply carbohydrate. If carbohydrate is consumed in fluid form, the ideal concentration of the sport drink should be less than 6% carbohydrate.[32] During intense exercise fluid absorption in the small intestine is encouraged by including a small amount of glucose and sodium with fluid ingested. Sport drink is the fluid of choice if activity time is expected to last more than an hour. The small amount of carbohydrate in sport drinks, when consumed at adequate levels, is enough to sustain an athlete's stamina and allow them to perform at optimal capacity for their entire activity time.

For children playing a sport that lasts less than an hour, water is all they require to perform at their best. For children who engage in vigorous sports ($\dot{V}O_2$ max >75%), or a sport where nonstop play is required, or a sport that takes place in very hot and humid conditions a sport drink may be more beneficial than plain water. The American Academy of Pediatrics recently released a statement supporting water over sport drinks for most children's exercise. They highlight the fact that if conditions of sport do not necessitate the need for added carbohydrate and sodium in sport drinks, consumption of sport drinks during sport or outside of sport contribute to obesity and tooth decay in children.[33]

Athletes may be tempted to pour fluid over their body while exercising in the heat. To avoid heat stroke or other heat-related illnesses, athletes should be advised that it is more important to put water inside their body to stay cooler. Every 1% loss of body mass caused by dehydration during exercise causes a 0.27°F to 0.36°F rise in core body temperature.[34] This is especially important if exercise takes place in a humid environment, which may limit cooling of the body through evaporation.

In all types of exercise, physical work capacity, time to exhaustion, time trial performance, power output, and sport-related motor skills are improved when fluid losses are kept less than 2% of body weight and carbohydrate is also consumed.[35] When exercise is intense or will last longer than 1 hour, taking in fluid or carbohydrate independently enhances performance. If hydration and glucose replenishment are properly achieved during such exercise, performance is enhanced above the individual performance effect of each nutrient.[36] For optimal sport performance proper hydration and carbohydrate maintenance throughout exercise are necessary.

FUELING FOR RECOVERY

Part of ensuring that athletes are properly fueled for their next practice or competition is making sure they refuel depleted energy, fluid, and electrolyte stores after competition or practice. It may take 24 hours to do this.[30] Rapid repletion of muscle glycogen is especially important after exercise if an athlete must exercise more than once within a 24-hour period. The body recovers best when an athlete begins refueling as soon as they finish exercise.

Rehydration

Replacing fluids lost through sweat is top priority for recovery. It is common for athletes to remain mildly dehydrated after exercise despite their efforts to replace fluids. This can impair exercise performance in subsequent exercise. The American Dietetic Association recommends 16 to 24 oz of fluid be consumed for every 1 lb lost.[13] This is a rate of 100% to 150% of total body fluid lost. Consuming this amount of fluid over a longer period of time improves rehydration. It can take about 6 hours to reachieve proper losses during exercise.[37] Rapid rehydration does not work because of obligatory urine losses. Fluids with electrolytes are the best choice. Electrolytes, specifically sodium, are critical for preventing insensible losses by way of urine and for effectively increasing plasma volume.[38] Because urine losses seem to positively correlate with the amount of fluid ingested, but decrease as sodium consumption is increased, it is wise to liberally include sodium and extra fluid in recovery fuel choices.

In a rehydration study by Shirreffs and colleagues,[39] 12 cyclists were brought to just greater than 2% dehydration by exercise on 4 separate weeks. On each occasion, every subject was given fluids either in the amount of 50%, 100%, 150%, or 200% of body mass lost after exercise. Each week, six of the subjects received 23 mmol/L sodium in their fluid and the other six received a 61 mmol/L sodium concentration. At 7.5 hours after exercise, blood and urine samples were remeasured. Rehydration was almost achieved for the subjects in the lower sodium concentration group when they consumed either the 150% or 200% amount of fluid. A total of 91% of starting body mass was achieved with ingestion of each of those volumes, compared with only 39% recovery for the subjects that drank only 50% of lost mass, and 60% recovery for the subjects that rehydrated with 100% of mass lost. Full rehydration was achieved by subjects that received the higher sodium concentrated fluid and either the volume of 150% (107% mass recovered) or 200% (127% mass recovered) of body mass lost. Despite the higher sodium content, the subjects that only received fluid in volumes of 50% (regained 38% mass lost) or 100% (regained 81% mass lost) of mass loss did not achieve full rehydration.

An exact sodium recommendation has not been developed, but evidence is clear regarding sodium's role in encouraging plasma and total body rehydration by increased fluid intake and retention after dehydrating exercise. Because the amount of fluid needed is likely to be in excess of 16 oz, it may be helpful to choose fluids that have flavor and sodium.[40] This encourages athletes to drink more. Chilled beverages after exercise are also more generously consumed and are favorable.[13] Fluids increase blood volume and help circulate water and other nutrients needed to lower the body's core temperature quickly and return the body to homeostasis.

Refueling

When carbohydrate is supplemented immediately after exercise the rate of glycogen synthesis is increased.[41] Athletes that have continuously exercised for 90 minutes or more need 1.5 g/kg body weight of carbohydrate within 30 minutes.[42] The short window of time after exercise is ideal for glycogen resynthesis because blood flow to the muscles is still copious and there is greater insulin sensitivity. High glycemic carbohydrates in fluid or solid form are most quickly absorbed and shuttled into cells for most rapid muscle glycogen restoration.[43] Fructose is not as effective for restoring muscle glycogen immediately after exercise because it is taken by the liver for hepatic glycogen storage.[44] Athletes with shorter duration or less intense exertion do not require a formal recovery drink with as many carbohydrates.

A moderate amount of protein should be combined with the fluid, electrolytes, and carbohydrates to promote muscle protein synthesis and enhance muscle glycogen availability.[45,46] Including a small amount (0.2 g/kg) improves muscle tissue repair more effectively than carbohydrate alone.[47] Choosing protein hydrolysates may further improve muscle uptake and use of protein immediately after exercise.[48,49] Moore and colleagues[50] found that ingesting 20 g of intact protein after resistance exercise was optimal for enhancing muscle and albumin protein synthesis. Protein consumed in greater amounts than this may promote irreversible oxidation and no further increase in protein synthesis.

If an athlete can consume fluid, electrolytes, 10 to 20 g protein, and 100 to 200 g carbohydrate (or specific amount according to their body weight, sport intensity, and duration) within 30 minutes of finishing exercise, they are most likely to limit fatigue and strain on their body. Choosing a drink rich in carbohydrates and moderate in protein, such as a fruit and yogurt smoothie, or low-fat chocolate milk, is an easy way to shuttle in the necessary nutrients for recovery.

The recovery drink should be followed by a complete meal or multiple snacks and ample fluids to achieve full recovery need repletion. If an athlete has 24 hours before their next exercise session, the meal, snack, and fluid choices can be consumed a few times in large quantities or in several smaller quantities, according to what is convenient and comfortable to the athlete. If exercise must be commenced again within 8 hours, a more structured schedule is advised to optimize necessary nutrient intake.[51] Including produce in meal and snack choices is a natural way to provide antioxidants, vitamins, and minerals to aid in tissue repair and recovery. What is most important is that the total food and fluid choices provide enough carbohydrate and fluid to sufficiently restore muscle glycogen and hydration status before the athlete's next exercise session.

Practical Considerations for Eating and Drinking After Exercise

Many athletes feel entitled to eat or drink whatever they desire after what they perceive as great effort in sport. This can often lead to postexercise recovery food and fluid choices to include fatty foods along with alcoholic beverages. Athletes should be warned that choosing beverages with greater than 4% alcohol content may delay physical recovery from exercise.[52] This is especially prudent for college athletes because they have a greater propensity compared with nonathletes to engage in drinking, especially binge drinking.[53] There is no evidence that including fat as part of sport recovery enhances recovery or further sport performance. Calories consumed in the form of alcohol or fat may take away from needed calories coming from carbohydrate, which are priority for proper muscle glycogen synthesis.

Table 3
Fueling sport performance summary

	Needs Before Exercise	Needs During Exercise	Needs for Recovery After Exercise
Exercise <75% Vo_2 max or <2 h			
Timing	<1–4 h prior	As needed throughout exercise	According to convenience of athlete
Amount of nutrient required	1 g CHO/kg body wt + 16–24 oz fluid for each hour before exercise start	Water and electrolytes in the amount equal to losses	Complete meal or snack that is high in carbohydrate and contains protein and electrolytes
Strength-based exercise			
Timing	Just before exercise start	As needed throughout exercise	According to convenience of athlete
Amount of nutrient required	10–20 g protein + 35 g CHO	Water equal to amount lost during exercise	Complete meal or snack that is high in carbohydrate and contains protein
Exercise >75% Vo_2 max or >2 h			
Timing	<1–4 h prior	Within 1 h of exercise start, and then every hour following	Within 30 min of finishing
Amount of nutrient required	1 g CHO/kg body wt + 16–24 oz fluid for each hour before exercise start	30–60 g CHO/hr + fluid and sodium to match losses (or at least within 2% of fluids lost)	1.5 g CHO/kg body wt + 10–20 g protein + 100%–150% body mass lost in fluids that contain electrolytes

Abbreviation: CHO, carbohydrate.

The sport nutrition supplement industry was a $27.8 billion dollar market in 2007. Its global market growth is expected to achieve $91.8 billion by 2013 (based on a compound annual growth rate of 24.1%).[54] Athletes are lured in by the promises of the latest and greatest to help them more easily achieve their best in athletic performance. Because much of physical adaptation occurs in the recovery process in response to the exercise performed,[55] the market is rife with specially engineered recovery powders, pills, and processed foods. Research shows that such products offer no advantage over whole food choices for recovery.[56] Getting the proper nutrients, whether from engineered or natural sources, is what is important. Engineered recovery products can offer convenience, but are considerably more expensive compared with the cost of getting the same nutrients by whole food.

SUMMARY

No matter the sport, the main principal for using sports nutrition to peak athletic performance is to avoid nutrition-related deficits (**Table 3**). This includes ensuring that day-to-day energy balance is met, hydration and glycogen stores are not deficient before and during exercise, and nutrition stores are restored at a rate consistent with demands of exercise.

REFERENCES

1. Mukika I, Burke L. Nutrition in team sports. Ann Nutr Metab 2010;57(Suppl 2): 26–35.
2. Kirwan JP, O'Gorman D, Evans WJ. A moderate glycemic meal before endurance exercise can enhance performance. J Appl Phys 1998;84(1):53–9.
3. Bergstrom J, Hermansen L, Hultman E, et al. Diet, muscle glycogen and physical performance. Acta Physiol Scand 1967;71(2–3):140–50.
4. Armstong LE, Costil DL, Fink WJ. Influence of diuretic-induced dehydration on competitive running performance. Med Sci Sports Exerc 1985;17(4):456–61.
5. Barr SI. Effects of dehydration on exercise performance. Can J Appl Physiol 1999;24(2):164–72.
6. Robinson TA, Hawley JA, Palmer GS, et al. Water ingestion does not improve 1-h cycling performance in moderate ambient temperatures. Eur J Appl Physiol 1995; 71(2–3):153–60.
7. Febbraio MA, Keenan J, Angus DJ, et al. Pre-exercise carbohydrate ingestion, glucose kinetics, and muscle glycogen use: effect of the glycemic index. J Appl Phys 2000;89:1845–51.
8. Kerksick C, Harvey T, Stout J, et al. International society of sports nutrition position stand: nutrient timing. J Int Soc Sports Nutr 2008;3:5–17.
9. Tipton KD, Wolfe RR. Exercise, protein metabolism, and muscle growth. Int J Sport Nutr Exerc Metab 2001;11(1):109–32.
10. Tipton KD, Elliott TA, Cree MG, et al. Stimulation of net muscle protein synthesis by whey protein ingestion before and after exercise. Am J Physiol Endocrinol Metab 2007;292(1):E71–6.
11. Hargreaves M, Hawley JA, Jeukendrup A. Pre-exercise carbohydrate and fat ingestion: effects on metabolism and performance. J Sports Sci 2004;22(1):31–8.
12. Hawley JA, Burke LM. Effect of meal frequency and timing on physical performance. Br J Nutr 1997;77(Suppl 1):S91–103.
13. Rodriguez NR, DiMarco NM, Langley S. Position of the American Dietetic Association, Dietitians of Canada, and the American College of Sports Medicine: nutrition and athletic performance. J Am Diet Assoc 2009;109:509–27.

14. Gonsalez-Alonso J, Calbet JA, Nielsen B. Muscle blood flow is reduced with dehydration during prolonged exercise in humans. J Physiol 1998;513(3):895–905.
15. Sawka MN. Physiological consequences of hypohydration: exercise performance and thermoregulation. Med Sci Sports Exerc 1992;24(6):657–70.
16. Maughen RJ. Impact of mild dehydration on wellness and on exercise performance. Eur J Clin Nutr 2003;57(Suppl 2):S19–23.
17. Shirreffs SM. The importance of good hydration for work and exercise performance. Nutr Rev 2005;63(Supppl 1):S14–21.
18. Bouchama A, Knochel JP. Heat stroke. N Engl J Med 2002;346:1978–88.
19. Sawka MN, Montain SJ, Latzka WA. Hydration effects on thermoregulation and performance in the heat. Comp Biochem Physiol A Mol Integr Physiol 2001; 128(4):679–90.
20. Convertino VA, Armstong LE, Coyle EF, et al. American College of Sports Medicine position stand. Exercise and fluid replacement. Med Sci Sports Exerc 1996;28(1):1–7.
21. Murray B. Hydration and physical performance. J Am Coll Nutr 2007;26(Suppl 5): s542–8.
22. Sanders B, Noakes TD, Dennis SC. Sodium replacement and fluid shifts during prolonged exercise in humans. Eur J Appl Physiol 2001;84(5):419–25.
23. Moses FM. Exercise-associated Intestinal Ischemia. Curr Sports Med Rep 2005; 4(2):91–5.
24. Geliebter A. Gastric distension and gastric capacity in relation to food intake in humans. Physiol Behav 1988;44(4–5):665–8.
25. Gisolfi CV. Is the GI system built for exercise? News Physiol Sci 2000;15(3):114–9.
26. Carrio I, Estorch M, Serra-Grima R, et al. Gastric emptying in marathon runners. Gut 1989;30:152–5.
27. Jeukendrup AE. Carbohydrate intake during exercise and performance. Nutrition 2004;20(7):669–77.
28. Burke LM, Hawley JA, Wong SH, et al. Carbohydrates for training and competition. J Sports Sci 2011;29(Suppl 1):s17–27.
29. McConell G, Klkoot K, Hargreaves M. Effect of timing of carbohydrate ingestion on endurance exercise performance. Med Sci Sports Exerc 1996;28(10):1300–4.
30. Coyle EF. Substrate utilization during exercise in active people. Am J Clin Nutr 1995;61(4):s968–79.
31. Karlsson J, Saltin B. Diet, muscle glycogen, and endurance performance. J Appl Phys 1971;31(2):203–6.
32. Ryan AJ, Lambert GP, Shi X, et al. Effect of hypohydration on gastric emptying and intestinal absorption during exercise. J Appl Phys 1998;84(5):1581–8.
33. American Academy of Pediatrics. Clinical report-sports drinks and energy drinks for children and adolescents: are they appropriate? Pediatrics 2011. http://dx.doi.org/10.1542/peds.2011-0965. Web Accessed July 28, 2012.
34. Coris EE, Ramirez AM, Van Durme DJ. Heat illness in athletes: the dangerous combination of heat, humidity and exercise. Sports Med 2004;34(1):9–16.
35. Casa DJ, Clarkson PM, Roberts WO. American College of Sports Medicine roundtable on hydration and physical activity: consensus statements. Curr Sports Med Rep 2005;4:115–27.
36. Below PR, Mora-Rodriguez R, Gonzalez-Alonso J, et al. Fluid and carbohydrate ingestion independently improve performance during 1 hour of intense exercise. Med Sci Sports Exerc 1995;27(2):200–10.
37. Kovacs EM, Schmahl RM, Senden JM, et al. Effect of high and low rates of fluid intake on post-exercise rehydration. Int J Sport Nutr Exerc Metab 2002;12(1):14–23.

38. Burke LM. Nutrition for post-exercise recovery. Aust J Sci Med Sport 1997;29(1): 3–10.
39. Shirreffs SM, Taylor AJ, Leiper JB, et al. Post-exercise rehydration in man: effects of volume consumed and drink sodium content. Med Sci Sports Exerc 1996; 28(10):1260–71.
40. Clapp AJ, Bishop PA, Smith JF, et al. Effects of carbohydrate-electrolyte content of beverages on voluntary hydration in simulated industrial environment. Am Ind Hyg Assoc J 2000;61(5):692–9.
41. Ivy JL, Katz AL, Cutler CL, et al. Muscle glycogen synthesis after exercise: effect of time of carbohydrate ingestion. J Appl Phys 1988;64(4):1480–5.
42. Ivy JL, Lee MC, Brozinick JT Jr, et al. Muscle glycogen storage after different amounts of carbohydrate ingestion. J Appl Phys 1988;65(5):2018–23.
43. Burke LM, Collier GR, Hargreaves M. Muscle glycogen storage after prolonged exercise: effect of the glycemic index of carbohydrate feedings. J Appl Phys 1993;75(2):1019–23.
44. Blom PC, Hostmark AT, Vaage O, et al. Effect of different post-exercise sugar diets on the rate of muscle glycogen synthesis. Med Sci Sports Exerc 1987;19(5): 491–6.
45. Zawadski KM, Yaspelkis BB III, Ivy JL. Carbohydrate-protein complex increases the rate of muscle glycogen storage after exercise. J Appl Phys 1992;72(5): 1854–9.
46. Ivy JL, Goforth HW Jr, Damon BM, et al. Early postexercise muscle glycogen recovery is enhanced with a carbohydrate-protein supplement. J Appl Phys 2002; 93(4):1337–44.
47. Ivy JL. Regulation of muscle glycogen repletion, muscle protein synthesis and repair following exercise. J Sports Sci Med 2004;3:131–8.
48. Manninen AH. Protein hydrolysates in sports and exercise: a brief review. J Sports Sci Med 2004;3:60–3.
49. Van Loon LJ, Saris WH, Kruijshoop M, et al. Maximizing postexercise muscle glycogen synthesis: carbohydrate supplementation and the application of amino acid or protein hydrolysate mixtures. Am J Clin Nutr 2000;72(1):106–11.
50. Moore DR, Robinson MJ, Fry JL, et al. Ingested protein dose response of muscle and albumin protein synthesis after resistance exercise in young men. Am J Clin Nutr 2009;89:161–8.
51. Burke LM, Kiens B, Ivy JL. Carbohydrates and fat for training and recovery. J Sports Sci 2004;22(1):15–30.
52. Shirreffs SM, Maughan RJ. Restoration of fluid balance after exercise-induced dehydration: effects of alcohol consumption. J Appl Phys 1997;83(4):1152–8.
53. Nelson TF, Wechsler H. Alcohol and college athletes. Med Sci Sports Exerc 2001; 33(1):43–7.
54. BCC Research Market Forecasting. Sports Nutrition and High Energy Supplements: the Global Market. Sept. 2008. Report Code: FOD043A. Available at: http://www.bccresearch.com/report/sports-nutrition-energy-supplements-fod043a.html. Accessed July 30, 2012.
55. Hawley JA, Tipton KD, Millard-Stafford ML. Promoting training adaptations through nutritional interventions. J Sports Sci 2006;24(7):709–21.
56. Cockburn E, Hayes PR, French DN, et al. Acute milk-based protein-cho supplementation attenuates exercise-induced muscle damage. Appl Physiol Nutr Metab 2008;33(4):775–83.

Nutritional Supplements and Ergogenic Aids

David G. Liddle, MD[a,b,*], Douglas J. Connor, MD[a]

KEYWORDS

- Nutritional supplements • Ergogenic aids • Performance enhancing drugs
- Anabolic steroids • Stimulants • Masking agents • Creatine • Stimulants

KEY POINTS

- Androgenic anabolic steroids increase muscle strength, muscle size, and lean body mass. They are also illegal and 99% of users report adverse side effects, some which are permanent and/or life threatening.
- Human growth hormone can affect body composition but there is no evidence that it increases strength, endurance, power, or workload capacity.
- Blood doping and erythropoietin increase endurance and $V_{O_{2Max}}$ but carry significant risk for cardiovascular complications and infectious diseases. These methods offer no performance benefit in power and anaerobic sports.
- Amphetamines and caffeine are stimulants that increase alertness, improve focus, decrease reaction time, and delay fatigue, allowing for an increased intensity and duration of training. Both are increasingly prevalent in sports while being associated with serious health risks and possible impairing performance.
- Creatine increases total and lean body mass and improves performance in repeated bouts of high-intensity exercise. There is no clear performance benefit on a single bout of exercise or event. It seems to be safe in previously healthy athletes when following the currently described dosing regimens.

INTRODUCTION AND OVERVIEW

In the so-called age of performance-enhancing drugs, there are both increasing pressures to compete and increasing means, both legal and illegal, by which athletes try to obtain a competitive edge (**Table 1**). Nutritional supplements and ergogenic aids have

[a] Department of Orthopedics and Rehabilitation, Vanderbilt Sports Medicine, Vanderbilt University Medical Center, 1215 21st Avenue South, 3200 MCE South Tower, Nashville, TN 37232, USA; [b] Department of Internal Medicine, Vanderbilt Sports Medicine, Vanderbilt University Medical Center, 1215 21st Avenue South, 3200 MCE South Tower, Nashville, TN 37232, USA
* Corresponding author. Department of Orthopedics and Rehabilitation, Vanderbilt University Medical Center, Vanderbilt Sports Medicine, 1215 21st Avenue South, 3200 MCE South Tower, Nashville, TN 37232.
E-mail address: david.g.liddle@vanderbilt.edu

Prim Care Clin Office Pract 40 (2013) 487–505
http://dx.doi.org/10.1016/j.pop.2013.02.009 primarycare.theclinics.com
0095-4543/13/$ – see front matter

Table 1
Usage and perceived benefits of nutritional supplements

What		Why	
Sport drinks	Protein	Improved performance	Health benefit
Energy drinks	Creatine	Energy boost	Parental support
Vitamins/minerals	Guarana	Improved immunity	Compensate for diet
Herbs	Coenzyme Q10	Illness prevention	Taste

Data from O'Dea JA. Consumption of nutritional supplements among adolescents: usage and perceived benefits. Health Educ Res 2003;18(1):98–107.

been used for centuries and are becoming ever more sophisticated and supported by science. Regardless of the level of athletes one cares for, these following general facts are important:

- Athletes of all ages and competition levels may use supplements and other substances for a variety of reasons.
- Improved sports performance is the most common motivation for use.[1,2]
- Male athletes are more likely that female athletes to use steroids and legal substances, but abuse occurs in both genders.[3]
- Purity and quality assurance of these substances are not regulated.
- Little evidence is available to evaluate the efficacy and safety of these substances at the doses and regimens that are actually used by athletes.
- Few studies provide long-term data on their use, effectiveness, and side effects.
- High-school sports participation increases the likelihood of supplement use, which, in turn, increases the likelihood of steroid use.[3]
- There are no data regarding the effects of supplements on children or adolescents.
- Forty percent to 65% of users list their coaches as the main influence of their use.[1,4]
- Greater knowledge of supplements and ergogenic aids can decrease use.[5]

SUPPLEMENTS AND ERGOGENIC AIDS

Anabolic-Androgenic Steroids

Overview

The use of androgenic anabolic steroids (AAS) has become a hot topic not only in sports medicine but also in the mainstream media. The use of AAS has left indelible images in our society from US congressional hearings to Olympic controversies. Initial accounts of AAS use in the Olympics have been traced back to the 1950s by Soviet weightlifters, who were alleged to have used testosterone to enhance their performance. The mentality is echoed in comments from 1956 Olympic hammer-throw Gold medalist Harold Connally, "any athlete should take any steps necessary, short of killing himself, to maximize his performance."[6] The use of testosterone and its derivatives has become a $400 million business with more than 100 different products available on the black market. In 1990, the US Congress passed the Anabolic Steroid Control Act, which makes the possession of AAS without a prescription punishable by law. The act was amended in 2004 to include prohormones and, currently, a bill has been proposed to expand the definition to designer steroids.

Multiple estimates on the extent of use exist, but likely underestimate the true incidence and prevalence. The first estimates of AAS use from the National Household

Survey on Drug Abuse suggested that at least one million people had used anabolic steroids in their lifetime with a prevalence of about 0.9% of men and 0.1% of women.[7] The 2011, estimates from *Monitoring the Future, National Results on Adolescent Drug Use* (**Table 2**) suggest a decline in the use of AAS among high-school students.[8] Surveys indicate that the use among National Collegiate Athletic Association (NCAA) athletes is approximately 5% to 14%.[9] The highest estimated use in the scientific literature is among recreational bodybuilders, who use AAS for both strength gain and cosmetic appearance. An interview of 500 Chicago gym members in 1984 revealed 44% admitted to using steroids at some time in their life.[10]

- A few themes span AAS steroid epidemiologic data: men are more likely to use anabolic steroids than women; higher levels of competition seem to have higher rates, and men bodybuilders are at highest risk
- The use of anabolic steroids is associated with current or past dependence on other illicit substances, like cocaine, heroin, and opioids.[11]

Preparations and dosages

Multiple preparations of AAS have been developed and new forms are made to avoid detection by screening and provide different means of administration. Testosterone is the classic endogenous anabolic steroid, whereas, recently, prohormones such as dehydroepiandrosterone and androstenedione are becoming more popular. Designer steroids, synthetic molecules that mimic prohormone physiologically, are nearly impossible to regulate because they are constantly evolving and have gained popularity in the past several years.

The modes of AAS administration that are currently available are oral, injectable, and transdermal. Transdermal forms have been used for many years in the treatment of hypogonadism. Oral forms are typically 17-α-alkyl derivatives, which are relatively resistant to hepatic degradation. The injectable agents are the most commonly abused form in sports. They have undergone esterification of the 17-β-hydroxy group to make them more soluble in lipids, leading to a slower release of the steroid into circulation. The doses used by athletes are reported to be 5 to 20 times the therapeutic dose, sometimes even higher. Furthermore, athletes who use AAS often use multiple other drugs for performance enhancement.[11] Complex dosing regimens are used, which are called "stacking" and "cycling." Cycling involves gradually increasing the dose over several weeks with subsequent tapering; most cycles last 8 to 12 weeks. Longer cycles are purported to have better gains but more risk of side effects. Stacking involves the use of other substances thought to enhance the AAS, such as aromatase inhibitors, estrogen receptor modulators, and peptide hormones. If an athlete requires hormone replacement, the treating physician should have expertise in the management of the condition with an ultimate goal of care being restoration of the normal endocrine physiology. Dosing can vary widely between individuals.

Table 2
Monitoring the future: National results on adolescent drug use 2011. Lifetime Prevalence of Anabolic Steroid Use Among High School Males

Grade Level	2001	2005	2011
8th	2.8%	1.7%	1.2%
10th	3.5%	2.0%	1.4%
12th	3.7%	2.6%	1.8%

Physiologic and performance effects

The primary benefits of AAS for performance enhancement are related to increased muscle strength, increased muscle size, and increased lean body mass.

- Multiple studies have shown that AAS will increase muscle size and strength in a dose-dependent relationship and independent of an exercise program.[12]
- Muscle size increase is typically found in the neck, thorax, shoulders, and upper arms. Size increase is due to muscle hypertrophy and formation of new muscle fibers.[13]
- Many athletes perceive faster recovery times after training. Indirect evidence has shown heart rate and lactate levels return to baseline faster with AAS.[14]

Adverse effects

- Ninety percent of users had at least one patient report side effects of acne, testicular atrophy, gynecomastia, cutaneous striae, or injection site pain (**Table 3**).[15]
- Life-threatening side effects include cardiovascular disease with impaired diastolic filling and arrhythmias, stroke, blood clots, and liver dysfunction or cancer.
- Perioperative planning for known or suspected steroid users requires special consideration because they are theoretically at an increased risk for postoperative complications. Expert opinion has suggested that preoperative workup should include an electrocardiogram, complete blood count, comprehensive metabolic panel, and a high index of suspicion for other illicit substances.[9]

Testing

- Screening: Urine immunoassay to determine testosterone:epitestosterone ratio. Epitestosterone is a minor metabolite and therefore its concentration does not increase with exogenous steroid use, leading to an elevated ratio.[16]
- Most ratios are less than 2:1; the World Anti-Doping Agency (WADA) has set the upper limit at 6:1.
- More recently, gas and liquid chromatography has led to the identification of specific chemical compounds and is used to identify newer designer steroids.

Peptide Hormones and Growth Factors

Human growth hormone

Overview Human growth hormone (HGH) is one of the hormones regulating human growth. It is secreted from the somatotrope cells of the anterior pituitary. In turn, it

Table 3
Adverse effects from anabolic androgenic steroid use

Self-Reported	Reproductive	Cardiovascular	Psychiatric	Hepatic
Acne	Testicular atrophy	Elevated blood pressure	Depression	Cholestasis
Increased body hair	Gynecomastia	Arrhythmia	Irritability and hostility	Impaired liver function
Male pattern baldness	Infertility	Atherogenesis, stroke, and pulmonary embolism	Muscle dysmorphism	Liver cancer
Fluid retention	Clitoromegaly	Cardiomyopathy	Insomnia	

Data from Hartgens F, Kuipers H. Effects of androgenic-anabolic steroids in athletes. Sports Med 2004;37(8):513–54.

stimulates release of insulinlike growth factor-1. These hormones cause a net increase in lipolysis and protein anabolism.[17] Exercise stimulates the release of growth hormone.[18] When endogenous growth hormone levels are too high and unregulated, acromegaly occurs, causing increased height, body weight, muscle mass, and bone mass, especially in the hands, feet, jaw, and skull. HGH is increasing in popularity as an ergogenic aid, including popularity among adolescents, where one study found that 5% of teens reported using HGH.[19] It is often used in combination with AAS as a means of "stacking" multiple ergogenic aids. Its use as an ergogenic aid began in the 1980s and has remained popular due, in part, to a lack of reliable tests for detection of use.[17]

Preparations and dosages

- Recombinant HGH (injectable)[17]
- Cadaveric HGH (injectable), which is available in Europe and on the black market.
  - Root cause of some cases of Creutzfeldt-Jacob disease
- HGH secretagogues, used to increase endogenous growth hormone production, are available as the injectable subcutaneous peptides hexarelin and ipamorelin. Oral forms (MK-0677 and NNC 26-0703) are in development.[20]

Physiologic and performance effects Athletes use HGH because it is thought that it will improve healing and increase muscle mass, muscle strength, and body size.[17] Data support that HGH does the following[21]:

- Increases lean body mass but not body weight or fat mass
- Increases basal metabolic rate
- Increases heart rate
- Shows no benefit in exercising respiratory exchange ratio or energy expenditure, bicycling speed, power output, or Vo_{2Max}
- Changes body composition but no performance benefit
- Shows no benefit in muscle strength, power, or workload capacity[18,22]

Use of HGH continues despite a lack of published research. Like many substances discussed in this article, HGH is studied at different doses than athletes use when they are looking for a performance advantage.

Adverse effects are listed in (**Table 4**).

Erythropoiesis stimulating agents and blood doping

Overview Blood doping was first, or at least most famously, discovered in competitive athletics in the 1976 Olympics in Montreal, Canada.[23] The rationale for this practice is a byproduct of the improved performance of athletes who live at high altitudes

Table 4
Adverse effects of human growth hormone use

Soft tissue edema	Irreversible facial, jaw, and skull bone growth	Impaired glucose tolerance and diabetes mellitus
Fatigue	Coarsened facial features	Hyperlipidemia
Arthralgias	Carpal tunnel syndrome	Cardiomyopathy
Muscle weakness	Erectile dysfunction	Death

Data from Stacy JJ, Terrell TR, Armsey TD. Ergogenic aids: human growth hormone. Curr Sports Med Rep 2004;3(4):229–233; and Pipe A. Effects of growth hormone on athletic performance: a review. Clin J Sport Med 2009;19(1):75–6.

and train at low altitudes. The lower oxygen tension of their environment stimulates erythropoiesis and increases their red blood cell mass and therefore their oxygen-carrying capacity.

Autologous blood doping is accomplished by first removing usually 2 units of blood. The blood is then stored at −80°C. This relative anemia stimulates the body to produce enough red blood cells to return to a normal level. The stored blood is then thawed and re-infused 1 week before the event. Homologous matched blood from other donors can also be used in a similar fashion.[24] The postinfusion hemoglobin should be less than 17 g/dL and the hematocrit should be less than 50%; otherwise, hyperviscosity can occur, which can result in decreased blood flow velocity as well as the other adverse effects noted in later discussion.[25]

Epothropoietin (EPO) is a hormone that is produced by the kidney that stimulates red blood cell production in the bone marrow. Recombinant human erythropoietin has a half-life of 20 hours when given subcutaneously but the red blood cell production that results continues for about 2 weeks. It is used medically to treat anemia that results from renal disease.[26] Athletes started using EPO to get the benefits of increased red blood cell mass without the complications and challenges of blood doping. Currently, there is no method to directly test for the use of exogenous EPO that is readily available or used consistently, which also makes this substance attractive to some athletes.

Physiologic and performance effects

- Increased red blood cell mass, hemoglobin, hematocrit, and, therefore, oxygen-carrying capacity
- Increased Vo_{2Max} and endurance[27]
- There are no data to support its use in power and anaerobic sports.
- There is no clear and predictable relationship between the level of rise in hemoglobin/hematocrit and improvement in Vo_{2Max}, aerobic capacity, and endurance performance, which suggests that although cardiac output and oxygen delivery can be increased, there may limits at the muscle level on oxygen use.[27]
- Current evidence does not support the logic that use of EPO is as effective as blood doping[25]

Adverse effects

- Complications of hyperviscosity include decreased cardiac output, intravascular thrombosis, heart failure, cerebrovascular and myocardial ischemia, pulmonary embolism, deep vein thrombosis, and death.
- Other complications include infection, phlebitis, septicemia, and transfusion-associated lung injury. Mismatched blood types with homologous doping can be further complicated by hemolytic reactions, renal failure, allergic reactions, and contracted blood-borne illnesses, including hepatitis C virus, hepatitis B virus, malaria, cytomegalovirus, and human immunodeficiency virus.[28]
- Decreased training and exercise capacity during the period between removal of blood and reestablishing normal red blood cell levels, and re-infusion of blood in autologous blood doping.[27]
- Re-infusion of blood that contains previously used banned substances that had been stopped to avoid detection and the increased blood levels are both potential means by which athletes that are doping and cheating may be discovered.[27]

Hormones and metabolic modulators

AAS are the most frequently abused drug in sports and testing is now better able to detect these agents, which have led to newer methods of androgenic doping. The endogenous production of testosterone is tightly regulated by the hypothalamus-pituitary-gonadal axis via negative feedback through the concentration of testosterone and estrogen. Indirect androgen doping takes advantage of this system to increase endogenous testosterone production.[29]

- Growth hormones, gonadotropins, metabolic modulators, and anti-estrogenic substances all can be classified under the concept of indirect doping and are banned.
- Chorionic gonadotropin and luteinizing hormones ultimately stimulate Leydig cells to increase the production of testosterone.[29]
- Estrogen receptor blockers and anti-estrogenic substances work by causing a false sense of low estrogen levels, which in turn is a potent stimulant of gonadotropin release.[29]

The extent of gonadotropin and anti-estrogenic substance use is currently unknown. Multiple studies on anabolic androgenic steroids have shown that many users combine multiple substances including chorionic gonadotropin/luteinizing hormone and estrogen blockade. No scientific evidence exists that gonadotropins or anti-estrogenic substances actually have benefits on exercise or performance, but biologically plausible evidence of elevated testosterone levels has led to WADA prohibiting these substances.

Special consideration for testing must be considered. Screening for human chorionic gonadotropin is not performed in women as this invades health privacy for possible pregnancy or recent miscarriage and no evidence exists for performance enhancement in women. Furthermore, a man who tests positive must be evaluated for testicular cancer, as this will cause elevated human chorionic gonadotropin levels.

Diuretics

The use of diuretics in sports has 2 following major functions: rapid weight loss and masking illegal substances. Diuretics were first banned in 1988 and remain on the in-competition and out-of-competition prohibited substance list. Athletes who participate in sports with weight categories have used diuretics to reduce body weight transiently to compete at lower weight classes, whereas athletes using a banned substance will attempt to dilute their urine, making detection more difficult.

- In 2010, diuretics and masking agents represented 7% of all adverse analytical findings reported by WADA laboratories.
- Diuretics were the second most commonly used nonprescription weight-loss product reported by Division I female athletes, who cited appearance enhancement as the number 1 reason for use.[30]

Diuretics work by increasing the volume of urinary water excretion through multiple mechanisms in the kidneys. The classes of diuretics used are thiazides, loops, carbonic anhydrase inhibitors, and mineralocorticoid receptor antagonists, with thiazides and loops accounting for nearly 70% of WADA positive tests. Special consideration must be taken for acetazolamide because it is the preferred medication for prophylaxis and treatment of acute altitude sickness.

- Diuretics may lead to dehydration, fatigue, electrolyte imbalances, and increased susceptibility to heat illness.
- No data exist to suggest that diuretics by themselves enhance performance and are most likely to impact exercise tolerance negatively.

Plasma volume expanders and intravenous fluid hyperhydration

Dehydration is a common problem encountered during training as well as competition. To combat this issue, athletes are recommended to maintain euhydration. The use of plasma volume expanders, such as glycerol and intravenous albumin, dextran, hydroxyethyl starch, and mannitol, is banned by WADA under the section of masking agents. No studies are currently available regarding the extent of use of volume expanders, but, in 2010, WADA reported 7 adverse analytical findings of hydroxyethyl starch.

A study on the prevalence of intravenous fluid (IVF) hyperhydration before National Football League football games recently found that 75% of National Football League teams used a pregame IVF in an average of 5 to 7 athletes. Although not a prohibited practice, half of the trainers reported a history of complications, including air emboli, pulmonary edema, arterial stick, provider needle stick, peripheral edema, and player dependence on IVF before games, raising a question of player safety when no benefit of intravenous over oral hydration or rehydration has been consistently found in the literature.[31]

The method in which athletes hydrate before, during, and after exercise has been studied extensively. The American College of Sports Medicine published a position statement on exercise and fluid replacement in 2007 with recommendations including the following[32]:

- Body weight changes can be used to calculate fluid replacement needs.
- Dehydration increases physiologic strain and perceived effort, resulting in degraded aerobic exercise performance, especially in warm to hot weather.
- Hyperhydration can be achieved by several methods, but provides equivocal benefits and has several disadvantages.
- Gylcerol is the most extensively studied plasma volume expander. A recent systematic review reported that most studies did not find a significant advantage in performance enhancement and that the documented benefits to exercise performance are inconsistent in the current scientific literature.[33]

β-blockers

Overview β-Blockers are a class of drugs that acts as β-agonist receptor inhibitors. β-Receptors are part of the autonomic nervous system and are common in the cardiac, vascular, and pulmonary tissues as well as skeletal muscles. The 2 main types of β-receptors are β_1 and β_2. β_1-Receptors are mainly found in cardiac muscle but also in the stomach and kidneys. β_2-Receptors are more widespread but are found in the bronchi and bronchioles, skeletal muscle and its arterioles, adipose tissue, gastrointestinal tract and salivary gland smooth muscle, and solid organs like the brain, liver, kidneys, and pancreas. When stimulated by the binding of the catecholamines, epinephrine and norepinephrine, these receptors trigger several downstream effects.

Cardiovascular effects include increases in heart rate, mean arterial pressure, and cardiac contractility as well as muscle bed vasodilation and splanchnic vasoconstriction. Increases in respiratory rate, tidal volume, and minute ventilation as well as bronchodilation also occur. Other effects include pupillary dilation, increasing body temperature, perspiration, glycogenolysis, gluconeogenesis, lipolysis, and insulin secretion. Nervous system effects include alertness, focus, euphoria, anxiety, irritability, and tremors. Adverse effects include dyspepsia, nausea, cardiac arrhythmias, palpitations, and bronchospasm.

β-Blockers serve to inhibit all of the physiologic responses listed above to β-stimulation. In medicine, these drugs are used commonly in cardiac and neurologic conditions, including acute myocardial infarction, heart failure, hypertension, and essential tremor. In sports, athletes whose sport requires control of anxiety and tremors, like archery, shooting, gymnastics, racing, and golf, use these drugs to control performance anxiety. In 2010, the WADA banned the use of β-blockers for these and all Olympic sports.

Preparations and dosages

- Selective β-blockers bind to β_1-receptors but not β_2-receptors
  - Includes atenolol, bisoprolol, metoprolol, and esmolol
- Nonselective β-blockers bind to both β_1-receptors and β_2-receptors
  - Includes labetalol, sotalol, propranolol, timilol, and carvedilol

Physiologic and performance effects

- Decreased anxiety and tremor
  - May have greater benefit to participants with less experience[34]

Adverse effects Significant interactions with antidepressants, oral diabetes medications, β-agonists, and other classes of antihypertensives also occur (**Table 5**).

Stimulants

Amphetamines

Overview Amphetamines are sympathomimetic drugs that have been used by athletes to increase alertness, delay fatigue, and provide a feeling of aggressiveness or well-being. They were first synthesized in the 1920s during the World War to combat fatigue in soldiers. More recently, amphetamines have been successful in the treatment of attention deficit-hyperactivity disorder (ADHD). The benefits in ADHD are many, but this has led to increased availability and abuse in sports. Major League Baseball has historically been associated with amphetamine abuse with informal player polls estimating more than half of current or past teammates having regularly used them.[16] This amphetamine abuse led to Major League Baseball banning amphetamines in 2005.

- Since 1993, the NCAA has surveyed student athletes regarding substance abuse. Unfortunately, the incidence of amphetamine use has risen in all 3 NCAA divisions (**Fig. 1**). The primary source of amphetamines seems to be from friends or relatives.[35]
- Stimulants represented 10% of WADA's adverse analytical findings in 2010, which is up from 6.4% in 2009. Stimulants have been the second most common reason for a positive test the past 3 years.

Table 5
Adverse effects of β-blocker use

Decreased performance in aerobic and anaerobic sport	Fluid retention, especially in extremities	Impaired glucose tolerance and poor glucose control
Psychomotor slowing	Heart failure	Fatigue and drowsiness
Bradycardia	Heart block	Dry mouth and eyes
Hypotension	Erectile dysfunction	Dizziness
Shortness of breath	Peripheral arterial disease	Weight gain

Data from Jonas AP, Sickles RT, Lombardo JA. Substance abuse. Clin Sports Med 1992;11:379–401.

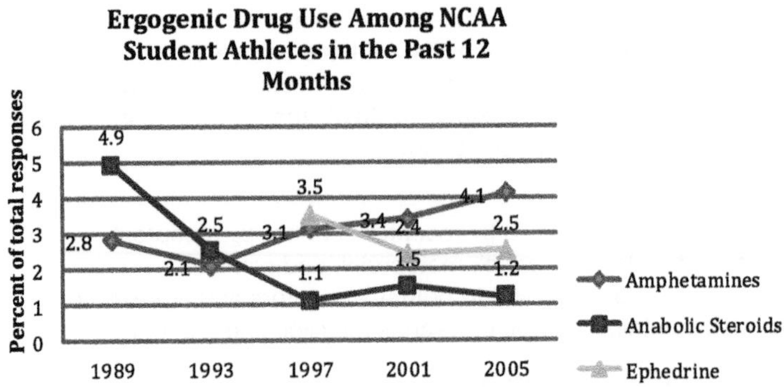

Fig. 1. Ergogenic drug abuse among college athletes.

Therapeutic use exemptions Therapeutic use exemptions (TUE) exist for the treatment of ADHD. Current estimates of the prevalence of ADHD are between 4% and 10% of children aged 5 to 18. Treating physicians are expected to make a clinical diagnosis of ADHD based on Diagnostic and Statistical Manual of Mental Disorders-IV criteria and use appropriate standardized rating scales (Conners, Adult ADHD Self-Report Scale [AASRS], Barkley Adult ADHD Rating Scale-IV [BAARS-IV], and others) before treatment with stimulant medications (**Table 6**) can be prescribed if an athlete is to qualify for a medical exemption.[36] After an appropriate diagnosis is made, the TUE may be granted for amphetamines (or any other banned substance or method) only if all of the following criteria met[37]:

- The athlete would experience significant impairment if the substance or method were withheld.
- The use of the substance or method would produce no additional enhancement of performance other than to return the athlete to a state of normal health.
- There is no reasonable alternative.
- The necessity of use cannot be a consequence of prior use without a TUE.

Once an exemption has been granted, proper documentation is critical. For example, the NCAA requires that institutions maintain records from the prescribing physician including the medical history, diagnosis, verification of standardized assessment forms and procedures, and dosing information in the student-athlete's on-campus medical records.[38]

Physiologic and performance effects

- Amphetamines increase dopamine/norepinephrine release and inhibit their reuptake, leading to central nervous system (CNS) stimulation
- Amphetamines seem to enhance athletic performance in anaerobic conditions[39,40]

Table 6
Prescription stimulants: Schedule II controlled substances

Amphetamine	Methamphetamine	Methylphenidate
• Dexedrine • Adderall • Procentra	• Desoxyn	• Ritalin • Concerta • Focalin • Methylin

- Improved reaction time
- Increased muscle strength and delayed muscle fatigue
- Increased acceleration
- Increased alertness and attention to task

Adverse effects

- Multiple side effects are associated with stimulant use[39,40]
  - Serious adverse reactions: Impaired heat tolerance, cardiac arrhythmias, dyskinesia, seizures, hallucinations, and tolerance leading to dependence/abuse
  - Common side effects: Restlessness, agitation, gastrointestinal upset and nausea, headaches, rebound fatigue

Testing

- Quantitative tests are able to detect the presence of amphetamines in urine and are used to screen for prohibited use.[19]

Caffeine

Overview Caffeine is a CNS stimulant that is readily available in a variety of forms, including coffee, tea, colas, soft drinks, energy drinks, tablets, and capsules, as well as many sports supplements (**Table 7**). For performance enhancement, the most often used dose is 6 mg/kg (ie, 420 mg for a 70-kg adult) 1 hour before an event.[41] However, there is no clear dose-response relationship and likely a plateau effect at 3 mg/kg (or 200 mg).[42–44]

Physiologic and performance effects

- Increases exercise capacity[45]
  - Delays fatigue by increasing use of fatty acids and thereby sparing body glycogen reserves
  - Increased translocation of Ca^{2+}, increasing its availability for muscle contraction and cation signaling

Table 7
Caffeine content in common foods, drinks, and over-the-counter drugs

Fixx Energy Drink	400 mg/16 oz.	Espresso	107 mg/16 oz.
Starbucks Breakfast Blend Coffee	327 mg/16 oz.	No Doz (Australia)	100 mg/1 Tab
Nos Energy Drink	260 mg/16 oz.	Mountain Dew	72 mg/16 oz.
Full Throttle Energy Drink	200 mg/16 oz.	Coca-Cola	62 mg/16 oz.
No Doz (USA) & Vivarin	200 mg/1 Tab	Dark chocolate	55 mg/2 oz. piece
Ammo Energy Shot	170 mg/1 oz.	Dr. Pepper	53 mg/16 oz.
Starbucks iced coffee	165 mg/16 oz.	Pepsi	48 mg/16 oz.
Brewed coffee	160 mg/16 oz.	Jolt Gum	33 mg/1 stick
Red Bull, Monster, Amp, Rock Star, and Jolt drinks	160 mg/16 oz.	PowerBar sports gel	25 mg/16 oz.
Instant coffee	120 mg/16 oz.	Tea	20–100/16 oz.
Frappuccino	114 mg/16 oz.		

16 oz. = 473 mL; 8 oz. = 250 mL; 1 oz. = 30 mL.
Data from Burke LM. Caffeine and sports performance. Appl Physiol Nutr Metab 2008;33:1319–34.

- Increases cyclic adenosine monophosphates by inhibition of phosphodiesterase
- Stimulates release and activity of adrenaline
- Alters to CNS affecting perception of effort and fatigue

- Increases alertness by blocking adenosine receptors
- Effective for a wide range of exercise types and durations[41,46]
- Unclear effects on a single exercise bout, especially events of short duration (seconds) or primarily dependent on strength or power[46]
- Unclear whether superior performance and mood represent direct net benefits or are due to reversal of adverse withdrawal symptoms[47]

Adverse effects are listed in **Table 8**.

Ephedra

Overview Also known as Ma Haung, this herb comes from an evergreen shrublike plant in Central Asia and Mongolia and has been used in China and India for thousands of years.[48] It has been used to treat cold and flu symptoms as well as asthma and headaches. Dried stems and leaves are crushed to form pills, tinctures, extracts, and teas.

Ephedrine, the active ingredient, is a CNS and cardiovascular stimulant and, as such, is a common ingredient in weight loss and energy products. Because of the unacceptable risk of cardiovascular and other complications, the Food and Drug Administration banned it in 2004 for use in dietary supplements.[49] It continues to be used in over-the-counter expectorant and asthma medications and other commercial products. There is no evidence that ephedra enhances athletic performance.

Adverse effects Systematic reviews have found that ephedra use carries an increased risk of the following:

- Cardiovascular disease complications, including hypertension, myocardial infarction, coronary artery aneurysm,[50] stroke, and sudden cardiac death (**Table 9**)
- Seizures in people with and without known seizure disorders
- Complications of diabetes and chronic kidney disease
- Combining ephedra with caffeine or other stimulants increases the risks of the above mentioned side effects.

Table 8
Adverse effects of caffeine use

Diuresis	Irritability	Tremor
Dehydration	Depression	Dyskinesias, especially Facial
Withdrawal	Distractibility	Hypertension
Headaches	Restlessness/jitteriness	Tachycardia
Fatigue	Tachypnea	Palpitations
Insomnia	Nausea/vomiting/dyspepsia	Death

Data from Stear SJ, Castell LM, Burke LM, et al. BJSM reviews: A–Z of nutritional supplements: dietary supplements, sports nutrition foods and ergogenic aids for health and performance. Part 6. Br J Sports Med 2010;44:297–8; and Knopp WD, Wang TW, Bach BR. Ergogenic drugs in sports. Clin Sports Med 1997;16(3):375–92.

Table 9
Other adverse effects of ephedra use

Headaches	Irritability	Insomnia
Xerostomia	Distractibility	Dyspepsia
Dysuria	Restlessness	Nausea
Tachycardia	Anxiety	Kidney stones
Arrhythmias	Depression	Tremor
Palpitations	Psychosis	

Data from Herbs At A Glance: Ephedra. In: National center for complementary and alternative medicine at the national institutes of health. 2010. Available at: http://nccam.nih.gov/health/ephedra. Accessed August 18, 2012.

Bitter Orange

Overview

Also known as Citrus Aurantium, this herb comes from bitter orange trees in eastern Africa and tropical Asia and has been used to treat nausea, indigestion, acid reflux, appetite stimulation, constipation, congestion, and weight loss.[51] It has also been used topically to treat fungal dermatoses. Dried fruit and peels are crushed to form pills and extracts. Oils are used topically.

Synephrine, the active chemical in bitter orange, is less potent than ephedrine, but is similar in its effects as a CNS and cardiovascular stimulant. For this reason, it is commonly used as a replacement for ephedra as an ingredient in weight loss and energy products, many of which are advertised as "ephedra-free." There is little evidence that it is safer than ephedra. There is no evidence that bitter orange enhances athletic performance.

Case reports have shown increased risk of cardiovascular disease complications, including syncope, hypertension, myocardial infarction, stroke, and intractable ventricular fibrillation[52] in otherwise healthy people. Combining bitter orange with ephedra, caffeine, or other stimulants increases the risks of the above-mentioned adverse effects. Topical use can increase the risk of sunburn.

Creatine

Overview

Creatine is one of the most common sports supplements currently used today with estimated sales around 400 million annually. It is currently not banned by any major sporting organizations. It first gained mainstream notoriety during the 1992 Barcelona Olympics after many elite athletes thought it enhanced their performance. Athletes use various dosing regimens (**Table 10**). It is a naturally occurring compound synthesized endogenously and is consumed in most diets. Normally about 2 g creatine is ingested for every pound of fish or meat. Most creatine is found in skeletal muscle and provides a rapid source of energy during short bouts of exercise.

Table 10
Creatine supplementation protocols

Loading with Maintenance	Cycling
• Load: 20–30 g for 5–7 d • Maintenance: 2–5 g/d	• Take loading doses for 3–5 d every 3–4 wk

- Creatine use has been reported in athletes as young as sixth grade.[53]
- High-school surveys estimate the prevalence of use between 5% and 30% with 12th-grade boys as high as 30% to 50%.[54,55]
- A survey at a prominent NCAA Division I school found that 28% of varsity athletes currently use creatine and every men's team except 2 had at least 30% of the athletes currently using creatine.[56]

Physiologic and performance effects

Creatine plays a major role in energy production during short bouts of anaerobic exercise. Phosphocreatine provides a rapidly available source of energy in the muscle capable of resynthesizing ATP from ADP. This reaction occurs in the absence of oxygen and does not produce lactic acid. This energy source is estimated to be used during the first 10 to 15 seconds of exercise.

- Nearly 50% of athletes have low creatine stores and lower baseline creatine stores were found to have a more robust response, up to a 50% increase in muscle phosphocreatine concentration, with creatine supplementation.[57]
- Creatine also seems to increase calcium reuptake into the sarcoplasmic reticulum, resulting in more rapid and forceful muscle contraction.[58]
- Creatine has been associated with decreased lactate production and increased lactate threshold in elite rowers.[58]

Multiple preparations of creatine exist that attempt to increase muscle absorption or decrease gastrointestinal side effects with insufficient evidence to suggest performance benefit of one form over another (**Table 11**).

Adverse effects

- Although long-term studies have not been performed and caution should be exercised in the setting of renal or liver disease, currently no significant adverse effect has stood the test of scientific rigor and therefore creatine is thought to be a safe ergogenic aid.[60]
- "Impure" creatine supplements have been traced to positive drug tests in athletes.[60]

Prevention

Education

ATLAS and ATHENA Athletes Training and Learning to Avoid Steroids (ATLAS) and Athletes Targeting Healthy Exercise and Nutrition Alternatives (ATHENA) are school-based, team-centered drug-prevention programs.[66] Although ATLAS is designed for high-school male athletes, ATHENA focuses on middle-school and high-school sports, dance, and cheer teams.

Table 11
Benefits of creatine supplementation

Body Composition	Performance
• Increase lean body mass • Increased total body mass	• Improved total work to fatigue, peak force, and peak power[59] • High-intensity power output[60,61] • Increased strength[62,63] • Improved in track mean sprint times and repeated short swimming sprint times[64,65]

Table 12
The 2012 prohibited list, World Anti-Doping Agency (January 2012)

Prohibited Substances In and Out-of-Competition	Prohibited Methods In and Out-of-Competition	Prohibited Substances In Competition	Prohibited Substances Particular Sports
Anabolic agents • Anabolic androgenic steroids • Other anabolic agents	Enhancement of oxygen transfer • Blood doping • Artificial enhancement of uptake, transport or delivery of oxygen	Stimulants • Nonspecific stimulants • Specific stimulants	Alcohol • Aeronautics, archery, automobile, karate, motorcycling, powerboating
Peptide hormones and growth factors • EPO • Chorionic gonadotropin, luteinizing hormone (men) • Insulins • Corticotropins • Growth hormone and growth factor	Chemical and physical manipulation • Tampering of samples • IV infusions or injections of 50 mL per 6 h • Sequential withdrawal, manipulation, and reintroduction of any blood	Narcotics	β-Blockers • Aeronautic, archery, automobile, billiards, boules, bridge, darts, golf, ninepin and tenpin bowling, power boating, shooting, skiing/snowboarding
β-2 agonists	Gene doping • Transfer of nucleic acids or nucleic acid sequences • Use of genetically modified cells	Cannabinoids	
Hormone and metabolic modulators • Aromatase inhibitors • Selective estrogen receptor modulators • Anti-estrogenic substances • Myostatin inhibitors • Metabolic modulators		Glucocorticosteroids	
Diuretics and masking agents • Diuretics • Plasma expanders • Desmopressin			

Data from WADA: The World Anti-Doping Code, The 2012 Prohibited List, International Standard. 2011. Available at: http://www.wada-ama.org/Documents/World_Anti-Doping_Program/WADP-Prohibited-list/2012/WADA_Prohibited_List_2012_EN.pdf. Accessed August 27, 2012.

These programs use coach and peer leaders to facilitate 45-minute, hands-on, interactive classroom and 3 exercise sessions to teach students about avoiding drugs. The sessions, 10 sessions for boys and 8 sessions for girls, are integrated into their usual sport-training activities. Topics include sports nutrition, exercise alternatives, effects of substance abuse, drug-refusal role-playing, and health promotion. The programs also focus on ways to reduce the risk of anabolic steroid and other drug use through athletic teams, healthy nutrition, and exercise as alternatives. They also work to reduce disordered eating, body shaping, and other drug abuse.

These programs are supported in partnership with the National Football League Youth Football Fund and are run through the Center for Health Promotion and Research at Oregon Health and Sciences University in Portland, Oregon. More information is available at http://www.atlasathena.org and http://www.ohsu.edu/hpsm/index.cfm.

Governing bodies/agencies

WADA Established in 1999, WADA is "an international agency composed and funded equally by the sport movement and governments of the world."[67] Through research, education, and development of antidoping capacities, the organization strives to develop and implement policies, referred to collectively as the World Anti-Doping Code, that unify and harmonize the antidoping efforts in all sports and all countries. It was founded in Lausanne, Switzerland and is headquartered in Montreal, Canada.

The organization's priorities are code-compliance monitoring (**Table 12**), cooperation with law enforcement, and research into identification and detection of doping substances. It also works to coordinate antidoping efforts through the Anti-Doping Development Management Systems web-based database system designed to be a central clearinghouse for storing data, test results, therapeutic use exemptions, and antidoping rules violations in an effort toward efficiency, transparency, and effectiveness. WADA also works to promote resource sharing through Regional Anti-Doping Organizations, education, and athlete outreach.

REFERENCES

1. Scofield DE, Unruh S. Dietary supplement use among adolescent athletes in central Nebraska. J Strength Cond Res 2006;20(2):452–5.
2. Sobal J, Marquart LF. Vitamin/mineral supplement use among high school athletes. Adolescence 1994;29(116):835–43.
3. Dodge TL, Jaccard JJ. The effect of high school sports participation on the use of performance-enhancing substances in young adulthood. J Adolesc Health 2006;39(3):367–73.
4. Nieper A. Nutritional supplement practices in UK junior national track and field athletes. Br J Sports Med 2005;39(9):645–9.
5. Massad SJ, Shier NW, Koceja DM, et al. High school athletes and nutritional supplements: a study of knowledge and use. Int J Sport Nutr 1995;5(3):232–45.
6. Todd T. Anabolic steroids: the gremlins of sport. J Sport Hist 1987;14(1):87–107.
7. Yesalis CE, Kennedy NJ, Kopstein AN. Anabolic-androgenic steroid use in the United States. JAMA 1993;270:1217–21.
8. Johnston LD, O'Malley PM, Bachman JG, et al. Montoring the future, national results on adolescent drug use: overview of key findings. Ann Arbor (MI): Institute for Social Research, The University of Michigan; 2011.
9. Evans NA. Current concepts in anabolic-androgenic steroids. Am J Sports Med 2004;32(2):534–42.

10. Frankle M, Cicero G, Payne J. Use of androgenic anabolic steroids by athletes. JAMA 1984;252:482.
11. Brennan BP, Kanayama G, Hudson JI, et al. Human growth hormone abuse in male weightlifters. Am J Addict 2001;20(1):9–13.
12. Hartgens F, Kuipers H. Effects of androgenic-anabolic steroids in athletes. Sports Med 2004;37(8):513–54.
13. Kadi F, Eriksson A, Holmner S, et al. Effects of anabolic steroids on the muscle cells of strength-trained athletes. Med Sci Sports Exerc 1999;31:1528–34.
14. Keul J, Deus B, Kindermann W. Anabolic steroids: damages, effects of performance, and on metabolism. Med Klin 1976;71(12):497–503 [in German].
15. Evans NA. Gym and tonic: a profile of 100 male steroid users. Br J Sports Med 1997;31:54–8.
16. Tokish JM, Kocker MS, Hawkins RJ. Ergogenic aids: review of basic science, performance, side effects, and status in sports. Am J Sports Med 2004;32(6): 1543–53.
17. Stacy JJ, Terrell TR, Armsey TD. Ergogenic aids: human growth hormone. Curr Sports Med Rep 2004;3(4):229–33.
18. Dean H. Does exogenous growth hormone improve athletic performance? Clin J Sport Med 2002;12:250–3.
19. Rickert VI, Pawlak-Morello C, Sheppard V, et al. Human growth hormone: a new substance of abuse among adolescents? Clin Pediatr (Phila) 1992;31:723–6.
20. Jenkins P. Growth hormone and exercise: physiology, use and abuse. Growth Horm IGF Res 2001;11(Suppl A):S71–7.
21. Pipe A. Effects of growth hormone on athletic performance: a review. Clin J Sport Med 2009;19(1):75–6.
22. Bidlingmaier M, Wu Z, Strasburger CJ. Doping with growth hormone. J Pediatr Endocrinol Metab 2001;14:1077–84.
23. Ghaphery NA. Performance-enhancing drugs. Orthop Clin North Am 1995;26: 433–42.
24. Knopp WD, Wang TW, Bach BR. Ergogenic drugs in sports. Clin Sports Med 1997;16(3):375–92.
25. Simon TL. Induced erythrocythemia and athletic performance. Semin Hematol 1994;31:128–33.
26. Wadler GI. Drug use update. Med Clin North Am 1994;78:439–55.
27. Jones M, Pedoe DS. Blood doping: a literature review. Br J Sports Med 1989;23: 84–8.
28. Smith DA, Perry PJ. The efficacy of ergogenic agents in athletic competition. Part II: other performance-enhancing agents. Ann Pharmacother 1992;26:653–9.
29. Handelsman DJ. Indirect androgen doping by oestrogen blockade in sports. Br J Pharmacol 2008;154:598–605.
30. Martin M, Schlabach G, Shibinksi K. The use of nonprescription weight loss products among female basketball, softball, and volleyball athletes from NCAA division 1 institutions: issues and concerns. J Athl Train 1998;33:41–4.
31. Fitzsimmons S, Tucker A, Martins D. Seventy-five percent of National Football League teams use pregame hyperhydation with intravenous fluids. Clin J Sport Med 2011;21(3):192–9.
32. Burke LM, Eichner RE, Maughan RJ, et al. Exercise and fluid replacement, ACSM Position Stand. Med Sci Sports Exerc 2007;39(2):377–90.
33. Van Rosendal SP, Osborne MA, Fassett RG, et al. Physiologic and performance effects of glycerol hyperhydration and rehydration. Nutr Rev 2009;67(12): 690–705.

34. Mottram DR. Drugs in sport. Champaign (IL): Human Kinetics Books; 1988. p. 111–6.
35. Green GA, Uryasz FD, Petr TA, et al. NCAA study of substance use and abuse habits of college student-athletes. Clin J Sport Med 2001;11(1):51–6.
36. Kuthcer JS. Treatment of attention-deficit hyperactivity disorder in athletes. Curr Sports Med Rep 2011;10(1):32–6.
37. WADA: the world anti-doping code, the therapeutic use exemptions, international standard. 2011. p. 14. Available at: http://www.wada-ama.org/Documents/World_Anti-Doping_Program/WADP-IS-TUE/2011/WADA_ISTUE_2011_revJanuary-2012_EN.pdf. Accessed October 28, 2012.
38. NCAA banned drugs and medial exemptions policy guidelines regarding medical reporting for student-athletes with attention deficit hyperactivity disorder (ADHD) taking prescribed stimulants. Available at: www.ncaa.org/wps/wcm/connect/00e85e004e0b8a619ae5-fa1ad6fc8b25/ADHD_QA2009.pdf. Accessed October 28, 2012.
39. Pelham WE, McBurnett K, Harper GW, et al. Methylphenidate and baseball playing in ADHD children: who's on first? J Consult Clin Psychol 1990;58:130–3.
40. Chandler JV, Blair SN. The effect of amphetamines on selected physiological components related to athletic success. Med Sci Sports Exerc 1980;12(1):65–9.
41. Graham TE. Caffeine and exercise: metabolism, endurance and performance. Sports Med 2001;31:785–807.
42. Cox GR, Desbrow B, Montgomery PG, et al. Effect of different protocols of caffeine intake on metabolism and endurance performance. J Appl Physiol 2002;93:990–9.
43. Kovacs EM, Stegen JH, Brouns F. Effect of caffeinated drinks on substrate metabolism, caffeine excretion, and performance. J Appl Physiol 1998;85:709–15.
44. Graham TE, Spriet LL. Metabolic, catecholamine, and exercise performance responses to various doses of caffeine. J Appl Physiol 1995;78:867–74.
45. Stear SJ, Castell LM, Burke LM, et al. BJSM reviews: A–Z of nutritional supplements: dietary supplements, sports nutrition foods and ergogenic aids for health and performance Part 6. Br J Sports Med 2010;44:297–8.
46. Burke LM. Caffeine and sports performance. Appl Physiol Nutr Metab 2008;33:1319–34.
47. James JE, Rogers PJ. Effects of caffeine on performance and mood: withdrawal reversal is the most plausible explanation. Psychopharmacology (Berl) 2005;182(1):1–8.
48. Herbs at a glance: ephedra. In: National Center for Complementary and Alternative Medicine at the National Institutes of Health. 2010. Available at: http://nccam.nih.gov/health/ephedra. Accessed August 18, 2012.
49. Newton MA. Ephedra. In: Blumenthal M, Goldberg A, Brinckman J, editors. Herbal medicine: expanded commission e monographs. Newton (MA): Lippincott Williams & Wilkins; 2000. p. 110–7.
50. Thomas JE, Munir JA, McIntyre PZ, et al. STEMI in a 24-year-old man after use of a synephrine-containing dietary supplement: a case report and review of the literature. Tex Heart Inst J 2009;36(6):586–90.
51. Herbs at a glance: bitter orange. In: National Center for Complementary and Alternative Medicine at the National Institutes of Health. 2010. Available at: http://nccam.nih.gov/health/bitterorange. Accessed August 18, 2012.
52. Srivatsa UN, Ebrahimi R, El-Bialy A, et al. Electrical storm: case series and review of management. J Cardiovasc Pharmacol Ther 2003;8(3):237–46.

53. Metzl JD, Small E, Levine SR, et al. Creatine use among young athletes. Pediatrics 2001;108(2):421–5.
54. McGuine TA, Sullivan JC, Bernhardt DT. Creatine supplementation in high school football players. Clin J Sport Med 2001;11(4):247–53.
55. McGuine TA, Sullivan JC, Bernhardt DA. Creatine supplementation in Wisconsin high school athletes. WMJ 2002;101(2):25–30.
56. LaBotz M, Smith BW. Creatine supplement use in an NCAA Division I athletic program. Clin J Sport Med 1999;9:167–9.
57. Rawson ES, Volek JS. The effects of creatine supplementation and resistance training on muscle strength and weight-lifting performance. J Strength Cond Res 2002;17:822–31.
58. Chwalbinska-Moneta J. Effect of creatine supplementation on aerobic performance and anaerobic capacity in elite rowers in the course of endurance training. Int J Sport Nutr Exerc Metab 2003;13(2):173–83.
59. Burke DG, Silver S, Holt LE, et al. The effect of continuous low dose creatine supplementation on force, power, and total work. Int J Sport Nutr Exerc Metab 2000;10:235–44.
60. Terjung RL, Clarkson P, Eichner RE, et al. The American College of Sports Medicine roundtable: the physiologic and health effects of oral creatine supplementation. Med Sci Sports Exerc 2000;32:706–17.
61. Kreider RB. Effects of creatine supplementation on performance and training adaptations. Mol Cell Biochem 2003;244(1):89–94.
62. Dempsey RL, Mazzone MF, Meurer LN. Does oral creatine supplementation improve strength? A meta-analysis. J Fam Pract 2002;51(11):945–51.
63. Volek JS, Duncan ND, Mazzetti SA, et al. Performance and muscle fiber adaptations to creatine supplementation and heavy resistance training. Med Sci Sports Exerc 1999;31(8):1147–56.
64. Leenders NM, Lamb DR, Nelson TE. Creatine supplementation and swimming performance. Int J Sport Nutr 1999;9:251–62.
65. Mujika I, Chatard JC, Lacoste L, et al. Creatine supplementation improves sprint performance in soccer players. Med Sci Sports Exerc 2000;32:518–25.
66. Available at: http://www.atlasathena.org. Accessed August 27, 2012.
67. Available at: http://www.wada-ama.org/en/. Accessed August 27, 2012.

The Potential Role of Sports Psychology in the Obesity Epidemic

Vincent Morelli, MD[a,*], Carolyn Davis, PhD[b]

KEYWORDS

• Sports psychology • Childhood obesity • Psychological disorders in athletes

KEY POINTS

- Sports psychologists play an important role in enhancing performance among athletes.
- Sports psychologists can also lend their expertise to assist with injury prevention and recovery, as well as compliance issues.
- Sports psychology also has a role in helping to reverse the growing obesity epidemic among school-aged children.
- These professionals, working with coaches, can increase children's levels of physical activity.
- Cognitive-behavioral techniques (eg, confidence building, anger management) could lead to enhanced enjoyment, increased participation, improved school performance, and a reduction in obesity.

DEFINING SPORTS PSYCHOLOGY

In psychology, there are many subfields with unique practices and specific areas of focus. Sport psychology is 1 such subfield, requiring the practicing professional to be appropriately educated, trained, and focused in this area of expertise. The definition from the American Psychological Association's (Exercise and Sport Psychology) Web site states: "Exercise and sport psychology is the scientific study of the psychological factors that are associated with participation and performance in sport, exercise, and other types of physical activity. It is important to note that although overlap exists, 'doing therapy' with a person who happens to be an athlete is *not* considered sport psychology."[1]

[a] Department of Family and Community Medicine, Meharry Medical College, 1005 Dr D. B. Todd Boulevard, Nashville, TN 37208, USA; [b] Department of Counseling Psychology, Walden University, 100 Washington Avenue, Suite 900, Minneapolis, MN 55401, USA
* Corresponding author.
E-mail address: morellivincent@yahoo.com

Prim Care Clin Office Pract 40 (2013) 507–523
http://dx.doi.org/10.1016/j.pop.2013.02.001 primarycare.theclinics.com
0095-4543/13/$ – see front matter

THE ROLE OF THE SPORTS PSYCHOLOGIST

Interest and involvement in sport psychology have grown tremendously in the last 15 to 20 years.[2] This change is, in part, a result of the increased awareness of how psychological and physiologic factors interact to enhance performance and how a balanced integration of these 2 facets can provide athletes with a winning edge.[3]

Although performance enhancement has heightened the awareness and popularity of sports psychology, there is still much about the role of the sports psychologist that needs to be emphasized to involved team physicians. Research has also shown that sports psychology can play an important role in injury prevention and healing (discussed later), in improving the athlete's self-care, improving mood, improving quality of life, and increasing the athlete's sense of internal control.[4] Physiologic advantages such as improvement in immune response, decreased postoperative pain and anxiety, shortened hospital stays, and decreased use of pain medications have also been proved to be enhanced by proper sports psychology intervention in athletes.[5]

Another area that is vital for team physicians to heed is recognition and management of psychological disorders in athletes (discussed later). Most current texts in sports psychology contain an abundance of information on cognitive-behavioral techniques, goal setting, imagery, and visualization for performance enhancement, but contain only limited discussions of the presence of psychological maladies in athletes and little examination of the dynamics at play inside the athlete's mind. There may be discussions between patients and team physicians about anxiety disorders or disordered eating, but mood or other personality disorders may be overlooked. It is possible that such disorders are more common in this population than is suspected.

For example, many of the behaviors associated with advanced or exceptional performance can be closely aligned with disordered personality diagnoses such as obsessive compulsive behavior patterns and perfectionist tendencies. Some individuals may even show characteristics of borderline personality and narcissistic personality disorders as a function of participation in their particular sport. Sports physicians and team psychologists need to be particularly aware of this potential for psychopathology in athletes to optimally manage such issues.

An area that may benefit the team physician is an awareness of the sports psychologist's role in recognizing the athletic identity: the degree with which an individual identifies with an athlete role.[6] This is an important self-concept that influences an individual's experiences, relationships with others, and pursuit of sport activity.[7] Strong athletic identification has been correlated with a firm sense of self-identity, more social interactions, increased confidence, and more positive athletic experiences.[8]

On the other hand, athletes who place too much emphasis on this identity may be at risk for psychological problems, particularly during sport transition periods such as adaptation to injury or retirement. The recognition of this overidentification by the sports psychologist or team physician may allow intervention to prevent transitional hardships for the athlete.[9]

SPORTS PSYCHOLOGIST AND SPORTS PHYSICIAN PARTNERSHIP

As discussed earlier, there are several areas in which a team physician and sports psychologist may work together to more effectively serve the athletes under their care. Such interaction may be used to address health issues such as stress, anxiety, depression, risky behavior, and unhealthy habits. Interactions with the sports psychologist and the team physician may also help athletes better deal with injury, maintain psychological well-being, and improve the athlete's performance to better prepare them for future life transitions. The following sections describe 5 specific areas of potential partnership.

Psychiatric Disorders in Athletes

Overall, the prevalence of psychiatric disorders in the athletic population is no different from that found in the general nonathletic population.[10–12] For example, the incidence of depression in college athletes (a significant 21%) is the same as that found in nonathletic college students.[13] Other maladies such as anxiety, obsessive compulsive disorder, and exercise addiction are much discussed in the sports psychology literature, but the incidence and prevalence of these disorders in athletics have been minimally studied. One caveat here is that there are increased incidences of certain disorders in certain types of athletics. For example, in aesthetic sports (eg, ballet, figure skating), 15% of athletes have been reported to suffer from anorexia or bulimia[14] compared with 1.2% to 2.3% in the general population.[15–18] In bulk/strength athletic endeavors, 23% of male athletes and up to 56% of female athletes taking anabolic steroids have reported major symptoms of mood disorders.[19,20]

With these points in mind, it is important for the team physician to be aware of the frequency of mood disorders, eating disorders, and other psychiatric conditions in the athletic population. A partnership between team physician and sports psychologist may heighten awareness, better educate coaching staff, and more effectively provide prompt therapeutic intervention when needed.

Overtraining

Overtraining syndrome is an ill-defined malady characterized by an increased perception of effort during sport, lack of energy, muscle soreness, sleep disturbances, loss of appetite, weight loss, mood disturbances, decreased self-confidence, inability to concentrate, and frequent upper respiratory tract infections.[21–23] These symptoms often overlap or are described as indistinguishable from depression/major mood disorders.[24]

Overtraining increases the incidence of injury and may also predispose some athletes to an increased incidence of long-term illness, such as diabetes in athletes who are continuingly bulking up; continued eating disorders in ballet dancers, skaters, gymnasts, and wrestlers; and long-term arthritis and other maladies in contact sports.

In addition to physical risks, overtrained athletes (especially elite athletes) may be more susceptible to a narrowed sense of identity[25] which has been linked with psychological stress and depression, especially when challenged by injury, failure, aging, or retirement.[26] In younger elite athletes, overtraining may lead to the development of a one-dimensional identity, unrealistic expectations, perceptions of conditional love, and perfectionistic traits.[27]

Elite athletes have a reported seasonal incidence of overtraining syndrome of 7% to 20%,[21] and younger elite athletes may be even more at risk with an incidence reported at 20% to 30%.[27] Still higher rates have been reported in basketball players during training camp (33%), professional soccer players during the season (50%), and in elite runners, with career prevalence rates of up to 60%.[28,29]

It is well for the sports physician to be aware of the frequency of overtraining syndrome, of groups that may be at particularly high risk, and of the signs and symptoms shown by affected athletes. Such awareness allows the team physician and sports psychologist to promptly address any physical or psychological issues, educate coaches, and prevent potential injury.

Injury Prevention

The American College of Sports Medicine Consensus Statement on psychological issues related to injuries in athletes notes that although there is no clear injury-prone personality type, (eg, perfectionist, introvert, extrovert), psychological factors can predispose athletes to injury and also play an important role in the rehabilitation and recovery from injury.[30,31] In particular, stress and stressful life events (eg, divorce, death, financial crisis) are clearly associated with increased injury rates, and a team physician should be aware of this, make coaches aware, and monitor athletes (as much as possible) for the occurrence of such events. When encountered by the team physician, stress reduction techniques and psychological support with a sports psychologist or mental health worker have proved effective.

Injury Rehabilitation

Psychological factors also play a role in the rehabilitation of athletes because during this time they can experience, medical, social, financial, sport-related, or personal stressors (eg, loss of identity, fear of reinjury, loss of confidence, mood swings, obsession with return-to-play issues).[32,33] All such emotional responses during rehabilitation can adversely affect recovery and future athletic participation. Just as patient mood and attitude have been proved to prolong surgical recovery times,[34] such factors should also be taken into consideration when setting goals and predicting recovery times for athletes in postinjury rehabilitation.

Team physicians should be mindful of the potential effect of psychological factors on injury and recovery and should be aware of the need for both physical and psychological rehabilitation.[30] The integration of a sports psychologist or other mental health provider into team dynamics can help with such issues of injury recovery.

Athletic Performance Enhancement

Although performance enhancement is an important and exciting area of sports psychology, such concerns usually lie outside the team physician's purview. Issues such as overcoming performance anxiety, building confidence, enhancing motivation, using imagery, decision making, anger management, resiliency, self-talk, team-building strategies, goal setting, peak performance, coach-athlete relationships, and so forth are more in the domain of coaches and sports psychologists rather than in the team physician's realm of overall health and wellness. Still, the team physician may wish to be aware of these programs and methods, both from general interest and as a method of relationship building with coaches and athletes.

Summary of Sports Psychologist and Sports Physician Partnership

With the increasing acceptance and widening use of sports psychology in professional and university settings,[35] team physicians need to be aware of the role that sports psychologists play in performance enhancement, injury prevention and recovery,[30,36] compliance, and the overall psychological and physical health of the athlete. The team physician must be aware of the role that life stressors play in increasing the risk of injury[37] and must help to recognize and address such issues when they arise. In addition, the team physician may play a role in helping to recognize pathologic personality disorders, risk-taking behavior, and unhealthy choices. In these instances, the team physician may aid in facilitating proper referral and treatment.

A partnership between the sports physician and the sports psychologist is vital if athletes and teams are to perform well, prevent and recover from injuries, promote overall health, maximize human potential, and contribute optimally to society.

NEW AND EMERGING TRENDS IN SPORTS PSYCHOLOGY

Although there is much ongoing and exciting research in performance enhancement and virtually every other area of sports psychology, we would like to propose 1 new area in which sports psychology could potentially be applied, an area that is important to the health of the nation.

A Potential Role for Sports Psychology in Affecting the Obesity Epidemic

Exercise effects on physical and mental health

In the United States, more than 250,000 deaths per year (12% of the total deaths/y) are attributable to a lack of regular physical activity.[38,39] It is well established that regular physical activity is protective against diabetes,[40] heart disease,[41] obesity, hypertension, and breast, prostate, and colon cancer, and results in a lower all-cause mortality.[42] Observational studies have also shown exercise to be protective against dementia and cognitive decline in elderly people.[43,44] In addition, exercise can benefit those with established heart disease, diabetes, hypertension, peripheral artery disease, heart failure, osteoarthritis, depression, anxiety, and several other chronic medical conditions.[45–48]

Studies also report that physical activity is associated with improvements in self-esteem,[49] well-being, satisfaction with appearance,[50] and symptoms of anxiety and depression.[51–53] It may protect against the development of depression as well.[45,54] Physical activity is believed to lessen depression and anxiety by both physiologic (increasing neurotransmitting amines and endorphins)[55,56] and psychological mechanisms (distracting patients from unpleasant situations, increasing social interaction, and increasing feelings of self-competence).[57,58]

It is clear that physical activity is vital to a healthy existence.

THE PROBLEM OF OBESITY

In the United States, roughly 60% of adults are overweight and 24% are obese.[59] Finkelstein and colleagues[60] estimated the total annual costs related to weight issues in the United States to be more than 78 billion dollars, accounting for 9.1% of total medical expenditures in 1998. Projections estimate that if these obesity trends continue, by 2030 costs will reach nearly 100 billion dollars and account for nearly 16% of total health care expenditures.

International studies indicate that obesity and obesity-related costs are global issues. Australia's adult overweight/obesity prevalence is 40%,[61] with an estimated annual cost of 21 billion dollars (2005),[62] and Canada's overweight/obesity prevalence is nearly 60%,[63] with direct costs estimated at 6 billion dollars. In Europe, an estimated 50% of adults are overweight or obese.[64] Global estimates in 2005 found that 23.2% of the world's adults were overweight (937 million people) and 9.8% were obese (396 million people).[65]

As stated earlier, the health and mental health effects of this epidemic are devastating both on an individual and societal level.

THE PROBLEM OF OBESITY IN CHILDREN

It is estimated that one-third of children and adolescents in the United States are overweight or obese[66] and, if trends continue, more than 40% will be obese by 2036.[67] Approximately 50% of obese 6-year-olds will remain so as adults,[68,69] whereas only 9% of normal-weight children will become obese as adults.[70] One long-term international study noted that more than 80% of obese children remained obese into adulthood when evaluated 23 years later.[71] There is also strong evidence that once obesity is established, it is difficult to reverse through interventions.[72]

As with adults, the health problems associated with childhood obesity are well known. However, it is important to keep in mind that childhood health risks associated with obesity are carried forward into adulthood, with a higher incidence of both childhood disease and adult medical conditions manifesting in these overweight and obese patients (eg, asthma, sleep apnea, hypertension, hyperlipidemia, coronary artery disease, diabetes, cancers).[73,74]

In addition to medical risks, overweight children can also experience psychological stressors, including discrimination from their peers, lowered self-esteem, depression, sadness, loneliness, nervousness, and other psychological maladies and psychosocial problems, which may persist into adulthood.[75,76]

If overweight or obese children normalize their body mass index (BMI) by adulthood, a marked reduction in these conditions is proved to occur. This is the goal of all intervention programs.[74]

Habits Started in Childhood

Childhood is a critical time for effective health promotion because children are more amenable to changing their habits, and because healthy habits acquired in childhood are more likely to persist into adulthood.[77–79] The transition from childhood to adolescence is a particularly crucial period when children are at increased risk for unnecessary weight gain.[80,81] During this time (age 10–12 years), children are afforded more dietary decision-making power (often choosing poorly) and more freedom as to how they spend their leisure time. They may also initiate unhealthy behaviors such as skipping breakfast, dropping out of organized sports, or increasing screen time/computer use.[82]

The Benefits of Physical Activity in Children

It is well established that physical activity aids in disease prevention, promotes mental health and well-being,[83] and enhances social skills.[84]

A report in 2010 from the Centers for Disease Control[85] concludes "there is substantial evidence that physical activity can help improve academic achievement, including grades and standardized test scores." These findings are corroborated by the most recent 2012 review,[86] which concludes, "physical activity is positively related to academic performance in children."

Physical activity in childhood and adolescence also predicts higher educational achievement[87,88] and greater socioeconomic success in adulthood.[89,90] These benefits are seen regardless of a child's socioeconomic background.

Recent Cuts in Physical Education Programs

Informed by these findings, the recent political trend to cut physical education (PE) programs and budgets[91] is misguided if long-term health and productivity are judged to be important by society. Currently, only 5 states (Illinois, Iowa, Massachusetts, New Mexico, and Vermont) require PE every year from kindergarten to 12th grade, and no federal law requires it be offered. However, in light of the current obesity epidemic, Congress may soon be forced to address the issue on a national level.[92]

Numbers of Children Participating in Physical Activity

Although the exact numbers and percentages of children engaging in school-based and after-school physical activity are not well documented, it is likely that these numbers have declined recently as obesity rates have increased. Childhood habits, carried forward into adulthood, likely contribute to the fact that only 37% of men and 24% of women in the United Kingdom engage in 30 minutes of exercise per day[93] and that only 50% of US adults do so.[94]

Reasons Why Children Participate

A 2006 review of reasons why children and adolescents participate in sports[95] examined 24 high-quality studies and concluded that among adolescents, weight management, social interaction, and enjoyment were common reasons for participation in sport and physical activity. More importantly, from our perspective, were the motivating factors and barriers to exercise in the younger age groups. These children were motivated by a love of experimentation, an interest in engaging in unusual activities, and parenteral involvement and support. Barriers included involvement in competitive sports or highly structured activity.

A Review of Obesity Prevention Programs: Models that Promote Behavioral Change

Weight gain, overweight, and obesity are a result of an imbalance between food intake, physical activity,[64] and a variety of genetic, behavioral, cultural, environmental, and economic factors.[96] In addition, in the United States and other developed countries, there is a significant tie between obesity and lower socioeconomic status, as well as a racial bias. In the United States, blacks and Hispanic children have a rate of obesity twice that of white/non-Hispanic children.[97]

Various multidisciplinary approaches to the problem of obesity and physical inactivity have been undertaken in the recent past, with varying results. For example, 1 program[98] was instituted in grammar schools in 2007 to 2008 in which professional educators taught kindergarteners to second-graders about health-related topics, including nutrition, physical activity, bullying, and germ prevention. Their interventions proved to significantly increase the knowledge of taught topics but failed to report significant effects on BMI. An extension of this pilot program called *Wholesome Routines* taught similar topics to third-graders to fifth-graders and included teachers, families, and food service providers to approach the issue from multiple angles. Results of the program interventions over the course of 1 year (2007–2008) revealed that 8.3% of students reduced BMI by 5% to 10%, and 39% of students reported increasing their physical activity by an hour per week. Although this result represents some progress, it is certainly not enough to recommend widespread program adaptation or to engender much enthusiasm.

Several other obesity prevention programs are currently in use (or are being investigated) in the United States and other developed countries. Whereas some programs report effectiveness, modest weight loss, (eg, CATCH [Coordinated Approach To Child Health],[99] HOP'N [Healthy Opportunities for Physical Activity and Nutrition][100]), increased physical activity, or decreased screen time, others do not.[101] Overall, only 50% of obesity intervention programs reviewed in 2006 were found to be effective.[102–104]

In reviewing the literature, a 2011 Cochrane meta-analysis of obesity prevention programs[105] evaluated 37 programs with 27,946 participating children (most between ages 6 and 12 years). The analysis concluded that overall, the programs, were "effective at reducing adiposity" and that children in the intervention groups experienced a mean difference in adiposity of 0.15 kg/m^2 or about a 180-g (0.4-pound) weight loss for an average 6-year-old or a 230-g (half-pound) weight loss for an average 12-year-old. Again, this result was not nearly significant enough to engender enthusiasm, especially because several of the interventions took place over several years.

The review noted that in assessing programs, common elements that contributed to effectiveness were: (1) a school-based curriculum that included healthy eating, physical activity, and body image; (2) increased sessions for physical activity and the development of movement skills; (3) improvements in the nutritional quality of foods supplied in schools; (4) environments and cultural practices that support children eating healthier foods and being active throughout each day; (5) support for teachers and other staff to implement health promotion strategies; and (6) parental support so that they may encourage these behaviors at home.

The Cochrane review's conclusion notes that, although positive, the results may be biased by the omission of smaller studies with negative outcomes. It also states that the data do not identify which components of which programs were most effective, and that the duration of the beneficial effects could not be shown over the long-term. This conclusion, along with the minimal amount of weight loss discussed earlier, is again hardly a ringing endorsement of current intervention programs.

The latest 2012 review of obesity prevention programs focused on children aged 4 to 6 years[106] and concluded that parental knowledge (eg, via informational handouts, newsletters) alone is insufficient in obesity prevention. Successful programs instead require parental engagement, including physical activity modeling, especially for male caregivers. It states that this strategy is vital and that parents/caregivers should be a major target of intervention programs.[107] The review recommends that physical and dietary behaviors be targeted together and that activity programs should encourage at least 120 minutes/d of physical activity (only 60 minutes/d is recommended by the US Centers for Disease Control [CDC]) and that dietary interventions should include child education, parental education and an examination of barriers to healthy food choices. Optimal programs should also limit leisure screen time to 1 hour per day and offer a variety of physical activities,[79] so that all children are encouraged to participate. The review also notes that forced competition can be counterproductive.

The Cochrane review, this review, and others[108–111] emphasize the importance of clear and simple messages. These messages must be grounded in scholarship, be designed to effect positive behavioral change, and be effectively communicated with all teachers, leaders, and parents involved in the programs.

The American Association of Pediatrics recommends that in treating and preventing obesity, physicians can help induce behavioral change by tracking weight and BMI, promoting a healthy diet, and encouraging increased activity.[112] However, despite these recommendations, many primary care physicians report that they believe that they lack skills to appropriately address the problem.[113] Therefore, current thinking holds that obesity is best approached in a multidisciplinary fashion, with physicians, allied health personnel, and behaviorists all involved and playing significant roles.

The literature supports family lifestyle intervention programs that emphasize education, parent and family involvement, goal formation, and monitoring. Such programs have been shown to be more effective than education-only programs.[114–116] Several studies have emphasized that parents must be included if interventions are to be successful, both because they can help offer children healthy alternatives and because of the importance of modeling.[117] A recent study found that parental confidence (in the ability of a program to effect change) was the strongest predictor of the success of a program.[118] Parents are also vital in discussions of barriers to weight loss and in identifying social networks (eg, peers, neighbors, family members) that could help or hinder weight loss efforts.[119] In addition to the important role that parents play, family intervention can also often assess factors that predict poor response to weight loss, such as depression, loneliness, teasing, and other social issues that the child may experience. Such intervention may also help identify appetite patterns such as poor satiety response, binge eating, or night eating syndrome.[120]

The most successful obesity interventions offer a socioenvironmental approach, one that recognizes the important inclusion of parents, family, the home environment, peers, and the community.[121–123] This model, rather than placing the responsibility for behavioral change solely on the individual and individual willpower, recognizes the role that the environment plays in both the problem and the solution. The socioenvironmental model requires parental involvement for the purpose of providing modeling, rule setting, and environmental interventions. Such environmental interventions include removing unhealthy choices (eg, excessive screen time, high-fat/high-sugar food choices) and making activity and healthful choices more accessible. In addition, this model incorporates positive peer influence and community resources whenever possible. This approach also requires that interventions be repetitive and intense enough to engrain new habits and patterns of behavior. Recent evidence supports this approach for sustainable weight loss.[121,122,124] As part of this approach, health care providers should schedule follow-up sessions with families and patients every 3 months to track weight and overall health, assess patient adaptation, compliance and attitudes, and to reinforce teachings and inculcate healthful habits.[125]

Many of the reviews discussed recommend that programs should have a common framework, but with enough flexibility built in to provide teachers/leaders with the opportunity to modify the program to account for cultural differences, community differences, and individual differences among participants.

A ROLE FOR SPORTS PSYCHOLOGY IN OBESITY PREVENTION

The shortcomings in obesity prevention programs beg for an innovative approach to the problem. One such innovative approach is to educate school coaches and PE teachers in sports psychology. Although many of the reviewed programs do have behavioral components, to the best of our knowledge, no programs to date have instituted sports psychology training in an attempt to increase participation, increase activity, and prevent obesity. We believe that this oversight demands to be addressed. Naturally, such a sports psychology component would be used in conjunction with successful components of established programs, as noted earlier. We believe that our novel sports psychology in obesity prevention program fits well into the socioenvironmental model and offers both a way to further positively affect the child's environment and a practical way to continue to teach and inculcate healthful values.

In addition, research has shown that athletes evaluate psychosocially trained coaches more positively than nontrained coaches[126,127] and that such coaches have been proved to increases athletes' self-esteem to a greater degree than nontrained coaches.[128,129] This situation, in turn, can lead to greater enjoyment and increased participation. Barnett and colleagues[129] found that 95% of youth who played for psychologically trained coaches returned to participate the following year, whereas only 74% of those who played for nontrained coaches returned.

An innovative advancement might be to incorporate a sports psychology component into an already proven prevention program, for the following reasons:

- Because physical inactivity has been reported as the most prevalent chronic disease risk factor, costing developed countries billions of dollars each year[130]
- Because sport is a major platform for encouraging the general population to become more physically active, and a key element of obesity reduction and health promotion strategies in developed countries[131]
- Because childhood habits are carried forward into adulthood[77–79]

- Because physical activity and childhood participation in activity are so vital to long-term health, school performance, and socioeconomic gain[89,90]
- Because decreased PE time in schools, insufficient safe areas for after-school play, and competing sedentary behaviors such as computers, TV and video games are making it more challenging to meet physical activity goals[132]
- Because coaches trained in sports psychology have been proved to increase children's participation in sport and increase participant enjoyment of physical activity[129]
- Because, as summarized earlier, existing obesity prevention programs have limited effectiveness on weight and physical activity in children
- Because to date, no obesity prevention programs have included educating elementary school coaches and PE teachers in sports psychology

This strategy could positively affect the outcomes of enhanced enjoyment, increased participation, improved school performance, and a reduction of overweight and obesity. It is certainly a question worth exploring.

REFERENCES

1. Aoyagi MW, Portenga ST. The role of positive ethics and virtues in the context of sport and performance psychology service delivery. Prof Psychol Res Pr 2010; 41(3):253–9.
2. Costa C. The status and future of sport management: a Delphi study. J Sport Manag 2005;19(2):117–42.
3. Buckworth J, Dishman RK. Determinants of exercise and physical activity. In: Buckworth J, Dishman RK, editors. Exercise psychology. Champaign (IL): Human Kinetics; 2002. p. 3–15.
4. Armatas V, Chondrou E, Yiannakos A. Psychological aspects of rehabilitation following serious athletic injuries with special reference to goal setting: a review study. Physical Training. 2007. Available at: http://ejmas.com/pt/ptframe.htm. Accessed October 14, 2012.
5. Dworsky D, Krane V. Using the mind to health body. Association for Applied Sport Psychology. Available at: http://www.appliedsportpsych.org/resource-center/injury-&-rehabilitation/articles/imagery. Accessed September 12, 2012.
6. Brewer BW, Cornelius AE. Self-protective changes in athletic identity following anterior cruciate ligament reconstruction. Psychol Sport Exerc 2010;11(1):1–5.
7. Cornelius A. The relationship between athletic identity, peer and faculty socialization, and college student development. J Coll Stud Dev 1995;36(6):560–73.
8. Griffith KA, Johnson KA. Athletic identity and life role of Division-I and Division-III collegiate athletes. 2002. Available at: http://murphylibrary.uwlax.edu/digital/jur/2002/griffith-johnson.pdf. Accessed September 12, 2012.
9. Brewer BW, Van Raalte JL, Linder DE. Athletic identity: Hercules' muscles or Achilles heel? Int J Sport Psychol 1993;24:237–54.
10. Markser VZ. Sport psychiatry and psychotherapy. Mental strains and disorders in professional sports. Challenge and answer to societal changes. Eur Arch Psychiatry Clin Neurosci 2011;261(Suppl 2):S182–5.
11. Yang J, Peek-Asa C, Corlette JD, et al. Prevalence of and risk factors associated with symptoms of depression in competitive collegiate students athletes. Clin J Sport Med 2007;17(6):481–7.
12. Donohue B, Covassin T, Lancer K, et al. Examination of psychiatric symptoms in student athletes. J Genet Psychol 2004;131:29–36.

13. Kelly WE, Kelly KE, Brown FC, et al. Gender differences in depression among college students: a multi-cultural perspective. Coll Student J 1999;33:72–6. Available at: http://www.freepatentsonline.com/article/College-Student-Journal/62894055.html. Accessed October 15, 2012.
14. Byrne S, McLean N. Elite athletes: effects of the pressure to be thin. J Sci Med Sport 2002;5:80–94.
15. Bulik CM, Sullivan PF, Tozzi F, et al. Prevalence, heritability, and prospective risk factors for anorexia nervosa. Arch Gen Psychiatry 2006;63:305–12.
16. Keski-Rahkonen A, Sihvola E, Raevuori A, et al. Reliability of self-reported eating disorders: optimizing population screening. Int J Eat Disord 2006; 39(8):754–62.
17. Hudson JI, Hiripi E, Pope HG Jr, et al. The prevalence and correlates of eating disorders in the National Comorbidity Survey Replication. Biol Psychiatry 2007; 61(3):348–58.
18. Keski-Rahkonen A, Hoek HW, Linna MS, et al. Incidence and outcomes of bulimia nervosa: a nationwide population-based study. Psychol Med 2009;39: 823–31.
19. Pope HG Jr, Katz DL. Psychiatric and medical effects of anabolic-androgenic steroid use. A controlled study of 160 athletes. Arch Gen Psychiatry 1994; 51(5):375–82.
20. Gruber AJ, Pope HG Jr. Psychiatric and medical effects of anabolic-androgenic steroid use in women. Psychother Psychosom 2000;69(1):19–26.
21. Morgan WP, Brown DR, Raglin JS, et al. Psychological monitoring of overtraining and staleness. Br J Sports Med 1987;21(3):107–14.
22. Hawley CJ, Schoene RB. Overtraining syndrome: why training too hard, too long, doesn't work. Phys Sportsmed 2003;31(6):47–8.
23. Budgett R, Newsholme E, Lehmann M, et al. Redefining the overtraining syndrome as the unexplained underperformance syndrome. Br J Sports Med 2000;34(1):67–8.
24. Schwenk TL. The stigmatization and denial of mental illness in athletes. Br J Sports Med 2000;34(1):4–5.
25. Cresswell SL, Eklund RC. Athlete burnout: a longitudinal qualitative investigation. Sport Psychol 2007;21:1–20.
26. Reardon CL, Factor RM. Sport psychiatry: a systematic review of diagnosis and medical treatment of mental illness in athletes. Sports Med 2010;40:61–80.
27. Winsley R, Matos N. Overtraining and elite young athletes. Med Sport Sci 2011; 56:97–105.
28. Morgan WP, O'Connor PJ, Sparling PB, et al. Psychologic characterization of the elite female distance runner. Int J Sports Med 1987;8(Suppl 2):124–31.
29. Morgan WP, O'Connor PJO, Ellickson KA, et al. Personality structure, mood states, and performance in elite male distance runners. Int J Sport Psychol 1988;19:247–63.
30. American College of Sports Medicine, American Academy of Family Physicians, American Academy of Orthopaedic Surgeons, et al. Psychological issues related to injury in athletes and the team physician: a consensus statement. Med Sci Sports Exerc 2006;38(11):2030–4.
31. Wiese-Bjornstal DM. Psychology and socioculture affect injury risk, response, and recovery in high-intensity athletes: a consensus statement. Scand J Med Sci Sports 2010;20(Suppl 2):103–11.
32. Evans L, Wadey R, Hanton S, et al. Stressors experienced by injured athletes. J Sports Sci 2012;30(9):917–27.

33. Podlog L, Dimmock J, Miller J. A review of return to sport concerns following injury rehabilitation: practitioner strategies for enhancing recovery outcomes. Phys Ther Sport 2011;12(1):36–42.
34. Rosenberger PH, Jokl P, Ickovics J, et al. Psychosocial factors and surgical outcomes: an evidence-based literature review. J Am Acad Orthop Surg 2006;14(7):397–405.
35. Williams JM. Sport psychology: past, present, future. In: Williams JM, editor. Applied sports psychology. 6th edition. Philadelphia: McGraw Hill Higher Education; 2009. p. 7–13.
36. Ahern DK, Lohr BA. Psychosocial factors in sports injury rehabilitation. Clin Sports Med 1997;16(4):755–68.
37. Williams JM, Andersen MB. Psychological antecedents of sport and injury: review and critique of the stress and injury model. J Appl Sport Psychol 1998;10:5–25.
38. Hahn RA, Teutsch SM, Rothenberg RB, et al. Excess deaths from nine chronic diseases in the United States. JAMA 1990;264:2654–9.
39. McGinnis JM, Foege WH. Actual causes of death in the United States. JAMA 1993;270:2207–12.
40. Helmrich SP, Ragland DR, Leung RW, et al. Physical activity and reduced occurrence of non-insulin-dependent diabetes mellitus. N Engl J Med 1991;325: 147–52.
41. Kodama S, Saito K, Tanaka S, et al. Cardiorespiratory fitness as a quantitative predictor of all-cause mortality and cardiovascular events in healthy men and women: a meta-analysis. JAMA 2009;301:2024.
42. Paffenbarger RS Jr, Hyde RT, Wing AL, et al. The association of changes in physical-activity level and other lifestyle characteristics with mortality among men. N Engl J Med 1993;328:538.
43. Simonsick EM. Fitness and cognition: encouraging findings and methodological considerations for future work. J Am Geriatr Soc 2003;51:570.
44. Coyle JT. Use it or lose it–do effortful mental activities protect against dementia? N Engl J Med 2003;348:2489.
45. Pate RR, Pratt M, Blair SN, et al. Physical activity and public health. A recommendation from the Centers for Disease Control and Prevention and the American College of Sports Medicine. JAMA 1995;273(5):402–7.
46. Martinsen EW. Physical activity and depression: clinical experience. Acta Psychiatr Scand 1994;377(Suppl):23–7.
47. Dimeo F, Bauer M, Varahram I, et al. Benefits from aerobic exercise in patients with major depression: a pilot study. Br J Sports Med 2001;35(2):114–7.
48. Dunn AL, Trivedi MH, O'Neal HA. Physical activity dose-response effects on outcomes of depression and anxiety. Med Sci Sports Exerc 2001;33(Suppl 6): 587–97.
49. Martinsen EW, Hoffart A, Solberg O. Aerobic and non-aerobic forms of exercise in the treatment of anxiety disorders. Stress Med 1989;5:115–20.
50. Paluska SA, Schwenk TL. Physical activity and mental health: current concepts. Sports Med 2000;29(3):167–80.
51. Mead GE, Morley W, Campbell P, et al. Exercise for depression. Cochrane Database Syst Rev 2009;(3):CD004366.
52. Krogh J, Nordentoft M, Sterne JA, et al. The effect of exercise in clinically depressed adults: systematic review and meta-analysis of randomized controlled trials. J Clin Psychiatry 2011;72(4):529–38.
53. Conn VS. Depressive symptom outcomes of physical activity interventions: meta-analysis findings. Ann Behav Med 2010;39(2):128–38.

54. Raglin JS. Exercise and mental health. Beneficial and detrimental effects. Sports Med 1990;9(6):323–9.
55. Ransford CP. A role for amines in the antidepressant effect of exercise: a review. Med Sci Sports Exerc 1982;4(1):1–10.
56. Morgan WP. Affective beneficence of vigorous physical activity. Med Sci Sports Exerc 1985;17:94–100.
57. North TC, McCullagh P, Tran ZV. Effect of exercise on depression. Exerc Sport Sci Rev 1990;18:379–415.
58. Peluso MA, Guerra de Andrade LH. Physical activity and mental health: the association between exercise and mood. Clinics (Sao Paulo) 2005;60(1):61–70.
59. Centers for Disease Control and Prevention (CDC). State-specific prevalence of obesity among adults–United States, 2005. MMWR Morb Mortal Wkly Rep 2006; 55(36):985–8.
60. Finkelstein E, Fiebelkorn I, Wang G. National medical expenditures attributable to overweight and obesity: how much and who's paying? Health Aff (Millwood) 2003;(Suppl Web Exclusives):W3-219-26.
61. Dunstan DR, Zimmet P, Welborn T, et al. Diabesity & associated disorders in Australia–2000: the accelerating epidemic. The Australian Diabetes, Obesity and Lifestyle Study (AusDiab). Melbourne (Victoria): International Diabetes Institute; 2001.
62. Colagiuri S, Lee CM, Colagiuri R, et al. The cost of overweight and obesity in Australia. Med J Aust 2010;192(5):260–4.
63. Anis AH, Zhang W, Bansback N, et al. Obesity and overweight in Canada: an updated cost-of-illness study. Obes Rev 2010;11(1):31–40.
64. Brug J, Lien N, Klepp KI, et al. Exploring overweight, obesity and their behavioural correlates among children and adolescents: results from the Health-promotion through Obesity Prevention across Europe project. Public Health Nutr 2010;13(10A):1676–9.
65. Kelly T, Yang W, Chen CS, et al. Global burden of obesity in 2005 and projections to 2030. Int J Obes (Lond) 2008;32(9):1431–7.
66. Ogden CL, Carroll MD, Kit BK, et al. Prevalence of obesity and trends in body mass index among US children and adolescents, 1999-2010. JAMA 2012;307:483.
67. Kopelman PG. Obesity as a medical problem. Nature 2000;404:635–43.
68. Whitaker RC, Wright JA, Pepe MS, et al. Predicting obesity in young adulthood from childhood and parental obesity. N Engl J Med 1997;337:869.
69. Singh AS, Chin A, Paw MJ, et al. Dutch obesity intervention in teenagers: effectiveness of a schoolbased program on body composition and behavior. Arch Pediatr Adolesc Med 2009;163(4):309–17.
70. Freedman DS, Khan LK, Serdula MK, et al. Racial differences in the tracking of childhood BMI to adulthood. Obes Res 2005;13(5):928–35.
71. Herman KM, Craig CL, Gauvin L, et al. Tracking of obesity and physical activity from childhood to adulthood: the Physical Activity Longitudinal Study. Int J Pediatr Obes 2009;4:281.
72. Oude Luttikhuis H, Baur L, Jansen H, et al. Interventions for treating obesity in children. Cochrane Database Syst Rev 2009;(1):CD001872.
73. Daniels SR. The consequences of childhood overweight and obesity. Future Child 2006;16(1):47–67.
74. Juonala M, Magnussen CG, Berenson GS, et al. Childhood adiposity, adult adiposity, and cardiovascular risk factors. N Engl J Med 2011;365:1876.
75. Strauss R. Childhood obesity and self-esteem. Pediatrics 2000;105:e15.

76. Dietz WH. Health consequences of obesity in youth: childhood predictors of adult disease. Pediatrics 1998;101(3 Pt 2):518–25.
77. Tripodi A, Severi S, Midili S, et al. "Community projects" in Modena (Italy): promote regular physical activity and healthy nutrition habits since childhood. Int J Pediatr Obes 2011;6(Suppl 2):54–6.
78. te Velde SJ, Twisk JW, Brug J. Tracking of fruit and vegetable consumption from adolescence into adulthood and its longitudinal association with overweight. Br J Nutr 2007;98(2):431–8.
79. Cleland V, Dwyer T, Venn A. Which domains of childhood physical activity predict physical activity in adulthood? A 20-year prospective tracking study. Br J Sports Med 2012;46(8):595–602.
80. Demory-Luce D, Morales M, Nicklas T, et al. Changes in food group consumption patterns from childhood to young adulthood: the Bogalusa Heart Study. J Am Diet Assoc 2004;104:1684–91.
81. Kimm SY, Glynn NW, Obarzanek E, et al. Relation between the changes in physical activity and body-mass index during adolescence: a multicentre longitudinal study. Lancet 2005;366:301–7.
82. Windle M, Grunbaum JA, Elliott M, et al. Healthy passages–a multilevel, multimethod longitudinal study of adolescent health. Am J Prev Med 2004;27: 164–72.
83. Biddle SJH, Fox KR. The way forward for physical activity and the promotion of psychological well-being. In: Biddle SJH, Fox KR, Boutcher SH, editors. Physical activity and psychological well-being. London: Routledge; 2000. p. 154–68.
84. Mahoney L, Carns B, Farmer T. Promoting interpersonal competence and educational success through extracurricular activity participation. J Educ Psychol 2003;95:409–18.
85. Rasberry CN, Lee SM, Robin L, et al. The association between school-based physical activity, including physical education, and academic performance: a systematic review of the literature. Prev Med 2011;52(Suppl 1):S10–20.
86. Singh A, Uijtdewilligen L, Twisk JW, et al. Physical activity and performance at school: a systematic review of the literature including a methodological quality assessment. Arch Pediatr Adolesc Med 2012;166(1):49–55.
87. Taras H. Physical activity and student performance at school. J Sch Health 2005;75:214–8.
88. Dwyer T, Sallis JF, Blizzard L. Relation of academic performance to physical activity and fitness in children. Pediatr Exerc Sci 2001;13:225–37.
89. Koivusilta LK, Nupponen H, Rimpelä AH. Adolescent physical activity predicts high education and socio-economic position in adulthood. Eur J Public Health 2012;22(2):203–9.
90. Aarnio M, Winter T, Kujala U, et al. Associations of health related behaviour, social relationships, and health status with persistent physical activity and inactivity: a study of Finnish adolescent twins. Br J Sports Med 2002;36:360–4.
91. Roslow Research Group. Physical education trends in our nation's schools a survey of practicing K-12 physical education teachers. National Association for Sport and Physical Education (NASPE); 2009. Available at: http://www.aahperd.org/naspe/about/announcements/upload/PE-Trends-Report.pdf. Accessed November 2, 2012.
92. Perna FM, Oh A, Chriqui JF, et al. The association of state law to physical education time allocation in US public schools. Am J Public Health 2012;102(8): 1594–9.

93. Joint Health Surveys Unit. Health survey for England 1998. London: HMSO; 1999.
94. Haskell WL, Lee IM, Pate RR, et al. Physical activity and public health updated recommendation for adults from the American College of Sports Medicine and the American Heart Association. Med Sci Sports Exerc 2007;39(8):1423–34.
95. Allender S, Cowburn G, Foster C. Understanding participation in sport and physical activity among children and adults: a review of qualitative studies. Health Educ Res 2006;21(6):826–35.
96. Lobstein T, Bauer L, Uauy R. Obesity in children and young people: a crisis in public health. Obes Rev 2004;5(Suppl 1):1–104.
97. Ogden CL, Flegal KM, Carroll MD, et al. Prevalence and trends in overweight among US children and adolescents, 1999–2000. JAMA 2002;288:1728–32.
98. Vinsel D. Shedding old habits to create a new future. Interactive program targets childhood obesity by teaching healthy lifestyle choices. Healthc Exec 2010; 25(3):70, 72.
99. Hoelscher DM, Springer AE, Ranjit N, et al. Reductions in child obesity among disadvantaged school children with community involvement: the Travis County CATCH Trial. Obesity (Silver Spring) 2010;18(Suppl 1):S36–44.
100. Dzewaltowski DA, Rosenkranz RR, Geller KS, et al. HOP'N after-school project: an obesity prevention randomized controlled trial. Int J Behav Nutr Phys Act 2010;7:90.
101. Croker H, Viner RM, Nicholls D, et al. Family-based behavioural treatment of childhood obesity in a UK National Health Service setting: randomized controlled trial. Int J Obes (Lond) 2012;36(1):16–26.
102. Doak CM, Visscher TL, Renders CM, et al. The prevention of overweight and obesity in children and adolescents: a review of interventions and programmes. Obes Rev 2006;7:111–36.
103. Campbell K, Waters E, O'Meara S, et al. Interventions for preventing obesity in childhood. A systematic review. Obes Rev 2001;2:149–57.
104. Hardeman W, Griffin S, Johnston M, et al. Interventions to prevent weight gain: a systematic review of psychological models and behaviour change methods. Int J Obes Relat Metab Disord 2000;24:131–43.
105. Waters E, de Silva-Sanigorski A, Hall BJ, et al. Interventions for preventing obesity in children. Cochrane Database Syst Rev 2011;(12):CD001871.
106. Summerbell CD, Moore HJ, Vögele C, et al. Evidence-based recommendations for the development of obesity prevention programs targeted at preschool children. ToyBox-study group. Obes Rev 2012;13(Suppl 1):129–32.
107. Doak C, Heitmann B, Summerbell C, et al. Prevention of childhood obesity–what type of evidence should we consider relevant? Obes Rev 2009;10:350–6.
108. Haerens L, Vereecken C, Maes L, et al. Relationship of physical activity and dietary habits with body mass index in the transition from childhood to adolescence: a 4-year longitudinal study. Public Health Nutr 2010;13(10A):1722–8.
109. Robinson TN. Television viewing and childhood obesity. Pediatr Clin North Am 2001;48:1017–25.
110. Gortmaker SL, Cheung LW, Peterson KE, et al. Impact of a school-based interdisciplinary intervention on diet and physical activity among urban primary school children: eat well and keep moving. Arch Pediatr Adolesc Med 1999; 153:975–83.
111. James J, Thomas P, Cavan D, et al. Preventing childhood obesity by reducing consumption of carbonated drinks: cluster randomized controlled trial. BMJ 2004;328:1237.

112. Krebs NF, Jacobson MS. Prevention of pediatric overweight and obesity. Pediatrics 2003;112(2):424–30.
113. Holt N, Schetzina KE, Dalton WT 3rd, et al. Primary care practice addressing child overweight and obesity: a survey of primary care physicians at four clinics in southern Appalachia. South Med J 2011;104(1):14–9.
114. American Dietetic Association (ADA). Position of the American Dietetic Association: individual-, family-, school-, and community-based interventions for pediatric overweight. J Am Diet Assoc 2006;106(6):925–45.
115. Latzer Y, Edmunds L, Fenig S, et al. Managing childhood overweight: behavior, family, pharmacology, and bariatric surgery interventions. Obesity 2008;17: 411–23.
116. Wilfley DE, Tibbs TL, Van Buren DJ, et al. Lifestyle interventions in the treatment of childhood overweight: a meta-analytic review of randomized controlled trials. Health Psychol 2007;26(5):521–32.
117. Young KM, Northern JJ, Lister KM, et al. A meta-analysis of family-behavioral weight-loss treatments for children. Clin Psychol Rev 2007;27:240–9.
118. Gunnarsdottir T, Njardvik U, Olafsdottir AS, et al. The role of parental motivation in family-based treatment for childhood obesity. Obesity (Silver Spring) 2011; 19(8):1654–62.
119. Wilfley DE, Kass AE, Kolko RP. Counseling and behavior change in pediatric obesity. Pediatr Clin North Am 2011;58(6):1403–24, x.
120. Vander Wal JS. Night eating syndrome: a critical review of the literature. Clin Psychol Rev 2012;32(1):49–59.
121. Glass TA, McAtee MJ. Behavioral science at the crossroads in public health: extending horizons, envisioning the future. Soc Sci Med 2006;62(7):1650–71.
122. Huang TT, Drewnosksi A, Kumanyika S, et al. A systems-oriented multilevel framework for addressing obesity in the 21st century. Prev Chronic Dis 2009; 6(3):A82.
123. Kumanyika SK, Obarzanek E, Stettler N, et al. Population-based prevention of obesity: the need for comprehensive promotion of healthful eating, physical activity, and energy balance: a scientific statement from American Heart Association Council on Epidemiology and Prevention, Interdisciplinary Committee for Prevention (formerly the Expert Panel on Population and Prevention Science). Circulation 2008;118(4):428–64.
124. Wilfley DE, Stein RI, Saelens BE, et al. Efficacy of maintenance treatment approaches for childhood overweight: a randomized controlled trial. JAMA 2007;298(14):1661–73.
125. Dorsey KB, Mauldon M, Magraw R, et al. Applying practice recommendations for the prevention and treatment of obesity in children and adolescents. Clin Pediatr (Phila) 2010;49(2):137–45.
126. Smith RE, Smoll FL, Curtis B. Coach effectiveness training: a cognitive-behavioral approach to enhancing relationship skills in youth sport coaches. J Sport Psychol 1979;1:59–75.
127. Smoll FL, Smith RE. Coaching behavior research and intervention in youth sports. In: Smoll FL, Smith RE, editors. Children and youth in sport: a biopsychosocial perspective. Dubuque (IA): Kendall-Hunt; 2002. p. 211–33.
128. Coatsworth JD, Conroy DE. Enhancing the self-esteem of youth swimmers through coach training: gender and age effects. Psychol Sport Exerc 2006;7: 173–92.
129. Barnett NP, Smoll FL, Smith RE. Effects of enhancing coach-athlete relationships on youth sport attrition. Sport Psychol 1992;6:111–27.

130. Allender S, Foster C, Scarborough P, et al. The burden of physical activity-related ill health in the UK. J Epidemiol Community Health 2007;61:344–8.
131. Hughes L, Leavey G. Setting the bar: athletes and vulnerability to mental illness. Br J Psychiatry 2012;200(2):95–6.
132. Telama R, Yang X. Decline of physical activity from youth to young adulthood in Finland. Med Sci Sports Exerc 2000;32:1617–22.

Medicolegal Aspects of Sports Medicine

Blake R. Boggess, DO[a], Jeffrey R. Bytomski, DO[b,*]

KEYWORDS

• Law • Liability • Sports medicine

KEY POINTS

- Legal issues in sports medicine are rapidly developing and establishing an important body of jurisprudence that defines the legal rights and duties of all those involved with protecting the health and safety of athletes.
- The law makes important distinctions between the relevant duty of care owed to high-school, college, and professional athletes because of the differing legal relationships that arise out of athletic participation at different levels of competition.

INTRODUCTION

The standards of care for providing medical services in sports medicine are rapidly evolving and expanding with each year. New position statements, updates of earlier position statements, new technologies, and new methods and modalities of treatment are introduced frequently. A variety of health care professionals are involved in sports medicine. These professionals include family physicians, orthopedic surgeons, internists, physiatrists, pediatricians, neurologists, physical therapists, athletic trainers, chiropractors, psychologists, dentists, nutritionists, dieticians, and physiologists. Although sports medicine services have been growing in recent years, so has the unprecedented growth of claims and lawsuits arising out of the practice of sports medicine. It behooves all members of the sports medicine team to become familiar with their potential legal and professional liabilities.

The recent tragic deaths of Minnesota Vikings offensive lineman Korey Stringer and Northwestern University football player Rashidi Wheeler raise important legal issues concerning the medical care provided to athletes. Since 1990, there has been a significant increase in sports medicine–related litigation.[1] Because of the increasing economic benefits of playing sports, such as college scholarships or multimillion-dollar professional contracts, injured athletes have a strong incentive

[a] Department of Orthopedics, Duke University Medical Center, 103 Cypress Mill Road, Morrisville, NC 27560, USA; [b] Department Community and Family Medicine, Duke University Medical Center, 103 Cypress Mill Road, Morrisville, NC 27560, USA
* Correponding author.
E-mail address: bytom001@mc.duke.edu

Prim Care Clin Office Pract 40 (2013) 525–535
http://dx.doi.org/10.1016/j.pop.2013.02.008 **primarycare.theclinics.com**
0095-4543/13/$ – see front matter

to seek compensation for harm caused by negligent sports medicine care rendered by team physicians, athletic trainers, and others.

DEFINITION OF SPORTS MEDICINE

Many consider the term sports medicine to apply to the health care professionals who provide professional services to those who participate in athletic activities. Sports medicine, a recognized medical subspecialty of the American Board of Medical Specialties, also includes prescribing exercise and recommending exercise equipment. The American Osteopathic Academy of Sports Medicine (AOASM) defines sports medicine as "that branch of the healing arts profession that uses an holistic, comprehensive team approach to the prevention, diagnosis, and adequate management (including medical, surgical and rehabilitative techniques) of sports and exercise-related injuries, disorders, dysfunctions, and exercise-related disease processes."

The sports medicine team is usually, and should be, composed of several members from a variety of backgrounds and training. Given the broad range of people involved, it is important to develop an organized structure of responsibilities and duties of each member. Each member should also know their limitations, the standard of care, and the limitations to their practice.

THE STANDARD OF CARE

Team physicians have a legal duty to conform to the standard of care corresponding to their specialty training. For example, an orthopedic surgeon should be held to the standard of an orthopedist certified in sports medicine if they are providing care for high-level athletes. A physician certified by the American Boards of Emergency Medicine, Internal Medicine, Family Practice, Pediatrics, or Physical Medicine and Rehabilitation may earn a certificate of added qualification in sports medicine by passing a written examination and is held to the standards conferred by this certification. Certification is tied to their primary board certification.

In malpractice suits involving a medical specialist, the trend is to apply a national standard of care because national specialty certification boards exist to ensure standardized training and certification procedures. A national standard of care for team physicians is preferable because appropriate sports medicine care and treatment should not vary depending on the area of practice. The applicable legal standard of physician conduct is good medical practice within the physician's type of practice. What is commonly done by physicians in the same specialty generally serves as the standard by which a physician's actions are measured. What should have been done under the circumstances, not what is commonly done, determines applicable standard. Physicians have a legal obligation to keep up to date on new guidelines and advances in sports medicine, and they may be liable for using outdated treatment methods that no longer have a sound medical basis or that do not currently constitute appropriate care.[2]

To determine acceptable medical practice, a medical expert may use their own education, training, and experience, as well as any relevant medical literature and medical association guidelines.

The standard of care may be difficult to establish, because of the many medical and allied health professionals caring for athletes. The standard at any time is influenced by various sources, including published statements from professional associations, government policies, and state and national government regulations.[3] The amount of research and development of new treatment and techniques makes it challenging for the sports medicine provider to stay up to date. Without knowledge of the most current standards and the incorporation of these into operating procedures and protocols, the sports medicine team may be at risk for legal issues coming from personal injury lawsuits.

MEMBERS OF THE SPORTS MEDICINE TEAM

Team Physician

The National Collegiate Athletic Association (NCAA) Sports Medicine Handbook outlines the role of the team physician as follows: "The team physician and athletic health care team should assume responsibility for developing an appropriate injury prevention program and providing quality sports medicine care to injured student-athletes."[4] The team physician is responsible for minimizing athletic injuries by thorough preparticipation screening, exemplary medical care using state-of-the-art technology, and careful evaluation of athletes before return to play is allowed.

The team physician is required to provide high-quality sports medicine care and to minimize personal and institutional liability. Specifically, the team physician's duties include determining: (1) the athlete's medical eligibility for participation; (2) the athlete's medical eligibility to resume athletic participation after injury; (3) the availability of medical services; (4) the supervision of personnel providing athletic health care services; (5) the selection of training practices with health implications; and (6) protection against legal liability.[5]

Expert testimony in sports medicine litigation usually focuses on whether the practitioner adhered to the proper professional standard of care and whether their care or advice was below the standard of care and thereby negligently led to injury.

Professional teams and colleges usually hire a physician or a group of physicians to provide medical care to their athletes. Many high schools also select a physician to provide preparticipation physical examinations and emergency medical care to athletes participating in athletics. A team physician provides medical services to athletes that are arranged, or paid for, at least in part, by an institution or entity other than the patient or their parent or guardian.[6] Team physicians may or may not receive monetary compensation for their time. The team physician's primary responsibility is to provide care for the athlete and be mindful of the best interest of the athlete. Specific responsibilities may include providing preseason physical examinations; providing medical clearance for an athlete to play the sport; and diagnosing, treating, and rehabilitating athletic injuries. The team physician may also be responsible for overseeing all sports medicine services provided to a team's athletes and for the supervision of physician assistants, athletic trainers, student assistants, physical therapists, and nurses providing medical care to athletes.

Although one of the team physician's responsibilities is to avoid the unnecessary restriction of sports participation, their foremost duty should be to protect the athlete's health. Team physicians may face pressure from parents, coaches, team management, fans, or the athlete to provide medical clearance to participate or treatment enabling immediate return to play. However, the team physician's judgment should be governed by current medical practice, instead of the team's need for the services of the player or the athlete's desire to play.

Physical Therapists and Chiropractors

Physical therapists often provide sports medicine care to athletes by screening or rehabilitating injuries. State licensing laws specifically define the authorized scope of physical therapy practice. If a physical therapist participates in the unauthorized practice of medicine and injures an athlete, they may be held to the standard of care required of a physician under similar circumstances.[7]

This was the case in Brown v Shyne. This case involved a chiropractor who claimed to be able to treat and diagnose conditions that were beyond the scope of his medical license. Shyne, a practicing chiropractor, treated Brown for laryngitis. Shyne did not have a license to practice medicine but claimed to possess skills necessary for diagnosis and treatment of disease. Shyne was convicted of a misdemeanor for practicing medicine without a license because Brown was harmed by Shyne's treatments.[7]

In most states, physical therapists are not licensed to diagnose an athletic injury or begin treatment without a prescription or referral from a physician. In Lavergne v Louisiana State Board of Medical Examiners,[8] a Louisiana appellate court made a distinction under the state's Physical Therapy Practice Act between permissible evaluation of the need for physical therapy and impermissible unauthorized medical diagnosis and treatment. Although voluntarily screening injuries incurred during athletic events for local high schools, a therapist examined a basketball player's injured ankle, performed a heel strike test, and concluded that his ankle was not broken. He advised the player to ice his ankle and seek treatment from a physician if he continued to experience pain. The Louisiana State Board of Medical Examiners placed the therapist on probation for 2 years for evaluating the athlete's injury before a physician examined the athlete. Although the State Board of Medical Examiners did sanction the therapist, the courts disagreed. The court found that the therapist's conduct did not constitute unauthorized medical diagnosis or treatment because he did not hold himself out as a physician, prescribe medication, suggest that the athlete needed physical therapy, or bandage or radiograph his ankle. The court concluded that instructing the athlete to keep ice on his ankle was permissible and appropriate advice by the therapist and invalidated the Board's disciplinary sanction. However, despite the court's overturn, the point remains that medical providers are legally at fault should they practice outside their realm of expertise.

The law permits physical therapists to establish the standard of care for rehabilitating injured athletes. In all areas of practice, a therapist must use the care and skill ordinarily possessed by competent members of the physical therapy profession. The American Physical Therapy Association allows a licensed physical therapist to receive certification as a specialist in sports physical therapy. Therapists who are certified in sports physical therapy may present themselves as having special expertise in treating athletic injuries and can be held to a higher standard of care than those in the general practice of physical therapy.

Athletic Trainers

Athletic trainers usually provide a variety of sports medicine services to athletes such as physical conditioning, injury prevention, emergency medical care, and injury rehabilitation. The National Athletic Trainers Association is the certifying body for athletic trainers. Many states require that athletic trainers be licensed, define the authorized scope of their practice, or otherwise regulate the profession. State law may require a physician to prescribe or supervise certain medical treatment provided to an athlete by an athletic trainer.

In Searles v Trustees of St Joseph's College, the Maine Supreme Court held that an athletic trainer "has the duty to conform to the standard of care required of an ordinary careful trainer" when providing care and treatment to athletes.[9] The court ruled that a trainer may incur negligence liability for failing to communicate the severity of a player's injuries to the team's coach, or for failing to advise an athlete that they should not continue playing with their medical condition. Team physicians should check with their particular state for the laws that govern physician trainer oversight and the scope of the trainer's ability to operate independently.

The following is an example of a supervision agreement between physician and athletic trainer from Pennsylvania[10]:

As team physician/consulting physician, I supervise the certified athletic trainer(s) named in their/his/her provision of athletic training services under my direction while employed by/working at (location).*

**Direction is defined by the PA Medical and Osteopathic Practice Acts, 49 PA. CODE, CHAPTERS 16, 18, AND 25 as… supervision over the actions of a certified athletic trainer by means of referral by prescription to treat conditions for a physically active person or written protocol approved by a supervising physician, or by direct consultation via radio, telephone, fax, email or other accepted means.*[11]

At all times, the certified athletic trainer(s) listed above will act within the scope of practice of his/her/their education and training as defined in the Rules and Regulations of the Pennsylvania Medical and Osteopathic Practice Acts: http://www.dos.state.pa.us/bpoa/cwp/view.asp?a=1104&q=432799 (see pages 5–7 of enclosure for further clarification of the State Boards' practice act) and as further delineated in the National Athletic Trainers' Association (NATA) Guide to Athletic Training Services: http://www.nata.org/sites/default/files/GuideToAthleticTrainingServices.pdf. The Certified Athletic Trainer will maintain communication with me, at defined intervals, via phone call, messaging, email, or face to face meeting.

In Jarreau v Orleans Parish School Board,[12] the Louisiana Court of Appeals upheld a jury finding that a high-school football team's trainer negligently failed to refer a player with a wrist injury to an orthopedist until after the season ended. The athlete complained that his wrist continued to hurt and was swollen, but he was not withheld from competition although his "play was adversely affected by the injury." The trainer's delay in referring the player for treatment of his fracture necessitated an extended period of treatment and caused a permanent disability.

Applying contributory negligence principles, the court found the player to be one-third at fault for failing to consult his own physician or requesting that he be referred to a school physician.

Naturally, team physicians are responsible for treatments they approve. One case showing this situation is the case of Marc Buoniconti, a former linebacker for The Citadel, who sued the university along with its team physician and athletic trainer, seeking damages for permanent paralysis suffered while making a tackle during a football game. Buoniconti had injured his neck during 3 previous games and had failed to recover completely with therapy.

Believing that Buoniconti had suffered an extension injury to his neck, the team's athletic trainer fixed a 25.4-cm (10-inch) elastic strap to the face guard of Buoniconti's helmet and connected it to the front of his shoulder pads. The device prevented Buoniconti's head from going back (essentially putting him in a spear tackling posture) and was approved by the team physician. While making a tackle with his head constrained by this device, Buoniconti broke his neck and was rendered a quadriplegic.

Buoniconti claimed that the team trainer and physician were negligent for permitting him to play with a serious neck injury and with equipment that placed his neck in a position at risk for being broken. Before trial, Buoniconti settled his claims against The Citadel and its trainer for $800,000.

In some instances, a negligence action against an athletic trainer employed by a public educational institution may be barred by state laws granting public employees qualified immunity. In Lennon v Petersen, the Alabama Supreme Court held that a college soccer player could not sue a university-employed athletic trainer for alleged negligent treatment of an injury. The court rejected the plaintiff's contention that the athletic trainer was not entitled to immunity because she exceeded her authority by practicing medicine without a license.

The court decided that as an athletic trainer, she had the responsibility to determine whether an athlete was faking or hiding an injury. She had to ascertain the source of the injury, the extent of the injury, and the treatment of the injury. She had to calculate whether the injury was adequately responding to treatment. She had the further responsibility of determining when an athlete should be restricted from play, referred to a doctor, or allowed to return to the field. Because all of these functions required the use of her judgment and discretion, she is entitled to discretionary functional immunity.

PRACTICE AND GAME COVERAGE: MEDICOLEGAL OBLIGATIONS

The medicolegal aspects of sport participation dictate appropriate game and practice coverage regarding the care of the athlete. The sports medicine team must be prepared to quickly take care of any injury or emergency that could compromise an athlete's health. All personnel who are associated with medical coverage of practices, competitions, skill instruction, and strength and conditioning should be at least minimally qualified through certification in cardiopulmonary resuscitation, first-aid techniques, and the prevention of disease transmission.[13]

According to the 2012 to 2013 NCAA Sports Medicine Handbook, an emergency action plan should be in place for each venue and should "incorporate roles and responsibilities of coaching staff, medical staff, spectators and others during injury evaluation/response on the field, to assure appropriate first response and medical evaluation. Institutions should have on file, and annually update, an emergency action plan for each athletics venue to respond to student-athlete catastrophic injuries and illnesses, including but not limited to: concussions, heat illness, spine injury, cardiac arrest, respiratory distress (eg, asthma), and Sickle Cell Trait (SCT) collapses. All athletics health care providers and coaches, including strength and conditioning coaches, sport coaches and all athletics personnel conducting activities with student-athletes should review and practice the plan at least annually."[4]

Although it may not be possible for a physician to be present at all workouts and practices, properly trained personnel, such as a certified athletic trainer, should provide prompt evaluation and emergency care when warranted. Oversight of these duties is the responsibility of the team physician.[14] The NCAA Sports Medicine Handbook specifically recommends that each scheduled practice or contest of an institution-sponsored intercollegiate athletics event, and all out of season practices and skills sessions, should include the presence of a person qualified and delegated to render emergency care to a stricken participant, and the presence or planned access to a physician for prompt medical evaluation of the situation, when warranted.

An example of an improperly implemented emergency plan is shown in the case of Mogabgab v Orleans Parish School Board.[15] In this case, a high-school player sustained prolonged heat stress during practice, which was not noted or treated by the coaches in a timely fashion and which led to his death. The facts reported in court were dramatic, in that no medical professionals were notified until an hour and

20 minutes after the athlete became unconscious. Medical treatment did not commence until approximately 2 hours after the boy became sick. This incident shows that all members of the sports medicine team, including coaches, must be prepared to deal promptly with health emergencies. Institutions sponsoring athletic events must ensure that they have a written emergency action plan, and the sports medicine team must be able to implement it in the event of an emergency.

University Legal Obligation to Provide Emergency Medical Coverage

Further discussion of this issue is seen in the case of Kleinknecht v Gettysburg College, which focused on whether a university should provide student-athletes with emergency medical care for serious injury incurred during participation in school-sponsored sports.[16] During practice, a lacrosse player suffered a cardiac arrest and subsequently died. A review of the incident showed that no certified athletic trainer or student athletic trainer was present, neither coach present was trained in cardiopulmonary resuscitation, and no radio or phone telephone was accessible on the practice field. The nearest telephone was 60 to 76 m (200–250 feet) away, with the shortest route requiring an individual to scale a 2.4-m-high (8-foot) fence. The court determined that the university had a legal obligation and responsibility to provide appropriate medical coverage to ensure prompt and effective treatment in the event of a life-threatening injury.

The plaintiff's case focused on the fact that the athlete was not engaged in personal activity, but rather was engaged in a school-sponsored activity, for which he had been recruited to advance the athletic success of the institution. Furthermore, it was decided that a foreseeable risk of serious or life-threatening injury exists for any student-athlete who is engaged in an intercollegiate athletic event. Therefore, colleges and universities must protect themselves against such risk by providing appropriate supervision and prompt and adequate emergency medical care. This case established a legal precedence, whereby adequate emergency medical care must be provided to student-athletes involved in any institutionally organized athletic activity.[13]

Risk Management Recommendations

Risk management is the key for preventing lawsuits in sports medicine. Risk management is a method intended to prevent financial, physical, property, and time loss for a group or organization. Factors proved to aid in risk management and liability reduction include maintaining clinical competence, keeping accurate medical records, and appropriate communication among sports medicine team members.[17] A well-designed risk management program should cover 4 essential elements: compassion, communication, competence, and charting.[18] Maintaining clinical competence and keeping accurate medical records are other important means to avoid liability for malpractice. Studies show that 70% of the medical litigations are caused by poor communication and attitude problems presented by physicians or trainers.[18]

Policies and Procedures

All sports medicine facilities and settings must have written policies and procedures that are reviewed and practiced regularly. These plans should correlate to the type of potential risk from the athletic event and at the particular location. Each program should have policies and procedures that provide a blueprint for actions that need to be taken by any member of the sports medicine team. The policies and procedures documents should be written in conjunction with legal council and appropriate medical and professional standards. The documents should include not only a hierarchical system for evaluation and treatment but also staffing and emergency response protocols and procedures.[4]

Informed Consent

Informed consent implies that the provider discloses the diagnosis, the nature and purpose of any proposed treatment, the risks and benefits of the treatment, any reasonably treatment alternatives, and the prognosis if the proposed treatment is not performed.[19] The landmark Canterbury case, and many of the cases decided in the 1970s regarding informed consent, called for disclosure of information beyond what physicians traditionally had provided for patients and what the law had required previously.[20] Despite the physician's required explanation of prognosis, a detailed statistical discussion of prognosis is not required, and the courts have not required physicians to provide detailed statistical information on a patient's prognosis or other aspects of the treatment that was performed.[21] The team physician is best protected by documenting the following points when performing an informed consent with a patient: (1) an oral review of all probable risks, and documentation signed by the patient indicating that these risks and benefits of the treatment were discussed; and (2) a catch-all provision to the informed consent that documents, in general terms, the additional or other potential risks or injuries that might occur and any reasonable treatment alternatives.[22] When proper informed consent is obtained with proper documentation, it generally protects the institution and physician from successful litigation.

Consent may be implied under certain circumstances, such as when an athlete is unconscious from a concussion and needs emergency medical treatment.[23] In these cases, the law generally assumes that if the injured athlete had not been injured, they would have authorized the treatment.

Preparticipation Examinations

The sports medicine practitioner traditionally conducts preparticipation physical examinations (PPEs) of athletes seeking medical clearance before participating in sports. The primary purpose of the PPE is to identify an athlete who may be at risk of injury to themselves or others before participation. The PPE has multiple objectives, including collecting basic medical data, determining athletic eligibility, serving as a primary examination for medically underserved populations, and enabling the detection of medical conditions that may not preclude the athlete's participation in sports but still require attention.[24]

The right to disqualify an athlete from athletic participation during a PPE has been upheld in the courts. This was the case in Knapp v Northwestern University.[25] In this case, Nicholas Knapp, a high-school senior, collapsed in cardiac arrest at the end of a pickup basketball game. He had documented ventricular fibrillation and returned to sinus rhythm after electrical defibrillation. An implantable cardioverter-defibrillator was placed 10 days after the cardiac arrest. Before the cardiac arrest, Knapp had accepted a basketball scholarship at Northwestern University. The university's team physicians disqualified him from participation shortly after Knapp enrolled in the autumn of 1995. The physicians determined that participation in college basketball would produce an unacceptable risk of sudden death and would be contrary to the 26th Bethesda Conference guidelines for participation with cardiovascular abnormalities. He was allowed to keep his full athletic scholarship for 4 years. Knapp filed suit that Northwestern University had violated the Rehabilitation Act of 1973, which prohibits discrimination against an athlete who is disabled yet has the capabilities to play a competitive sport. The court ruled in favor of Northwestern University and emphasized that it is proper for the team physician to rely on medical guidelines and recommendations such as the Bethesda guidelines in clearing an athlete for participation.

The Medicolegal Aspects of Returning to Play

After an athlete is injured, it is within the team physician's medical judgment to decide whether the athlete can return to athletic participation safely. The team physician has the primary duty to protect the athlete and is charged with this responsibility because of their relationship with the athlete and association with the representative institution.[22]

Litigation may arise when a team physician releases an athlete to return to play and subsequently the athlete sustains an additional injury. The athlete may hold the physician responsible, contending that they should have been withheld from athletic participation.[26]

In their 1990 lawsuit, Hank Gathers' heirs alleged that the team physician and consulting specialists improperly cleared him to resume playing college basketball with a serious heart condition. Plaintiffs also alleged that the defendant physicians not only negligently diagnosed and treated Gathers but also that the defendants conspired to intentionally fail to inform Gathers of the seriousness of his heart condition and of the dangers of continuing to play competitive basketball.

Some athletes have sued physicians for refusing to provide them with medical clearance to play a sport. In Penny v Sands, Anthony Penny claimed that a cardiologist was negligent for withholding his medical clearance to play college basketball with a potentially life-threatening heart condition.[27] The defendant cardiologist diagnosed Penny as having hypertrophic cardiomyopathy and disqualified him from participation in college basketball. Two other cardiologists were consulted and agreed with the opinion. Central Connecticut State University refused to allow Penny participate in its basketball program for 2 years. Penny eventually got clearance to play basketball from 2 other cardiologists. Penny claimed economic harm to his potential professional basketball career because he missed out from 2 seasons of college basketball. Penny subsequently collapsed and died suddenly while playing in a 1990 professional basketball game in England. Although the malpractice suit was voluntarily dismissed after his death, it is unlikely that a court would have awarded Penny's survivors compensation for economic loss after team officials accepted a physician's prudent recommendation that an athlete with established cardiac disease should be disqualified from competitive sports to reduce the risk of sudden death.[28]

Dispensing Medications to Athletes

When prescribing drugs to athletes, team physicians should comply with all laws regarding dispensation and record keeping and should follow accepted medical practices regarding the appropriate type and dosage of pharmaceutical treatment.[29] Team physicians may be liable for negligently prescribing anesthetics or painkillers to athletes to accelerate return to play.[17]

Confidentiality

The Health Insurance Portability and Accountability Act (HIPAA) regulates the way the team physicians and members of the health care team communicate and handle patient medical information. Two categories in the final rules of the HIPAA statutes that most likely affect the sports medicine practitioner are consent for treatment and authorization to release information. It is imperative that the team physician becomes familiar with these, and all, regulations. Any final interpretations of this act should be left to the institution's legal counsel and reviewed under applicable state law.[23]

Unauthorized disclosure of information about an athlete's medical condition to third parties such as the media violates a physician's ethical obligation to maintain patient confidences.[30] In addition, such unauthorized disclosure may expose the physician to legal liability for invasion of privacy and for defamation or intentional infliction of emotional distress if the information is false.[31]

In Chuy v Philadelphia Eagles Football Club, a football player alleged that the team physician defamed him by falsely informing the media that he had a potentially fatal blood disease and also caused him to suffer severe emotional distress.[31]

At the beginning of each season, many institutions require athletes to sign a waiver to seek permission to communicate the medical management of an athlete's injury between the athletic trainers, coaching staff, team physician, and the rest of the sports medicine team. This waiver does not allow for discussion with individuals not involved in the management of the athlete's health care such as media, sports information departments, and so forth.

SUMMARY

Legal issues in sports medicine are rapidly developing and establishing an important body of jurisprudence that defines the legal rights and duties of all those involved with protecting the health and safety of athletes. The law makes important distinctions between the relevant duty of care owed to high-school, college, and professional athletes, because of the differing legal relationships that arise out of athletic participation at different levels of competition.

REFERENCES

1. Isaacs CA. Comment. Conflicts of interest for team physicians: a retrospective in light of Gathers v. Loyola Marymount University. Albany Law J Sci Technol 1992;2: 147–63.
2. Nowatske v Osterloh, 543 NW2d 265, 271–74 (Wisc 1996).
3. AOSSM: ACSM, AMSSM, AAOS, AAFP, AOASM. Team Physician Consensus Statement. From the project-based alliance for the advancement of clinical sports medicine, comprised of the American Academy of Family Physicians, the American Academy of Orthopaedic Surgeons, the American College of Sports Medicine, the American Medical Society for Sports Medicine, the American Orthopaedic Society for Sports Medicine, and the American Osteopathic Academy of Sports Medicine. 2001. Available at: http://www.sportsmed.org/uploadedFiles/Content/Medical_Professionals/Professional_Educational_Resources/Publications_and_Resources/Consensus_Statements/CS_TeamPhysician.pdf. Accessed December 2, 2012.
4. NCAA 2011–2012 sports medicine handbook. 22nd edition. 2011. Available at: http://www.ncaapublications.com/productdownloads/MD11.pdf. Accessed December 1, 2012.
5. Bottomley M. Athletes at an overseas venue: the role of the team doctor. In: Payne S, editor. Medicine, sport and the law. Oxford (United Kingdom): Blackwell Scientific Publications; 1990. p. 158–65.
6. King JH. The duty and standard of care for team physicians. Houst Law Rev 1981;18(4):657–705.
7. Brown v Shyne, 151 NE 197, 199 (NY 1926).
8. 539 So2d 656 (La Ct App 1989).

9. Paul Searles v. Trustees of St Joseph's College, et al. Maine Supreme Judicial Court Reporter of Decisions. 1997. Available at: http://www.courts.state.me.us/opinions_orders/opinions/documents/97me128s.htm. Accessed December 1, 2012.
10. Pennsylvania Athletic Trainers Organization. Essential information and resources. Athletic trainer written physician supervising agreement. 2010. Available at: http://gopats.org/legisl-info/resources.htm. Accessed December 2, 2012.
11. The PA Code. Subchapter H. Athletic trainers. Available at: http://www.pacode.com/secure/data/049/chapter18/subchapHtoc.html. Accessed December 2, 2012.
12. Osborne B. Principles of liability for athletic trainers: managing sport-related concussion. J Athl Train 2001;36(3):316–21.
13. Anderson J, Courson R, Kleiner D, et al. National athletic trainers association position statement: emergency planning in athletes. J Athl Train 2002;37:99–104.
14. Herbert D. Medico-legal concerns and risk management suggestions for medical directors of exercise rehabilitation and maintenance programs. Exerc Stand Malprac Rep 1989;3:44–8.
15. Mogabgab v Orleans Parish School Board, 239 So2d 456 (Court of Appeals, Los Angeles, 1970).
16. Kleinknecht v Gettysburg College, US Court of Appeals, 989 F2d 1360 (3rd Cir 1993).
17. Herbert DL. Legal aspects of sports medicine. 2nd edition. PRC Publishing; 1995.
18. Gallup EM. Law and the team physician. Champaign (IL): Human Kinetics; 1995.
19. Rosoff A. Informed consent in the electronic age. Am J Law Med 1999;25:367–86.
20. Canterbury v Spence, 464 F2nd 772, 780n 15 (DC Cir 1972).
21. Appenzeller H. Managing sports and risk management strategies. Durham (NC): Carolina Academic Press; 1993. p. 99–110.
22. Pearsall AW IV, Kovaleski JE, Madanagopal SG. Medicolegal issues affecting sports medicine practitioners. Clin Orthop Relat Res 2005;(433):50–7.
23. US Department of Health and Human Services. Health information privacy. The Health Insurance Portability and Accountability Act of 1996 (HIPAA) privacy and security rules. Available at: http://www.hhs.gov/ocr/privacy/. Accessed November 29, 2012.
24. Glover DW, Maron BJ. Profile of preparticipation cardiovascular screening for high school athletes. JAMA 1998;279:1817–9.
25. Knapp v Northwestern University, 101 F3d 473 (7th Cir 1996).
26. Herbert DL. The death of Hank Gathers: an examination of the legal issues. Sports Med Stand Malprac Rep 1991;2(3):41–6.
27. Penny v Sands (D Conn Filed May 3, 1989) (No. H89–280).
28. Paterick TE, Paterick TJ, Fletcher GF, et al. Medical and legal issues in the cardiovascular evaluation of competitive athletes. JAMA 2005;294(23):3011–8.
29. Wallace v Broyles, 961 SW2d 712, 719 (Ark 1998).
30. Home v Patton, 287 So2d 824 (Ala 1973).
31. Chuy v Phila Eagles Football Club, 595 F2d 1265, 1273–81 (3d Cir 1979).

Index

Note: Page numbers of article titles are in **boldface** type.

Prim Care Clin Office Pract 40 (2013) 537–556
http://dx.doi.org/10.1016/S0095-4543(13)00040-7 primarycare.theclinics.com
0095-4543/13/$ – see front matter

L

M

S

U

V

W

Z

Printed and bound by CPI Group (UK) Ltd, Croydon, CR0 4YY
03/10/2024
01040441-0009